Awareness During Anesthesia

For SHAMS, OMAR, and NATASHA

Commissioning editor: Susan Pioli
Production controller: Debbie Clark
Desk editor: Angela Davies
Cover designer: Alan Studholme

Awareness During Anesthesia

Edited by

Mohamed M. Ghoneim, MD

Professor, Department of Anesthesia, College of Medicine,
University of Iowa, Iowa City, Iowa, USA

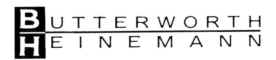

Oxford   Auckland   Boston   Johannesburg   Melbourne   New Delhi

Butterworth-Heinemann
Linacre House, Jordan Hill, Oxford OX2 8DP
225 Wildwood Avenue, Woburn, MA 01801-2041
A division of Reed Educational and Professional Publishing Ltd

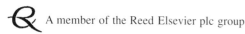 A member of the Reed Elsevier plc group

First published 2001

British Library Cataloguing in Publication Data
A catalogue record for this book is available from the British Library

Library of Congress Cataloging in Publication Data
A catalogue record for this book is available from the
Library of Congress

ISBN 0 7506 7201 3

Typeset at Replika Press Pvt Ltd, 100% EOU, Delhi 110 040, India
Printed and bound in Great Britain

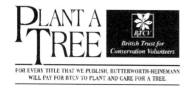

PLANT A TREE
British Trust for Conservation Volunteers

FOR EVERY TITLE THAT WE PUBLISH, BUTTERWORTH-HEINEMANN
WILL PAY FOR BTCV TO PLANT AND CARE FOR A TREE.

Contents

Acknowledgments

I thank my colleagues, the contributors to this book, who have been responsive to my requests for revisions and additions. I am also indebted to the staff at Butterworth-Heinemann Company, specifically Susan Pioli, Cheri Dellelo, Angela Davies, Joan Ryan, and Jodie Allen for their skills in editing the book and for their grace and enthusiasm. Teresa Block coped with my handwriting, my penchant for revisions, and numerous correspondences with professionalism and dedication.

M. M. Ghoneim, MD

Preface

This is, to our knowledge, the first book ever written on learning and memory during anesthesia (JG Jones edited a booklet in International Anesthesiology Clinics of 1993 on depth of anesthesia[1]). It is an explanation of what we know about learning and memory during anesthesia, written by carefully selected contributors who are widely accepted as experts in their topics as well as good communicators and talented writers through years of experience in scientific writing. They represent many of the finest institutions of North America and Europe, which have been at the cutting edge of research in this area. This allows an international presentation of the current information. Learning and memory during anesthesia are important topics for their clinical significance and potential impact on the theoretical interactions between the sciences of consciousness and learning and memory. Modern anesthesia has accomplished impressive gains in enhancing the safety of the surgical patient through a variety of mechanisms, including improved monitoring techniques, teaching and research. The last few years have also seen unprecedented steps taken to discover how the brain learns and remembers. It would be very rewarding for all the authors of this book if it contributes, even in a small way, to the advances on these two fronts.

The book should appeal to a wide variety of readers, including anesthesiologists, nurse anesthetists, intensivists, cognitive psychologists, clinical psychologists, psychiatrists and some hospital-based dentists. Surgeons, operating room nurses, other members of the operating room team, and physicians who occasionally work with the anesthetized patient, e.g. some radiologists, may also be interested in a problem which may occur in their patients, and to the occurrence of which they may inadvertently contribute.

The hospital nurse and aide who care for the postoperative patient may like to know about a problem which may affect the course of the patient's recovery, and the best way to deal with the patient under such conditions. Hospital lawyers and lawyers who work for health insurance agencies, as well as others, may find some parts of the book of interest to them in their professional work. Engineers and other personnel involved in development of monitors in the operating room and intensive care unit may also find parts of this book of interest. We hope all these groups will find the book a valuable and reliable resource.

Most good research in the area of learning and memory has been the result of a fruitful collaboration between anesthesiologists and psychologists, and this book is no exception. Each discipline has its own methodology, conceptual apparatus, scientific language and specific terminologies. It is a challenge to write a book which is easy to read, appreciate and comprehend, where jargon is cut to a minimum, and terminologies are well defined and explained. However, it would not be in the best interest of the scientific endeavor to cross the line between scientific rigor and oversimplification for the mere sake of accessibility. We think the authors have met the challenge and have not crossed this dividing line. To help them in this respect, the editor has allowed the author(s) of each chapter the freedom to discuss all aspects of the topic of that chapter. Obviously, some degree of repetition among chapters was expected and was tolerated so long as it enhanced the understanding of difficult or controversial concepts through explanations from different angles and presentations from different perspectives. Each chapter starts by identifying the topics that are covered and contains many figures, illustrations and tables, which should help in understanding the text and enhance its clarity.

The book contains nine chapters, which cover various aspects of the subject. We assumed that no single author possesses the breadth and depth of understanding of all subjects covered in this book; therefore, we chose for each chapter an author(s) who is expert in that area. In this introduction, we introduce the author(s) of each chapter in a few sentences, give an overview of the chapter, identify its main themes, and make brief comments on its contents and what binds it to other chapters in one cohesive unit. We hope that it will become apparent that, although the contributors may express different views on specific areas and may write in different styles, they share and agree on many fundamentals which support the science and practice of the whole area.

The book begins with two extensive up-to-date reviews of the literature by Ghoneim. The chapter on awareness during anesthesia discusses distinctions between implicit and explicit memory, one of the most prominent topics in modern memory research; definitions of awareness, consciousness, wakefulness, and learning during anesthesia, as well as postoperative memory of events during anesthesia and related concepts; the history of descriptions and studies of these phenomena; methods of postoperative interview and incidences of awareness and dreaming during anesthesia; causes of awareness during anesthesia, such as overly light anesthesia, increased anesthetic requirements of some patients, and equipment problems or misuse; clinical consequences of awareness during anesthesia, such as post-traumatic stress disorder, together with potential medicolegal consequences; management of incidents of awareness during anesthesia; and methods to prevent such incidents from occurring.

The second chapter by Ghoneim consists of a review of the literature concerning implicit memory for events occurring during anesthesia. This topic has generated considerable interest among anesthesia researchers in recent years. First, some early reports pertinent to the topic are discussed. Then, the distinction between implicit versus explicit memory, which parallels to some extent the notion of 'unconscious' versus 'conscious' learning during anesthesia, is described. Research concerning the possible occurrence of unconscious learning during anesthesia is then reviewed, including consideration of methods for distinguishing between implicit and explicit memory, other pertinent methodological distinctions (e.g. between perceptual versus conceptual priming), and factors such as anesthetic regimens that may affect the occurrence of implicit memory. One important conclusion, which is echoed in other chapters, is that many studies did not match the level of difficulty of implicit and explicit tasks, incorporate methods to ensure that the implicit task was not contaminated by explicit retrieval, or monitor the depth of anesthesia.

Several other pertinent avenues of research are also considered: behavioral suggestions administered during anesthesia to engage in some observable behavior, such as touching one's ear during a post-anesthesia interview; studies of the efficacy of administering therapeutic suggestions during anesthesia predicting a rapid and smooth postoperative recovery; studies of implicit memory during administration of drugs (usually in subanesthetic concentrations) to healthy volunteers; studies of learning during anesthesia in animals; and reports of cases of psychosomatic disorders that may possibly be related to unconscious learning during anesthesia. The potential clinical significance of implicit memory for events occurring during anesthesia, methods for preventing such implicit memory, and some shortcomings of the research that has been done in this area are discussed.

These two introductory chapters provide a synopsis of many of the topics covered in the book, which are discussed in more detail and from different angles in the intellectually stimulating chapters which follow. These chapters elaborate not only on facts and outcomes, but on the 'why' and 'how' of learning and memory during anesthesia. After finishing these chapters, readers will be connoisseurs of the literature and some may even be inspired to become investigators in this fascinating and complex area of research.

Despite a 154-year history of anesthesia, assessment of anesthetic depth and adequacy remains elusive. One author[2] suggested that the search for a monitor to measure anesthetic depth resembles the search for the Philosopher's stone. While we and other contributors to this book may not share this unwarranted pessimism, one has to confess to the difficulties involved in developing a monitor with good sensitivity and specificity which directly relates to the state of consciousness of the patient and allows titrating the administration of anesthetic agents.

Jones and his group have pioneered the use of the auditory evoked responses (AERs) as a possible monitor, investigated learning and memory during anesthesia, and written extensively on the subject of depth of anesthesia. While several authors have reviewed the latter subject in the past, arguably none is better suited to tackle the subject than Jones. In their chapter, Jones and Aggarwal share their extensive knowledge with the reader. They review definitions of awareness during anesthesia and types of memories of intraoperative events. Their terms – conscious awareness, conscious awareness without explicit memory, and subconscious awareness – are different from those used by Ghoneim. They assert that cases of awareness with distressing sequelae sufficient to lead to legal action are extremely rare and that patients experiencing some vaguer memories of intraoperative events indicative of awareness are more common, although still very infrequent. However, as Domino and Aitkenhead state in their chapter, awareness results in no litigation for most patients. They also discuss sociocultural factors and other influences that determine whether an adverse outcome results in malpractice litigation. This makes reliance on the incidence of legal claims an unsatisfactory route to assess the true incidence of awareness, although the figures quoted by Jones and Aggarwal are of great interest regarding the incidence of litigation attributable to this complication. (Incidentally, their figures are similar to those in a large USA hospital in which the authors of this chapter work.) It is also to Jones and Aggarwal's credit that they recognize the difficulty of relying on legal claims to assess the incidence of awareness, which was necessitated by the poor quality or absence of critical incident recording. Even a system of mandatory reporting of medical errors or complications is unlikely to be satisfactory. It would need an army of auditors to verify the reporting. Large prospective studies in anesthetized surgical patients are probably the only avenue to assess the true incidence. Domino and Aitkenhead tabulate all the studies that are available in the literature in their chapter. It is interesting that with the exception of one study, all have been done in Europe.

Ghoneim cites in his chapter four reasons for the need to update figures on the incidence of awareness. Implicit in the discussion is an assumption that future figures, if obtained in the manner envisaged, may prove to be higher or at least the same as current figures. Russell, in his chapter, confirms that sometimes patients recall at a later postoperative time what they have denied earlier, soon after surgery, and discusses the effects of prompting patients and 'jogging' their memories in increasing reports of awareness. It is safe to conclude that all the authors who have been quoted above agree about the uncertainty of the current figures and the need for an update.

Jones and Aggarwal outline stages of anesthesia based on memory and consciousness. A suitable monitoring device, they state, should show graded changes with increasing depth of anesthetic, be independent of neuromuscular block and anesthetic agent, show appropriate response to surgical stimulation, and reflect the level of consciousness.

Jones and Aggarwal consider changes in memory to be the most sensitive indicator of depth during conscious sedation. For monitoring depth of general anesthesia, they discuss clinical signs, the isolated forearm technique (IFT), electro-encephalographic (EEG) methods, and non-EEG physiological indicators such as esophageal motility, frontalis EMG, and respiratory sinus arrhythmia. The EEG methods discussed include power spectrum measures, bispectral analysis (BIS), and auditory, visual, and somatosensory evoked responses. Relations of some of these potential measures of depth of anesthesia to memory, responsiveness, and consciousness are reviewed. Jones and Aggarwal regard certain EEG methods – BIS, AERs, and the coherent frequency of steady state AERs – as the most promising methods to date for monitoring depth of anesthesia within clinically relevant depths. Nevertheless, these methods have some limitations, e.g. they indicate that both BIS and AERs are insensitive to the effects of nitrous oxide and opioids.

The authors end their chapter by outlining pertinent, common-sense conclusions, which include their belief that the cost effectiveness of routine EEG monitoring is such that it is more expensive than interventions commonly accepted, if used solely for detecting cases of awareness, and that standardized comparisons between the different monitoring methods are needed. With regard to the effectiveness of using depth of anesthesia monitors to decrease perioperative costs, it has been reported that titration of anesthetic dose using the BIS can decrease agent use and may allow patients to recover sufficiently fast to permit bypass of the phase I postanesthesia care unit.[3,4] Although the latter may decrease labor requirements, it may be harder to realize overall labor cost savings.[5–7]

Of course, these considerations would apply to all EEG and related monitors, current and future. We believe that one of the attractive features of using such a monitor in the operating room is the confidence that it may give the anesthesia provider, when light anesthesia has to be used, that the patient is not conscious. Such confidence may allay the clinician's concerns. One hopes that if the monitor does not give a warning of impending consciousness, it would at least give a warning soon, once the patient is awake, allowing the anesthesia provider to deepen the anesthetic immediately, and thus avoid a prolonged period of potential suffering to the patient and perhaps also provide amnesia for the awake episode. However, these assumptions remain to be validated in the future. Lastly, Domino and Aitkenhead mention in their chapter the possible bad news that the commercial availability of such monitors may be an incentive for litigation by attorneys and a basis for higher payments. They even consider the possibility that such a monitor may *increase* the incidence of awareness.

Two monitors are currently being developed for introduction into the market. The FACE monitor measures the voltages in facial muscles involved in the expression of arousal and pain during anesthesia. It has been developed by Dr Henry Bennett of the Patient Comfort Company (Madison, NJ) to monitor both the adequacy of the hypnotic and the analgesic components of anesthesia. Work is in progress at the time of writing to determine the outcome differences when the monitor is used, e.g. decreasing the dose of anesthetic used and allowing faster recovery (personal communication from Dr Bennett). Such studies seem to have been mandated by the Food and Drug Administration (FDA) in the USA as a prerequisite before approval of depth of anesthesia monitors. The Patient State Analyzer (PSA 4000) is an EEG monitor which has been developed by Physiometrix Company (N. Billerica, MA) using an EEG algorithm as a monitor of anesthetic adequacy. At the time of writing, the company has finished collecting the results of the mandated outcome studies and has applied to the FDA for approval before launching the monitor into the marketplace (personal communication from Mr John Williams). The BIS monitor itself (Aspect Medical Systems, Newton, MA), the only monitor which has been approved by the FDA for assessment of anesthetic effect, has undergone seven software upgrades (v1.0–v3.4) so far, to improve its performance and decrease the effects of artefacts. More upgrades are expected.[8] It is hoped that future competition will enhance the technology as well as lower the costs of monitoring.

Dr Andrade is a cognitive psychologist who has done an impressive amount of research on learning during anesthesia, which meshes with her interest in the scientific study of consciousness, a very important topic of cognitive psychology. In her chapter, Andrade discusses the possibility that learning during anesthesia and conscious sedation may not decrease monotonically with increasing doses of anesthetics, but instead may be significantly influenced by other factors, such as surgical stimuli. In her own work, she examined learning during anesthesia and sedation with propofol as the primary agent. One experiment involved sedation in healthy volunteers; one focused on sedation, anesthesia and intubation in patients about to undergo surgery; and a third examined surgery with sedation or anesthesia.

In her studies, memory tests provided no strong evidence for learning during anesthesia or even during sedation, although the third experiment, through the use of the process dissociation procedure,[9] provided some evidence of explicit learning during surgery, albeit somewhat weak. The latter finding was surprising because learning did not correlate with the depth of sedation/anesthesia, and because strong amnesic effects of propofol were observed in the first two experiments. Although comparison among the experiments is hampered by the use of different memory tests, Andrade points out some parallelism between her results and a seemingly paradoxical pattern of findings in the literature. The literature indicates that 'deep' sedation in volunteers appears to eliminate more consistently implicit learning than does general anesthesia in patients undergoing surgery. Andrade hypothesizes that the stress of surgery and surgical stimuli enable learning in conditions that would otherwise prevent it, possibly due to increases in epinephrine or norepinephrine levels. This hypothesis may explain the otherwise bewildering array of positive and null results in the literature and can be tested in the future.

Kerssens has been active in investigating memory for events during anesthesia while using the BIS to control the hypnotic state of the patients. She works in an institution with a long tradition of solid contributions to the literature on the subject of learning and memory during anesthesia. Dr Sebel has been involved with investigating the clinical utility of the BIS since its original development. He has also significantly contributed to the literature on learning and memory during anesthesia through his extensive research and organization of the Second International Symposium on Memory and Awareness in Anesthesia. All the authors of the book agree that it is important to control the depth of anesthesia for any future investigation of learning and memory during anesthesia and, with the commercial availability of the BIS monitor, this has become feasible. The chapter by these two experts takes stock of where we currently stand in the literature of BIS and memory during anesthesia and maps for us some future strategies for studies.

The authors review the basic concepts of EEG and processed EEG measures, the BIS, AERs, and the IFT – with primary emphasis on the BIS. They contend that the BIS correlates rather well with level of sedation/hypnosis. It may be superior to some other processed EEG variables in this respect, as well as having greater generality over varying anesthesia methods and depths of anesthesia. The accuracy of the BIS in predicting consciousness is good at high values, whereas patient variation in consciousness tends to increase at lower BIS values, a fact which has been alluded to by Jones and Aggarwal as well as Russell, in their chapters. Its accuracy as an indicator of the potential for explicit memory is similar. However, it may be of more limited value as an indicator of the potential for implicit memory; studies of this issue to date have been few and have produced somewhat inconsistent results. The extent, if any, to which implicit memory may be preserved in some patients at BIS levels considered to represent adequate anesthesia, i.e. BIS levels of 40 to 60, requires clarification. As Andrade points out in her chapter, in Lubke *et al.*'s fascinating study, which found learning with BIS between 40 and 60, the correlation between BIS and memory was weak (r = 0.35), suggesting a weak relationship between depth of anesthesia and learning.

Kerssens and Sebel suggest several directions for future research. Among these directions, they suggest that presentation of auditory information during anesthesia should be time-locked to CNS signals. This would limit the use of auditory-based monitors, like AERs. The authors also point to two other limitations of research. First, BIS was not designed to monitor memory function during anesthesia. Second, the dichotomy between conscious (explicit) memory and unconscious (implicit) memory may be too crude.

The latter limitation refers to results of studies that have used the Process Dissociation Procedure (PDP). The combination of word stem completion and PDP in studies in the anesthesia literature is discussed in the chapters by Ghoneim and Andrade, in addition to that of Kerssens and Sebel. As explained there, the PDP has been used widely in the psychology literature to estimate conscious and unconscious influences on memory by manipulation of test instructions. The chapter by Kerssens and Sebel describes two of the studies of their group. In one study in trauma patients, there was evidence of unconsciously mediated memory effects, while in another study in patients undergoing cesarean section, patients seemed to control their responses postoperatively. In the chapter by Andrade, she refers to a study during propofol administration in which there was also some evidence of explicit learning. Although the PDP method is an ingenious approach for tackling a difficult problem and is likely to be used more frequently in the future in the anesthesia literature, it has its difficulties. Some critics have argued that inclusion–exclusion instructions are too complicated for subjects to comprehend.[10] This could be a problem for the postoperative patient. Subjects may exclude responses on the basis of: (a) intentionally recollecting the item and excluding it, or (b) unintentionally retrieving the word and then recognizing and excluding it. In the latter case, explicit memory would be overestimated and implicit memory underestimated. The use of PDP with the inclusion – exclusion test instructions also relies on several assumptions that have been controversial.[11,12] For example, the assumption of the independence of explicit and implicit memory underlies the formulas for the calculation of explicit and implicit scores. Some of the problems may be avoided by the use of a variant of the procedure[13] that uses differences in congruence with prior training rather than the use of the inclusion – exclusion test instructions. However, this variant of the procedure may be difficult to adapt to studies during anesthesia.

The reader will find somewhat different perspectives from those of Kerssens and Sebel on the utility of the BIS as a depth of anesthesia monitor in the chapters by Ghoneim, Jones and Aggarwal, Russell, and Domino and Aitkenhead.

Dr Thornton, with her group, has pioneered the development of AERs to monitor anesthetic depth. Their impressive research has set the pace for the research to be expected on any provisional monitor of anesthetic depth. Dr Sharpe has contributed to this research. In their chapter, Thornton and Sharpe discuss AERs and memory during anesthesia or sedation. After reviewing basic concepts of memory and memory testing, they discuss characteristics of AERs, their anatomical significance, and their relationship to cognitive processes such as selective attention. The different waves of 'transient' evoked responses are considered, as are the '40 Hz steady state' response and the coherent frequency.

Thornton and Sharpe review the fairly small number of studies conducted by their own group and other investigators that are directly pertinent to the relationship of AERs to memory during anesthesia or sedation. In their own work, increased Nb latencies have been associated with loss of response to commands. Some studies have detected associations between AER measures and explicit or implicit memory, while others have not. Thornton and Sharpe find little evidence to date of specific relationships of AERs to memory, i.e. relationships that are independent of other covarying factors in these studies, such as drug concentrations and levels of consciousness. They conclude that a specific AER correlate of memory impairment remains elusive, but that AERs can be useful in preventing explicit memory after anesthesia because of its capability to distinguish consciousness from unconsciousness. For somewhat different perspectives on AERs as a monitor, the reader is referred to chapters by Jones and Aggarwal, and Kerssens and Sebel.

Tunstall, in 1977, introduced the IFT, which involves inflating a tourniquet around one arm prior to administration of muscle relaxants, so that the patient, if conscious, can respond to commands with the isolated forearm. Russell developed the technique, allowing it to be used for any length of surgery, and pioneered its use to detect responsiveness in the anesthetized patient both in clinical practice and research. Yet, he is a lonely hunter. Most of the work in this area has been done by him, frequently as the sole author (a refreshing change in these days of multi-authored articles). In his chapter, Dr Russell argues that responsiveness to command is the accepted indicator of the threshold between consciousness and unconsciousness, and that, when muscle relaxants are administered, the only method of assessing responsiveness to command is the IFT. Jones and Aggarwal in their chapter suggest that the method is 'arguably the nearest we have to a gold standard' for measuring the depth of anesthesia.

Russell attributes the lack of widespread use of the method to various criticisms and misconceptions, which he attempts to dispel. Contrary to various critics, he argues that (1) the imperfect correlation between IFT responses and the traditional clinical signs of light anesthesia that has been noted points toward the inadequacy of the traditional clinical signs. (2) His modification of Tunstall's original technique allows the IFT to be used for long surgery. (3) It is feasible to distinguish purposeful from reflex movements of the isolated forearm. (4) Responsiveness to command provides sufficient grounds for inferring that a patient is conscious. (5) An imperfect correlation between IFT responses and recall is to be expected, inasmuch as consciousness is not a sufficient condition for recall, i.e. higher anesthetic concentrations are required to suppress responsiveness than to suppress recall. (6) The IFT is not complex to use. (7) Consciousness correlates strongly with IFT responses, i.e. only rarely does a patient who is conscious fail to respond. (8) No serious adverse effects have been associated with use of the IFT.

Russell summarizes a number of studies of obstetric anesthesia that utilized the IFT. These demonstrated that a high percentage of patients (43%) were responsive at some point during surgery (usually between the intravenous induction and the establishment of adequate inhalational anesthesia), but less than 2% of these patients experienced recall. The IFT has also been used with other surgeries and with a variety of anesthetic techniques. A fairly high percentage of patients in these studies showed IFT responses, and these responses were generally not associated with recall or clinical signs of inadequate anesthesia. The IFT has also been used in a number of studies of volunteers to whom inhalational or intravenous anesthetics were administered. Results supported the generalization, mentioned above and echoed by several authors in this book, that higher anesthetic concentrations are required to suppress responsiveness than recall.

Russell argues that, while postoperative recall rarely occurs in the absence of IFT responses during anesthesia, responsiveness during anesthesia is much more common than recall. He criticizes studies of implicit memory during general anesthesia which assume that patients are unconscious throughout anesthesia without documenting their unresponsiveness using the IFT, arguing that some patients in such studies may have been presented with stimuli for postoperative memory tests during periods of awareness during anesthesia. We think that all authors of this book are currently in agreement that adequacy of anesthesia needs to be established by investigators before claiming that implicit learning has occurred. Russell contends that adequacy of anesthesia can best be documented by providing evidence of unresponsiveness using the IFT. The method is cost-effective and, in his opinion as its strongest advocate, compares favorably with the BIS monitor, a more expensive and sophisticated monitoring method.

Dr Wang, to our knowledge, is the only person who is currently managing patients with psychological problems following awareness, as well as studying learning and memory during anesthesia (in collaboration with Dr Russell). He has developed an impressive experience in both areas. In his chapter, Wang examines the psychological consequences of explicit and implicit memories of intraoperative events. Reports indicate that there is a clear possibility of post-traumatic stress disorder, other anxiety disorders, depression, or other psychiatric problems following consciously recalled memories of events that occurred during surgery. This risk may be heightened when these events included pain or other distressing perceptions, such as the experience of complete paralysis in patients with whom the use of muscle relaxants was not discussed preoperatively. He introduces the reader to two other groups of patients with postoperative psychiatric disturbances, which he contends are more frequent than the usual cases of consciously recalled intraoperative memories. The first group consists of patients who are unaware of intraoperative distress, yet in whom psychological disturbances develop because of subsequent postoperative emotional processing of the meaning of an intraoperative memory. The second group consists of patients with implicit emotional learning during anesthesia.

Wang discusses the difficulties of investigating groups of cases with consciously recalled memories of intraoperative events who suffer psychopathology, e.g. biased samples and absence of control groups. He also discusses the management of these cases and points out the need to study the best way to treat them.

Wang also reviews reports of postoperative psychiatric problems that may possibly be attributable to implicit learning during anesthesia, in the absence of conscious postoperative recall. He argues that such occurrences may be a real concern, although much of the evidence is anecdotal, and both the occurrence of such implicit learning, and its association with postoperative psychiatric problems, are difficult to demonstrate with scientific rigor.

There is a universal agreement among researchers in the field about the need to investigate the clinical significance of implicit memory following anesthesia. Ghoneim, in his chapter on implicit memory, cited the editorial by Andrade and Jones[14] which suggested that future research should be directed at the emotional impact of light anesthesia in well-controlled studies, to see if it would do any harm (assuming that affective priming would be more likely during light than adequate anesthesia). Ghoneim cautioned about possible difficulties with such studies because of the multifactorial causes of psychological complications following surgery and ethical concerns that might be raised about the use of light anesthesia.

Russell, in his chapter, suggested studies in patients who undergo general anesthesia for cesarean section, where light anesthesia is used as a rule. Researchers would look for differences in the recovery profiles of women who are unconscious during surgeries (i.e. make no response during the use of the IFT); women who do respond, but are not in pain; and women who respond and are in pain. This is an interesting proposition, but one has also to bear in mind that the postpartum period is a high-risk time for development of mental disorders, whose causal factors are not well understood.[15,16]

It is, therefore, exciting that Wang describes, at least briefly, the pioneering and intriguing studies which he and Russell have been doing investigating the psychological consequences of implicit emotional learning. Their preliminary results suggest that there may be a cause for concern, and may bolster Wang's conclusion that it is unsafe to conclude that episodes of intraoperative wakefulness in the absence of explicit recall are of no consequence.

Dr Domino is a member of the American Society of Anesthesiologists Closed Claims Analysis group. She is known primarily for her research in this area and has recently used her exceptional expertise to investigate the medicolegal aspects of awareness during anesthesia. Dr Aitkenhead has also been interested in the medicolegal aspects of awareness on the other side of the large pond and has also significantly contributed to the literature of learning and memory during anesthesia through research and authoring fine reviews and editorials on the subject. The collaboration of the two authors adds richness to the book and provides an international perspective. Alas, we are in total ignorance about the situation regarding awareness (i.e. incidence, causes, consequences, etc.) outside the USA and Europe. We need to know more, if we are to help our colleagues practicing in other parts of the global village.

In their chapter, Domino and Aitkenhead discuss medicolegal consequences of awareness during anesthesia. Like most patients who experience adverse outcomes from medical treatments (97% or more of patients who suffer negligent injury do not sue), patients who experience awareness during anesthesia usually do not file medical malpractice claims. Some do, however. Dissatisfaction with physician–patient communication is a key factor promoting malpractice claims. Patients who suffer medical injury have three main desires.[17] First, they want a full explanation of what occurred and why. Second, they want an acknowledgment or apology from the caregiver. And third, they want to know what steps will be taken to ensure that what happened to them will not happen to them again or to someone else. These desires can and should be satisfied. Ghoneim describes appropriate procedures in the section on Management of Awareness in the first chapter. Litigation is very expensive, and plaintiff's attorneys are reluctant to take cases unless there is potential for high damages, and a high likelihood of success. Claims for intraoperative awareness may not be pursued by attorneys because the injury is emotional rather than physical, and settlements involving only emotional injury are typically associated with lower payments than those involving substantial physical injury.

Domino and Aitkenhead review data concerning awareness during anesthesia from the ASA Closed Claims Project database. Awareness accounted for 1.9% of claims in this database. The severity of injury in claims for awareness was lower than the severity of the other claims. The claims concerning awareness were categorized as awake paralysis or more typical cases of recall under general anesthesia. Female gender and nitrous-narcotic-relaxant techniques without use of a volatile anesthetic increased the relative frequency of claims for recall under general anesthesia. Claims for awareness frequently resulted in compensation, although the magnitude of payment was usually relatively low. There has been an increase over time in the proportion of claims for awareness, i.e. in the 1990s, compared to the 1970s.

According to Domino and Aitkenhead, differences between the legal systems of the USA and European countries have affected patterns of litigation related to awareness. A dramatic increase in the UK in such litigation occurred in 1985, because of publicity surrounding one particular case. The frequency of litigation concerning awareness does not appear to have changed substantially in the last decade in the UK, whereas such claims have remained low in the rest of Europe. Such claims are much more frequent as a proportion of all claims against anesthesiologists in the UK than the USA. The authors provide details of common causes of litigation in the UK. Awareness has been commonly associated with faulty anesthetic technique or failure to check equipment. The reader who goes over this material, together with what has been written by Ghoneim in the first chapter, will have a compendium of almost all etiologies and will be in the best possible position to predict and prevent this catastrophe in most cases.

The authors end their fascinating chapter with a glimpse into the twenty-first century. Their expectations seem to be adequately reasoned. Their first prediction is of great concern. They expect a plateau in the number of cases in the UK, but an increase in the quantity and payment in the USA. The current financial and political climates in the USA seem to support the authors' view. These milieus have fostered adversarial posturing among those who receive and deliver health services. (At the time of writing, an example is the proposed Patient's Bill of Rights, with its insistence on a right to sue one's managed care organization.) The sad truths are: (1) medical errors are unlikely to be solved by litigation; (2) for patients, litigation is expensive and hard to win; and (3) for physicians, it is a traumatic and nightmarish experience. Their second prediction is that the introduction of a monitor of anesthetic depth into the marketplace may increase the risk of litigation and magnitude of payment. It may even increase the incidence of awareness because of the use of reduced anesthetic dosages. (To date, there have been approximately 1.3 million uses of BIS, with 41 awareness cases reported to Aspect Medical Systems, an incidence of 0.003%. BIS was 70 or above in cases where documentation was available (Paul Manberg, Aspect Medical Systems – personal communication). The reported number is well below the current expected incidence of awareness; however, a loose system of voluntary reporting would be expected to underestimate the true number of cases.) The authors' conclusion is that the frequency of litigation related to awareness could drop in the future, if there is improved education and training of anesthesiologists. Reading and understanding the contents of this book would be a giant step in this desirable direction.

We hope that this introduction to the contents of the book will help the reader to appreciate the contributions of these talented authors, which follow. These contributions are based on an enduring interest and fascination with the subject, which they have pursued for years.

M.M. Ghoneim, MD; Robert I. Block, PhD

References

1. Jones JG (ed.) Depth of anesthesia. *International Anesthesiol Clin* 1993; **31**: 1–141.
2. Prys-Roberts C. Anaesthesia: A practical or impractical construct? (Editorial). *Br J Anaesth* 1987; **59**:1341–1345.
3. Gan TJ, Glass PS, Windsor A, *et al*. Bispectral index monitoring allows faster emergence and improved recovery from propofol, alfentanil and nitrous oxide anesthesia. BIS Utility Study Group. *Anesthesiology* 1997; **87**:808–815.
4. Song D, van Vlymen J, White PF. Is the bispectral index useful in predicting fast-track eligibility after ambulatory anesthesia with propofol and desflurane? *Anesth Analg* 1998; **86**:267–273.
5. Dexter F, Macario A, Manberg PJ, Lubarsky DA. Computer simulation to determine how rapid anesthetic recovery protocols to decrease the time for emergence or increase the phase I postanesthesia care unit bypass rate affect staffing of an ambulatory surgery center. *Anesth Analg* 1999; **88**:1053–1063.
6. Dexter F, Macario A. Decrease in case duration required to complete an additional case during regularly scheduled hours in an operating room suite: A computer simulation study. *Anesth Analg* 1999; **88**:72–76.
7. Dexter F, Coffin S, Tinker JH. Decreases in anaesthesia-controlled time cannot permit one additional surgical operation to be reliably scheduled during the workday. *Anesth Analg* 1995; **81**:1263–1268.
8. Johansen JW, Sebel PS. Development and clinical application of EEG bispectrum monitoring. *Anesthesiology*, In Press.
9. Jacoby LL. A process-dissociation framework: Separating automatic from intentional uses of memory. *J Mem Language* 1991; **30**:513–541.
10. Graf P, Komatsu S. PDP: Handle with caution! *Europ J Cogn Psychol* 1994; **6**:113–129.
11. Roediger HL, McDermott KB. Implicit memory in normal human subjects. In Spinnler H, Boller F (eds). Memory, Dementia, Perception of Time, Music and Faces. *Handbook Neuropsychol* 1993; **8**:63–131.
12. Schmitter-Edgecombe M. Effects of divided attention on perceptual and conceptual memory tests: An analysis using a process-dissociation approach. *Mem Cogn* 1999; **27**:512–525.
13. Hay JF, Jacoby LL. Separating habit and recollection: Memory slips, process dissociations and probability matching. *J Exp Psychol (Learn Mem Cogn)* 1996; **22**:1323–1335.

14. Andrade J, Jones JG. Is amnesia for intraoperative events good enough? (Editorial) *Br J Anaesth* 1998; **80**:575–576.

15. O'Hara MW. Postpartum mental disorders. In Sciarra JJ (ed.) *Gynecology and Obstetrics*. New York: Lippincott Williams & Wilkins 1999; vol. 6 (ch. 84): 1–19.

16. O'Hara MW, Stuart S. Pregnancy and postpartum. In Robinson RG, Yates WR (eds). *Psychiatric Treatment of the Medically Ill*. New York: Marcel Dekker 1999; 253–277.

17. Dauer E, Marcus LJ. Adapting mediation to link the resolution of medical malpractice disputes with health care quality improvement. *Law and Contemporary Problems* 1997; **60**:185–218.

Contributing Authors

Sanjay Kumar Aggarwal, MA, MB, BChir
Foundation Scholar, Queen's College, Cambridge University, UK; Senior House
Officer, Department of Medicine, Leeds General Infirmary, Leeds, UK

Alan R. Aitkenhead, BSc, MB CLB, MD, FRCA
Professor, Anaesthesia and Intensive Care Department, University of Nottingham,
UK

Jackie Andrade, PhD
Lecturer in Psychology, Department of Psychology, University of Sheffield, Sheffield,
UK

Robert I. Block, PhD
Associate Professor, Department of Anesthesia, University of Iowa, Iowa City,
Iowa, USA

Karen B. Domino, MD, MPH
Professor of Anesthesiology, University of Washington Medical Center, Seattle;
Department of Anesthesiology, Harborview Medical Center, Seattle, Washington,
USA

M. M. Ghoneim, MD
Professor of Anesthesia, College of Medicine, University of Iowa, Iowa City;
Department of Anesthesia, University of Iowa Hospitals, Iowa City, Iowa, USA

J. G. Jones, MD, FRCP, FRCA
Professor of Anaesthesia, University of Cambridge, Cambridge, UK; Professor and
Head of Anaesthesia Department, Addenbrooke's Hospital, Cambridge, UK

Chantal Kerssens, MA
PhD Student of Medical Psychology and Psychotherapy, Erasmus University,
Rotterdam, The Netherlands; PhD Student of Anesthesiology, Academic Hospital,
Rotterdam, The Netherlands

Ian F. Russell, MB, ChB, BMedBiol(Hon), FRCA
Honorary Senior Lecturer of Obstetrics, University of Hull, Kingston upon Hull, UK; Consultant Anaesthetist, Hull Royal Infirmary, Kingston upon Hull, UK

Peter S. Sebel, MB, BS, PhD, MBA
Professor of Anesthesiology, Deputy Chair of Clinical Services, Department of Anesthesiology, Emory University School of Medicine, Atlanta, Georgia; Professor of Anesthesiology, Grady Memorial Hospital and Crawford Long Hospital, Atlanta, Georgia, USA

Roger M. Sharpe, BSc, MB, BS, FRCA
Consultant Anaesthetist and Honorary Clinical Senior Lecturer of Anaesthesia, Imperial College School of Medicine, Northwick Park Hospital, Harrow, Middlesex, UK

Christine Thornton, MSc, PhD
Principal Research Fellow, Academic Department of Anaesthesia, Imperial College School of Medicine, Northwick Park Hospital, Harrow, Middlesex, UK

Michael Wang, BSc(Hons), MSc, PhD, CPsychol, FBPsS
Clinical Director and Head of Clinical Psychology Department, University of Hull School of Medicine, Kingston upon Hull, East Yorkshire, UK; Honorary Consultant and Clinical Psychologist, Hull and Holderness Community Healthcare Trust, Kingston upon Hull, East Yorkshire, UK

Chapter 1

Awareness during anesthesia

M. M. Ghoneim

Contents

Introduction

Memory is not a single entity but is composed of multiple systems. The description of these systems started in the 1970s.[1,2] An essential classification of memory distinguishes between two types, explicit or conscious memory and implicit or unconscious memory.[3,4] *Explicit memory* refers to intentional or conscious recollection of prior experiences as assessed by tests of recall or recognition, which are also called *direct* memory tests. *Implicit memory*, by contrast, refers to changes in performance or behavior that are produced by prior experiences on tests that do not require any intentional or conscious recollection of those experiences.[5]

Several other distinctions in the literature are similar to the implicit/explicit distinction, including the contrast between declarative and nondeclarative memory,[6,7] and direct and indirect tests of memory.[8] In this chapter, I use the terms explicit or conscious or declarative memory and implicit or unconscious or nondeclarative or procedural memory as synonyms. The basic distinction between explicit or direct tests and implicit or indirect tests involves

1

the nature of the instructions given to the person being tested. In a direct test, participants are asked to recall or recognize events that may have occurred during anesthesia. In an indirect test, the instructions make no reference to events during the operation.

Explicit memory refers to the everyday uses of such terms as 'remembering' (e.g. can you remember what you did last Tuesday evening?). In the case of an anesthetized patient, you can ask the patient in the postoperative period questions such as 'can you remember hearing any words or sounds during your operation?' (i.e. a recall test) or 'which of the following words were played to you during surgery?' (a recognition test). I shall explain and discuss implicit memory in the next chapter.

Definitions

Awareness, memory and recall

We wrote before[9] about the confusion in anesthesia literature because of the unfortunate *use of the words 'awareness' and 'memory' or 'recall' in an interchangeable fashion.* 'Awareness is the quality or state of being aware; i.e. watchful, vigilant, informed, cognizant, or conscious.'[10] As we shall see, patients can respond to commands under anesthesia with no recall postoperatively and the opposite is also possible; i.e. patients may not follow commands but may show some evidence of implicit memory without being 'aware' or able to 'monitor' their environment. On the other hand, many patients with organic amnesias display nearly normal implicit memory and severe problems with long-term retention of new explicit memories, but without awareness deficit. Awareness is often associated with or equated to short-term or working memory; i.e. a limited-capacity memory that lasts only for seconds and contains whatever an individual is currently thinking about; this, however, should not be confused with long-term memory, which is what most people think of when they think of memory. Thus, the word 'awareness' as used in this context is anesthetic jargon and may interfere with our ability to communicate with clarity and conciseness with the disciplines of neuropsychology and cognitive psychology. Payne[11] also thought that the term 'awareness during general anesthesia' is semantically illogical because a patient under general anesthesia cannot be aware and an aware patient is not anesthetized.

Despite these arguments to use the terms 'memory' and 'awareness' separately, anesthesiologists have continued to use the term awareness as describing learning and memory during anesthesia. The term was used earlier than the initial distinction between explicit and implicit memory and its convenience of use as a simple word perhaps made it entrenched in the anesthesia literature. We have, therefore, decided to use it in the first two chapters to describe explicit memory after anesthesia.

Learning and memory

There is also some confusion in the anesthesia literature about *the use of the words 'learning' and 'memory' without adequate justification.* Sometimes the two words are combined together and in some others one word or the other is used. It is therefore important to distinguish between the two words. For convenience, one may think of learning and memory as two separate processes' – acquisition and retention. Acquisition and retention are not quite synonymous with learning and memory, but both are always required in order to demonstrate that learning and memory have occurred. The labels of learning and memory reflect different emphases on the processes of acquisition and retention. Generally, when we speak of learning, we place major emphasis on the investigation of the problems of acquisition. When we study memory, we are concentrating primarily upon the problems of retention. However, it must be recognized that every test of acquisition also involves a test of retention and every test of retention also necessitates some prior adequate acquisition. For learning to be demonstrated, some new information must be acquired and retained until tested. Similarly, for memory to be examined, some information must first be acquired.[12] In practice, the term learning is more often used when referring to experiments involving multiple presentations of stimuli than a single presentation. The distinction between learning and memory is of special interest when considering studies of patients during anesthesia that investigate explicit and implicit learning and memory, as will become apparent in the next chapter on implicit memory for events during anesthesia.

Consciousness, awareness and wakefulness

A third issue concerns the *use of the words 'consciousness', 'awareness' and 'wakefulness' interchangeably*. A complete definition of consciousness and its theories, functions, mechanisms, etc. are beyond the scope of this review,[13,14] but we will use here the term consciousness as defining a state of awareness of the outside world, as when we talk of someone 'losing consciousness after induction of anesthesia and regaining it after the end of the operation'. Thus, we will equate consciousness with wakefulness. Awareness can be dissociated from wakefulness in both normal subjects and neurologic patients. A normal subject can be awake but unaware of certain aspects of his or her environment. The neurovegetative patient can be awake but totally unaware.[15] Also, because a patient during anesthesia may be awake as indicated by response to commands, yet may be amnesic postoperatively to this experience (see below), this would contradict our definition of awareness in this review as synonymous with explicit memory. We will, therefore, distinguish awareness from wakefulness and consciousness.

Historical perspective

Early history

The history of memory for events under anesthesia is as old as the history of anesthesia itself (Table 1.1). Horace Wells failed to demonstrate the anesthetic properties of nitrous oxide at the Massachusetts General Hospital in 1845 when the patient screamed out in pain during dental extraction, even though later admitting to no recollection of pain.[16] One year later, William Morton, at the same hospital, succeeded in anesthetizing Gilbert Abbott with diethyl ether; Abbott later reported that he had been aware of the surgery but had experienced no pain.[17] Thus, it seems that Wells' patient was aware of the procedure but had no postoperative recall, while Morton's patient had some postoperative recall but there was no memory of pain. A little over a month after Morton's successful demonstration, a patient was reported who, following amputation of an arm, 'thought she had got a reaping hook in her arm and that she heard the noise of sawing wood.'[18] In 1873, Richardson[19]

Table 1.1. Milestones on the history of awareness during general anesthesia

1845	Wells' patient was aware during demonstration of anesthetic properties of nitrous oxide but had no postoperative recall.[16]
1846	Morton's patient had some postoperative recall during demonstration of anesthetic properties of diethyl ether.[17]
1847	Snow described five degrees of anesthesia.[42]
1937	Guedel published his classification of stages of anesthesia.[43]
1942	Griffith and Johnson introduced d-tubocurarine in anesthesia practice.[22]
1950	Winterbottom reported the first case of awareness during the use of muscle relaxants as anesthetic adjuvants.[25] Faulconer and Bickford began studies of the EEG effects of anesthetics.[47]
1953	Steinberg studied the memory and cognitive effects of subanesthetic concentrations of nitrous oxide.[28–30]
1954	Artusio used Guedel's first stage of ether anesthesia during cardiac surgery.[39,40]
1960	Hutchinson investigated the incidence of awareness.[26]
1965	Eger and his colleagues introduced the concept of MAC.[44]
1977	Tunstall described the isolated forearm technique.[45]
1981	Thornton group under the leadership of JG Jones began studies of the effects of anesthetics on the auditory evoked responses.[48]
1989	The First International Symposium on Memory and Awareness in Anaesthesia was held in Glasgow, Scotland[52]
1994	First abstract which linked the bispectral index of the EEG to the hypnotic state.[50] The technology was developed by Chamoun and his associates.

described his awareness of an operation performed on him using nitrous oxide as the anesthetic, 'I had no pain – still, I knew when the tumor was punctured.' George Crile,[20] the pioneer surgeon, described vivid memory and recall in one of his patients who had received nitrous oxide anesthesia in 1908. Three years later, a similar incident with the same anesthetic was reported.[21]

Introduction of muscle relaxants in anesthesia practice

However, despite these infrequent reports, a significant

'problem of awareness during anesthesia' only appeared after the introduction of muscle relaxants in anesthesia practice by Griffith and Johnson[22] in 1942. Patients can become conscious while totally paralyzed because there is no measurement that guarantees unconsciousness in the paralyzed patient. It is interesting that the plight and misery of these unfortunate patients were prophesied by Claude Bernard in 1878 (as quoted by Blacher[23]) while discussing the effects of curare: 'In all ages, poetic fictions which seek to arouse our pity have presented us with sensitive beings locked in immobile bodies. Our imagination cannot conceive of anything more unhappy than beings provided with sensation, that is to say of being able to feel pleasure and pain, when they are deprived of the power to flee the one and yearn toward the other. The torture which the imaginations of poets have invented can be found produced in nature by the action of the American poison. We can even say that the fiction falls short of reality.'

In 1947, Harroun et al.[24] suggested that the use of curare during anesthesia may allow some patients to wake up during surgery and remember intraoperative events without being able to communicate their distress to the anesthesiologists. Indeed, the case report by Winterbottom[25] in 1950 was followed by a voluminous literature on the subject, which consisted mainly of case reports and clinical studies. Hutchinson[26] was the first to investigate the magnitude of the problem through a prospective study by interviewing patients postoperatively. He reported that eight of 656 patients (1.2%) had recall of some events of their surgery. Other similar studies[27] assessing the incidence under various premedicant and anesthetic regimens, and after different types of surgery followed.

Studies of the effects of subanesthetic concentrations of anesthetics on memory

Serious objective studies of effects of subanesthetic concentrations of anesthetics on memory and behavior started with Steinberg's work[28–30] in the early 1950s on nitrous oxide. This was preceded by numerous clinical and incidental observations of the effects of this gas on behavior; e.g. the observations of James.[31] The work of Parkhouse et al.[32] appeared several years later. More interest in the subject was rekindled in the 1970s and early

1980s by studies of the residual effects of anesthetics on behavior, including the effects of pollution on operating rooms with trace concentrations of anesthetics[33–35] and illegal recreational use of these drugs.[36–38] At the same time that Steinberg was studying the effects of nitrous oxide, Artusio[39,40] was investigating Guedel's first stage of ether anesthesia for use during cardiac surgery. He divided it into three planes, in the deepest (plane 3) of which response to spoken commands was present together with total analgesia and absence of postoperative recall. Recent work has continued with a few groups of investigators mainly trying to define the concentrations of anesthetics that abolish learning and memory, and seeking correlations between electroencephalographic parameters and learning.[41]

Assessment of depth of anesthesia

Attempts to assess the depth of anesthesia date back as early as 1847 when John Snow[42] described five degrees of narcotism. Guedel's classification,[43] published in 1937, provided a more sophisticated approach to assessment of depth of anesthesia during induction and maintenance with inhalation anesthesia (diethyl ether). However, the use of muscle relaxants eliminates many of the signs upon which Guedel's classification depended. Eger and his colleagues[44] introduced the concept of MAC – the minimum alveolar concentration, which prevents movements in response to surgical incision in 50% of the patients – in 1965 as a measure of anesthetic potency. Anesthesia providers came to rely on the values of MAC for the different inhalation agents to calculate the doses of these drugs which they administer during surgery.

Tunstall,[45] in 1977, introduced the isolated forearm technique as a method to assess directly the presence of information processing during anesthesia. He isolated one forearm from the circulation before injection of muscle relaxants by inflating a pneumatic tourniquet. He then verbally instructed the anesthetized patient to move the non-paralyzed arm. The method has been used by some investigators, notably Russell,[46] to report on intra-operative consciousness during general anesthesia.

Intensive study of the electroencephalographic effects of general anesthetics began around 1950 by Faulconer and Bickford and their colleagues.[47]

They reported that all general anesthetics produced a basically similar dose-dependent sequence of six different electroencephalographic patterns. However, they cautioned that some anesthetics did not produce every pattern in the basic sequence and that a particular pattern did not necessarily signal the same clinical anesthesia state for different drugs. Thus, there were shortcomings to the use of the EEG as a uniform measure of anesthetic depth. The mid-latency auditory evoked responses and the bispectral index of the electroencephalograph are being currently investigated as monitors for measuring the depth of anesthesia. Thornton group under the leadership of J.G. Jones[48] was the first to systematically evaluate the effects of anesthetics on the auditory evoked responses with the aim of using the latter to monitor the depth of anesthesia. Aspect Medial Systems Company (Newton, MA) under the direction of N. Chamoun,[49] developed the bispectral index (BIS) technology starting in 1987. The first publication that linked the BIS to hypnotic state of anesthetics[50] appeared in 1994 and the monitor was approved by the FDA in 1996.

Scientific meetings on awareness

Scientific meetings provide good venues for presentations of research findings, discussions, exchanges of ideas, and education. A workshop on awareness was arranged in 1986 in Cardiff, Wales.[51] The First International Symposium on Memory and Awareness in Anaesthesia[52] was held in Glasgow, Scotland in 1989. The second symposium was held in Atlanta, Georgia[53] in 1992, the third in Rotterdam, The Netherlands[54] in 1995, and the fourth in London, England[55] in 1998. Arrangements are being made to hold the fifth symposium in New York City in 2001. These meetings have been specifically useful in bringing together participants from different disciplines, including anesthesiology, psychology, psychiatry, and others who share a common interest and hail from different parts of the world, in relatively modest size gatherings. Reading through the proceedings of these meetings gives the reader a valuable insight into the interest generated by the subject of memory and awareness in anesthesia, the quality of the scientific offerings at the time, and the directions of future research.

Incidence

The minimum of four questions that need to be routinely asked

The incidence of recall of events during anesthesia has been estimated by interviewing patients postoperatively. Asking the patient four simple questions – What was the last thing you remember before you went to sleep? What was the first thing you remember when you woke up? Can you remember anything in between these two periods? Did you dream during your operation?[56] – is *the minimum* required for such purpose and should also be part of the anesthesiologist's routine postoperative interview. This should allow the anesthesiologist to deal with this potentially traumatic experience at an appropriately early time. Evidence in the literature[57,58] and personal experience of those who lecture or talk frequently to the public media on the subject[59] (personal notes) suggest that some patients, particularly those who were not unduly disturbed by their experiences of awareness, may not voluntarily report them at the time without being specifically and directly asked. On the other hand, patients who had been significantly traumatized may avoid medical care and medical personnel (see Chapter 8). Some patients may also be reluctant or afraid to mention their episodes spontaneously to their surgical team for fear of appearing ungrateful or insane.[60] The current medical practice of day surgery and short lengths of stay may prevent the patients from communicating with their physicians about what happened to them.

Current figures

The incidence in *general surgical* cases has been estimated to be 0.2–0.7%.[57,61,]* The incidence is similar after *total intravenous anesthesia*.[62] It is higher, however, when light anesthesia is used. The incidence in *cardiac surgery*[63,64] ranges from 1.14

---

*An incidence of 0.15% has been reported recently (Sandin RH, Enlund G, Samuelsson P, Lenmarken C. Awareness during anesthesia: A prospective case study. *Lancet* 2000:**355**:707–711.)

to 1.5% with a balanced anesthetic technique consisting of benzodiazepines, low-dose fentanyl and a volatile agent. A higher incidence has also been reported for *obstetric cases*[65] (0.4%) and *major trauma cases*[66] (11–43%), and this incidence varies according to the dose of anesthetic administered. Lubke *et al.*,[67] in a recent study of trauma patients, found no evidence of explicit memory. (One patient claimed to have heard voices during surgery. This patient had had no anesthetic agent for a period of approximately 5 minutes. However, the patient could not recall any of the words presented during surgery.) The difference from the earlier results of Bogetz and Katz[66] can be explained by two reasons. First, the sample of Lubke *et al.*[67] included a wide variety of injuries ranging from minor to serious trauma, while Bogetz and Katz sample included only major trauma cases. Secondly, Lubke *et al.* suggested that there might have been a substantial improvement of the resuscitation of trauma patients in the field since the earlier study in 1984, which resulted in an increased tolerance for administration of anesthetic agents. Indeed, the mean bispectral index (BIS) for the patients in Lubke *et al.* study was 54, which is assumed to represent adequate anesthesia. In contrast, the patients in Bogetz and Katz study had a mean period of 57 consecutive minutes during which they received no anesthetic.

The incidence of intraoperative recall is 2% when 70% N_2O alone is used for anesthetic maintenance.[68] This incidence is not reduced by supplementing *nitrous oxide with opioid bolus doses.*[69] Jones[59] estimates that only 0.01% of patients report suffering from *pain* while being aware. It is probable that adequate doses of opioids together with the N_2O provide for most of the analgesic component of anesthesia, thus decreasing the complaints from pain.

Dreams

When light anesthesia is used, the patient may recall dreams that appear to be associated with the anesthetic.[56] Some of the dreams are disturbing. Dreams may be recalled more often than actual events, e.g. in Utting's[68] series of 500 patients anesthetized with nitrous oxide, the incidence of dreams that the patients thought were the worst features of their perioperative experiences was 7% *versus* 2% for recall of intraoperative events. In a recent study[69] of 100 patients anesthetized with N_2O supplemented with an opioid bolus regimen, 8% reported dreaming during anesthesia without explicit recall. Two of the dreams were related to the intraoperative events, but the remaining dreams were pleasant with predominant positive emotions. In a series of 1000 patients investigated by Liu *et al.*[57] (the anesthetic techniques have not been described), the incidence of dreams was 0.9% and none of the dreams was unpleasant or related to intraoperative events.

Utting[68] has suggested that there could be a continuum, with adequate anesthesia resulting in complete amnesia, lighter anesthesia resulting in dream recall, and still lighter anesthesia resulting in recall of actual events. Utting's comments probably concern dreams related to intraoperative events and usually are unpleasant. Other dreams may not fall into this category and may not be associated with evidence of light anesthesia as monitored by the auditory evoked responses.[69] Of course, there is no proof that dreaming reported to an interviewer postoperatively actually took place while the patient was anesthetized; it might have happened during recovery from the anesthetic.

It should be noted that some investigators object to the sleep metaphor of anesthesia. Bennett[70] suggested that historically the sleep metaphor has done more damage to aware patients than any other; patients were told that they 'had a bad dream' and were left with a sense of personal responsibility for what happened. Also, sleep and anesthesia have little to do with each other and recovery from anesthesia is unlike awakening refreshed and restored from a night's sleep. Thus, referring to 'dreams' during anesthesia unjustifiably implies a resemblance to the dreams of normal sleep. These experiences may be better described as altered states of awareness that are characterized by vivid thoughts and images.

A need for update

There is a need to update the above mentioned figures, for the following reasons:

1 There have been some *changes in the practice of anesthesia* in terms of use of new short-acting anesthetic drugs and dosages and more concern about the problem among anesthesiologists

and patients that may affect the incidence of awareness.

2   The optimum *time for testing recall* may vary. If patients are interviewed in the immediate postoperative period, the residual effects of anesthetics may impair their cognitive functions. On the other hand, delaying the interview too long may have the risk of degradation of the specific memory trace. The retention interval has a well-recognized effect on memory. Macleod and Maycock[71] and Russell and Wang[72] reported patients who denied awareness when interviewed immediately after surgery, but confirmed it later on. Nordström *et al.*[73] and Sanden and Lenmarken (personal communication)* reported patients who only reported recall 1–2 weeks after surgery. The trauma of intraoperative awareness may also lead to dissociation.[74] Dissociation causes memory to be organized as sensory fragments and intense emotional states and interfere with the ability to develop a narrative of the event.[75] Later on, in the postoperative period, there may be a gradual emergence of memories and formation of a narrative of the experience. Osterman and van der Kolk[76] suggest that assessment for awareness should be an ongoing process since these memories may gradually emerge over time. Assessment should begin in the recovery room and end at the standard 7–10 day postoperative visit to the surgery clinic.

3   *The interview may need to contain more details* than the four simple questions mentioned above. In a recent study,[69] we interviewed patients postoperatively for 20 minutes asking them many questions in an effort to probe and 'jog' their memories for the intraoperative experience. The interview started with the question 'Tell me everything you remember about your experience of anesthesia and surgery' and included the four questions commonly asked – 'What was the last thing you remember before you went to sleep?' 'What was the first thing you remember when you woke up?' 'Can you remember anything in between these two periods?' and 'Did you dream during your operation?' Some patients who did not give evidence of awareness based on their

answers to these questions, subsequently, with additional questioning, became more confident of their memories at the end of the interview. Russell and Wang[72] also reported on patients who, in response to the standard questions, gave no evidence of awareness. However, with specific prompting cue questions, similar to our study, the patients provided evidence of explicit recall. It is interesting that none of the patients in either study was aware of pain or seemed to be unduly concerned or disturbed by their experiences. (See also Chapter 7.)

4   *The trauma of the intraoperative memories may cause amnesia* for these events and may lead the patients to avoid reminders of the trauma, such as medical care and hospitals, which may prevent them from seeking treatment and discussing their awareness with the anesthesia or surgical teams.[75] These memories may be retrieved under hypnosis (see next chapter on implicit memory for more details).

Causes

When a patient experiences awareness during general anesthesia, usually one of three events has occurred (Figure 1.1).

Overly light anesthesia

For certain operations, such as Cesarean section, and for some patients, such as hypovolemic trauma patients or patients with minimal cardiac reserve, the anesthesiologist may aim at light anesthesia. The provision of light anesthesia in other situations hastens patient recovery, which permits a rapid return to 'street fitness' with early discharge home following ambulatory surgery. It also facilitates operating room turnover and may enable a greater number of procedures to be performed. This may result in lower health costs. Sometimes this light anesthesia may progress too far, to the point of consciousness and recall, which may not be surprising considering that judgments of depth of anesthesia are neither quantitatively precise nor infallible.

---

*An updated reference is: Sandin RH, Enlund G, Samuelsson P, Lenmarken C. Awareness during anaesthesia: A prospective case study. *Lancet* 2000; **355**:707–711.

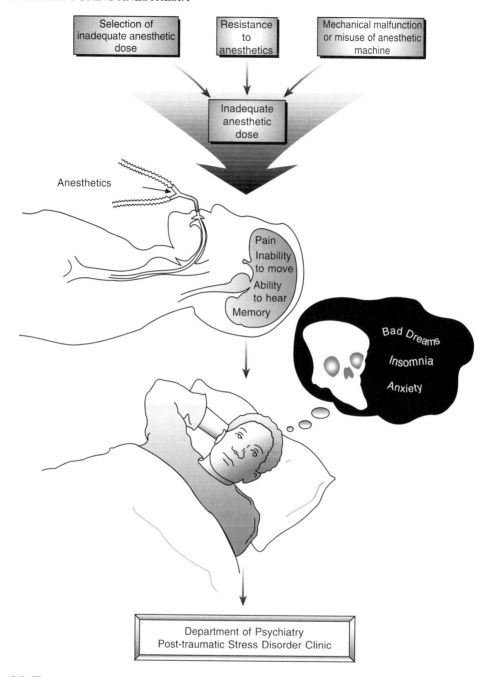

Figure 1.1. The causes and consequences of awareness during anesthesia. (Reprinted with permission from Ghoneim MM. Awareness during anesthesia. *Anesthesiology* 2000; **92**:597–602.)

The introduction of muscle relaxants in anesthesia practice introduced the problem of the unintentional too light anesthesia where unknown to the anesthesiologist the patient regains consciousness while remaining motionless due to paralysis. This is probably the commonest cause of awareness, therefore in a sense, awareness is essentially an iatrogenic mishap caused by the use of muscle relaxants. An inadequately anesthetized patient who is not paralyzed will usually (but not invariably) communicate his or her awakeness by movement, which alerts the anesthesiologist to deepen the anesthetic and thus prevents recall. The concentrations of anesthetics that block explicit memory are less than those which prevent motor responses to surgical stimuli.[77,78] Thus, when the patient first moves, he or she is still amnesic and deepening the anesthetic at this stage will usually prevent awareness. While current knowledge suggests that movement responses to noxious stimuli arise from the spinal cord,[79,80] and consciousness, learning and memory depend on interactions between various brain areas,[81,82] the depth of anesthesia that prevents movement response to noxious stimuli is fortunately greater than that needed for unconsciousness and amnesia. Chortkoff *et al.*[83] observed in their studies that MAC-awake appears to coincide with the anesthetic concentration that abolishes learning and memory, thereby potentially providing a surrogate end-point for amnesia.

Conscious recall of intraoperative events is therefore usually a dose-related phenomenon; however, the precise concentrations of anesthetic agents required to prevent recall are unknown in the usual clinical setting where the anesthesiologist uses a mixture of different drugs for induction and maintenance of anesthesia.

Heier and Steen[84] cite some theoretical reasons why total intravenous anesthesia may be associated with more awareness than volatile anesthetics:

- There is significant interindividual variability in the pharmacokinetics of intravenous anesthetics,[85–90] and during routine anesthesia the plasma drug concentration cannot adequately be predicted from the dose administered. Even with a computer-controlled infusion pump, using population-based pharmacokinetic data for drug delivery, the plasma concentration can deviate significantly from the target,[87] often resulting in too low plasma drug concentration. On-line plasma drug concentration determination is not yet available. For volatile anesthetics, the brain drug concentrations can be adequately estimated intraoperatively using continuous end-tidal concentration measurements.
- The interindividual variability in drug concentration needed to prevent movement response to noxious stimulation may be less with volatile than with total intravenous anesthesia.[87] Ausems *et al.*[91] reported that the required supplemental dose of alfentanil to nitrous oxide that controlled hemodynamic responses to noxious stimuli varied

more than fourfold (Figure 1.2). It is possible that this variability in pharmacodynamic effects may extend to effects on consciousness and recall. Despite these reasons, which predict more difficulty with maintenance of an adequate level of anesthesia with intravenous rather than volatile agents there is no evidence that the incidence of awareness is higher with total intravenous regimens.[62]

Increased anesthetic requirement of some patients

It is not unreasonable to expect that some patients may be more 'resistant' to the effects of anesthetics than others, analogous to the variability of responses seen with most drugs. Younger age, tobacco smoking, chronic use of drugs, such as alcohol, opiates, amphetamines, sedatives and tranquilizers,[92–100] and prior exposure to anesthetic agents,[101] may increase the anesthetic dose needed to produce unconsciousness. Guerra[102] suggested that there may be a higher incidence of consciousness and recall in obese patients because of the use of higher concentrations of oxygen in nitrous oxide–oxygen mixtures, the often prolonged time needed for endotracheal intubation, and the administration of lower doses of drugs to avoid excessive postoperative respiratory depression. The effects of obesity on the pharmacokinetics and pharmacodynamics of anesthetic drugs need to be adequately studied.

A machine malfunction or misuse

A machine malfunction or misuse may result in an inadequate concentration of anesthetic being delivered to the patient. This may be due to an empty vaporizer, leaks in the anesthesia machine, a malfunctioning or erroneous setting of a pump for intravenous anesthetics, or blockade or disconnection of its line to the vein, empty cylinder of nitrous oxide, or entrapment of air by a ventilator. Equipment failure or misuse are less common nowadays, particularly in developed countries, but they still happen despite the sophistication of modern anesthesia equipment.

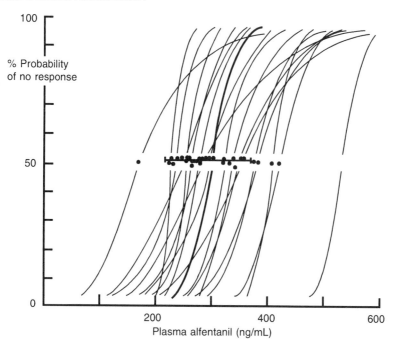

Figure 1.2. Alfentanil concentration *versus* effect curves for each patient receiving alfentanil and 66% nitrous oxide in oxygen during intra-abdominal surgery. The Cp_{50} (dots; the plasma concentration at which there is a 50% probability of suppressing a response to a specific stimulus) and slope of each curve was defined from multiple quantal responses of each patient using logistic regression. The heavy dark line represents the average response relationship for all patients (n = 34).--indicates $\pm$ SD of the mean Cp_{50}. (Reprinted with permission from Ausems ME, Vuyk J, Hug CC, Stanski DR. Comparison of a computer-assisted infusion *versus* intermittent bolus administration of alfentanil as a supplement to nitrous oxide for lower abdominal surgery. *Anesthesiology* 1988; **68**:851–861.)

Consequences

Patient's complaints

'The pain was like that of a tooth drilled without local anesthetic – when the drill hits a nerve. Multiply this pain so that the area involved would equal a thumb-print, then pour a steady stream of molten lead into it.'

The above quotation is from a physician describing her almost unbearable pain when she was aware during a Cesarean section.[103] There is no doubt that pain when present during surgery is the most distressing feature of awareness. Other frequent complaints of patients are ability to hear events during surgery, sensations of weakness or paralysis and feelings of helplessness, anxiety, panic, and impending death (see Figure 1.1). It seems that patients particularly recall conversations or remarks that are of a negative nature concerning themselves or their medical conditions.[104,105]

Patients may be unable to communicate their distress after surgery. This may be caused by the medical staff's disbelieving the patient or avoiding discussion of the issue, perhaps because of feelings of guilt or embarrassment and/or possible future litigation. Some lay people, like patients' families and friends, despite recent publicity about awareness during anesthesia, may not believe that consciousness can happen during a planned general anesthetic. The patients may also be tormented, if they were in an obtunded state, by doubts as to whether what they experienced really happened or whether there is something wrong with their minds.[23,106,107]

Temporary after-effects and post-traumatic stress disorder

For some patients, the experience of awareness may cause temporary after-effects, including sleep disturbances, nightmares and day-time anxiety that subside with time after surgery. For almost all patients though, there remains a nagging fear that awareness may happen again if they require anesthesia in the future.[108,109] However, some others develop post-traumatic stress disorder, marked by repetitive nightmares (usually poorly disguised replays of an operative situation), anxiety and irritability, a preoccupation with death, and a concern with sanity that make the patients reluctant to discuss their symptoms.[23] It is not readily apparent why some patients develop a post-traumatic stress disorder and others do not. Guerra[106] suggested that the patient's personality, emotional response to the illness and reason for the surgery may be factors. Blacher[23] claimed that patients who are wide awake, although they may suffer greatly during the procedure, may have fewer traumatic symptoms afterward than those who are in an obtunded state, perhaps because while awake what happens is not in doubt. However, this contradicts the current literature that suggests that most patients who suffer prolonged after-effects have experienced pain during the awareness episode.[59,76,84,105,110]

Osterman and van der Kolk[76] have suggested that the diagnosis of awareness induced post-traumatic stress disorder must be considered for all patients who present for mental health treatment following surgery. The following is a quotation from the report of a patient who suffered disabling after-effects following her awareness episode.[111]

'My awareness during surgery has dramatically changed my whole life. Not a minute goes by that I don't remember the horror of my surgery. In many respects my life has been a nightmare since my surgery. It's very difficult to talk about because I know of no one who has experienced what I have experienced.' (See Chapter 8 for more details.)

Medicolegal consequences

In addition to the medical consequences of awareness that are suffered by patients, there are medicolegal consequences that the anesthesia providers may have to face. Domino *et al.*[112] recently analyzed claims from the American Society of Anesthesiologists Closed Claims Project. Claims for awareness during anesthesia were 2% of all claims. This incidence was similar to rates of claims for such familiar complications after anesthesia, such as aspiration pneumonia and myocardial infarction. Claims were more likely in females and with nitrous oxide–opioid–relaxant technique. The latter is consistent with the increased incidence of awareness during light anesthesia. The issue of gender is unclear. Perhaps women are more likely than men to sue for emotional injury. The amount of compensation was rather modest, a median of $18,000. Payments for awareness claims show also some interesting variability from one country to another. While sizable payments have been reported in the United Kingdom, low payments have been reported in Finland. Social or cultural factors or others may be important. (See Chapter 9 for a complete discussion.)

Management

Five memoranda

If a patient complains of awareness, a detailed account of the patient's experience should be obtained (Table 1.2). This should include everything the patient heard or felt. Recall of conversations, particular sounds of instruments specific to the operation, specific events during the surgery, e.g. suturing, splitting the sternum, sensations of pain, paralysis, and others should be particularly noted and recorded. While there have been cases of fraudulent claims[113] and mistaken recall of events during emergence from anesthesia or dreaming at this time being interpreted as intraoperative events,[105] most claims are genuine[114] and their credibility can be easily established.

Table 1.2. Management: five memoranda

- Detailed interview with the patient
    Verify the patient's account
    Sympathize with the patient
    Try to explain what happened
    Reassure the patient about non-repetition in the future
    Apologize
    Offer psychological support
- Interview should be recorded in the patient's chart
- Inform the patient's surgeon, nurse and hospital lawyer
- Visit the patient daily during hospital stay and keep in contact by telephone afterwards
- Don't delay referral to a psychologist or psychiatrist

(Reprinted with permission from Ghoneim MM. Awareness during anesthesia. *Anesthesiology* 2000; **92**:597–602.)

The patient should be assured that the anesthesiologist believes their account and sympathizes with their suffering. Denial of the authenticity of the patient's experience may adversely influence the patient's psychological recovery and may turn him or her toward litigation.[102,113,115] Some explanation of what happened to the patient and its reasons should be given; e.g. necessity to administer light anesthesia in the presence of significant cardiovascular instability. The patient should be reassured about non-repetition of the same mishap with future anesthetics because the details will be in the patient's records and will guide the anesthesiologist managing subsequent anesthetics. An apology should be given and it is possible to apologize without admitting liability. The patient should be offered psychological or psychiatric support.

The details of the interview should be recorded in the patient's chart, and the surgeon, the patient's nurse and the hospital lawyer or the physician's insurer should be notified. Subsequently, the patient should be visited daily during hospital stay to look for and treat any psychological sequelae; e.g. sleep disturbances, day-time anxiety, intrusive thoughts of the surgery, etc. After the patient is discharged, frequent contacts through the telephone should be made until the patient is judged to be fully recovered. Referral to a psychiatrist or psychologist should not be delayed because there is some anecdotal evidence that early counseling may reduce the incidence of post-traumatic stress disorder.[71,76,116,117]

Prevention

Ten suggestions

Prevention of recall of events during anesthesia should be feasible in most cases (Table 1.3):

1 *Premedicate patients with amnesic drugs; e.g. benzodiazepines or scopolamine, particularly when light anesthesia is anticipated.* Benzodiazepines impair acquisition or encoding of new information, anterograde amnesia, while leaving the retrieval of previously learned material intact. They impair many types of explicit memory. The drugs impair episodic memory but not semantic memory. They do not impair short-term memory. They impair conscious effortful cognitive processes but do

Table 1.3. Prevention: ten suggestions

- Consider premedicating with amnesics
- Give adequate doses of induction agents
- Avoid muscle paralysis unless it is needed and even then avoid total paralysis
- Supplement N_2O and opioid anesthesia with at least 0.6 MAC of volatile agent
- Administer at least 0.8–1 MAC when volatile agents are used alone
- Use amnesics when light anesthesia is the only regimen that can be tolerated by the patient
- Check the delivery of anesthetic agents to the patient
- Inform the patient about the possibility of awareness and prevent hearing of operating room sounds
- Teaching and research
- Development of an awareness monitor

(Reprinted with permission from Ghoneim MM. Awareness during anesthesia. *Anesthesiology* 2000; **92**:597–602.)

not impair learning of skills or procedures.[118] Scopolamine also impairs acquisition, similar to the benzodiazepines. The types of explicit memory that are impaired are similar to those affected by the benzodiazepines, although scopolamine tends to impair short-term memory and some retrieval from semantic memory.[119–121]

The degree and duration of memory impairment progressively increase as the dose of each drug is increased. Figure 1.3 shows the results of an immediate free recall task administered at various times before and after oral administration of placebo, 0.1, 0.2 and 0.3 mg/kg diazepam.[122] In this task, subjects were asked to remember lists consisting of 24 words. Immediately after the last word of each list was presented, subjects were asked to write as many of the words as they could remember. One can see a progressive impairment of memory and parallel delayed recovery as the dose of the drug was increased. Similar results have been found with other benzodiazepines and with scopolamine.

Another point to emphasize regarding amnesia with the benzodiazepines is the specific drug given.[118] Some drugs are more potent as amnesics compared to others. Midazolam, triazolam and lorazepam are more potent in this respect. The dose of the drug to be given to produce maximal amnesia has to be counterbalanced by the potential side effects;

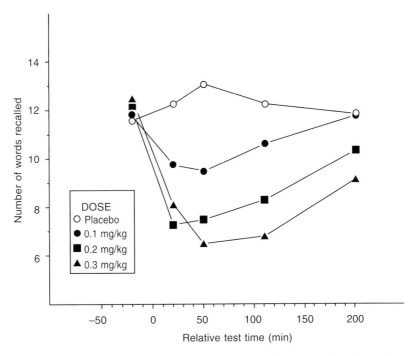

Figure 1.3. The mean number of words recalled in an immediate recall task as a function of test time relative to diazepam administration. Zero was the time of drug administration. (Reprinted with permission from Ghoneim MM, Hinrichs JV, Mewaldt SP. Dose-response analysis of the behavioral effects of diazepam: I. Learning and memory. *Psychopharmacology* 1984; **82**:291–295.)

e.g. dry mouth and postoperative delirium after scopolamine, and prolonged postoperative sedation after the benzodiazepines. An oral dose of diazepam, 0.2–0.3 mg/kg given 60–75 minutes before anesthesia produces anxiolytic and sedative effects in addition to the amnesia, and is usually well tolerated by most patients. Equivalent doses of other benzodiazepines can be used. Scopolamine 0.3–0.6 mg administered intramuscularly to adults is acceptable. Perhaps its use should be avoided in the elderly who seem to be sensitive to its undesirable CNS effects; i.e. delirium and prolonged somnolence. (It should be remembered that the exact dose of a benzodiazepine or scopolamine, which would *guarantee* absence of awareness in the patient during surgery, if such a dose exists, is unknown and is unlikely to be determined. Studies with these drugs, like the one shown in Figure 1.3, usually use volunteers who are presented neutral or non-threatening stimuli and aim to avoid doses which produce a 'floor' effect. To do a prospective dose-response study for investigating memory for intraoperative events during very light anesthesia would be fraught with ethical hazards as well as other problems.)

2 *Administer more than a 'sleep dose' of induction agents if they will be followed immediately by tracheal intubation.* The rapid redistribution of induction agents out of the brain and the strong stimuli of laryngoscopy and intubation tend to awaken the patients if an inadequate dose has been administered. The frequent report of cases of awareness associated with endo-tracheal intubation[105,112,123] should be a reminder to the anesthesiologist in everyday practice. Supplemental doses of induction agents should also be given when a difficult intubation is accompanied by a protracted period of intubation attempts. This important precautionary measure is frequently forgotten while the anesthesiologist is struggling to provide a patent airway to the patient.

3 *Avoid muscle paralysis unless it is needed for intubation and/or surgery and even then avoid total paralysis.* As we mentioned previously, awareness is essentially an iatrogenic mishap caused by the use of muscle relaxants. Auto-nomic responses to noxious stimuli during light

anesthesia; i.e. tachycardia, hypertension, sweating, lacrimation, and pupillary dilatation and reaction are unreliable indicators of anesthetic depth. They are affected by treatment with cardiovascular active drugs, changes in blood volume and cardiac contractility, acid–base disturbances and other factors.[124] Moerman et al.[105] reported that inspection of anesthetic records of awareness cases for relevant parameters, such as heart rate and blood pressure, could not be reliably distinguished from controls by experienced anesthesiologists. Schwender et al.[125] found no correlation between cardiovascular parameters and motor signs of wakefulness during general anesthesia supplemented by epidural analgesia, which may further obtund any sympathetic response to light anesthesia. Russell,[126] using the isolated forearm technique found that changes in blood pressure, heart rate, sweating and lacrimation could not be used to predict when a patient was awake. Thus, observation of voluntary movements or movement responses to noxious stimuli is the best clinical measure available for detecting wakefulness or its impendency during surgery. It is not infallible, but is the best we currently have. (Few non-paralyzed patients have been reported to be awake during surgery.[109,127] They felt comfortable, otherwise they would have moved; therefore, there is no reason to expect serious psychological sequelae in the non-paralyzed patient.) It is, therefore, necessary to use a nerve stimulator when administering a muscle relaxant to allow titration of the dose to preserve the patient's ability to some limb movement, if possible. It is also obvious that if the patient moves, administration of more muscle relaxant and not more anesthetic would be an illogical choice of drugs.

4   *Supplement nitrous oxide and opioid anesthesia with volatile agents to maintain their end-tidal concentrations at least at 0.6% MAC.*[128,129] The incidence of intraoperative recall is 2% when 70% N_2O alone is used for anesthetic maintenance.[68] In a recent study[69] with N_2O supplemented with opioid bolus doses: 7.5 microgram/kg fentanyl at induction and supplemental doses of 2.5 microgram/kg whenever the systolic arterial pressure or heart rate increased more than 15% above the preanesthetic values, the incidence of intraoperative recall was 6%. Thus, this method of supplementation of nitrous oxide does not reduce the risk of awareness compared with a pure nitrous oxide anesthetic. Perhaps, this is not surprising considering that administration of fentanyl to healthy volunteers does not affect learning and recall.[130,131] Also opioids, even in high doses, do not reliably produce unconsciousness.[132] Nitrous oxide has weaker memory and cognitive effects than equipotent concentrations of isoflurane.[78,133] Explicit memory was prevented in volunteers by 0.45 MAC isoflurane, but not completely prevented by 0.6 MAC N_2O (the ED_{50} was 0.2 MAC for isoflurane and 0.5 MAC for N_2O).[78]

5   *When inhalation agents are used alone, at least 0.8–1 MAC should be administered.*[77] These figures and those in the previous paragraph should be considered as tentative and may need to be reconsidered in the future. Data, which were obtained from healthy volunteers and in patients before surgery, may underestimate the concentrations needed during surgery. Until then, a prudent anesthesiologist may elect to use higher doses whenever feasible.

6   *In cases where light anesthesia is deemed necessary, the use of even small doses of amnesic drugs, e.g. scopolamine, midazolam, subanesthetic doses of ketamine, or inhalational agents and/or regional anesthesia should be considered.* In obstetric practice after induction of anesthesia with a drug like thiopental 3–5 mg/kg intravenously, anesthesia should be maintained with 50% N_2O in oxygen and 0.5–0.6 MAC of a volatile anesthetic. This low dose of volatile anesthetic usually ensures maternal unconsciousness without increasing maternal blood loss, altering the response of the uterus to oxytocin, or producing neonatal depression. It is advisable to monitor the output of the vaporizer and to add scopolamine as a premedicant in cases where awareness has been reported before by the patient. After delivery, anesthesia can be supplemented with additional volatile drugs or opioids.[134,135] Other situations where light anesthesia may need to be used include emergence from cardiac bypass, trauma surgery, hypovolemic patients, patients with severe cardiovascular disease and old patients with multiple organ pathologies.

Scopolamine's cardiovascular effects are restricted to a moderate and short-lived tachycardia. CNS toxicity manifested as delirium or prolonged postoperative somnolence, particularly in the elderly may occur but can be antagonized by physostigmine. Midazolam's effects on the cardiovascular system are relatively mild compared with other anesthetics and the severity of a patient's cardiovascular disease does not appear to influence significantly the hemodynamic responses.[136] There is synergism between benzodiazepines and volatile anesthetics when used in combination.[137,138] This interaction could be beneficial in reducing the required dose of benzodiazepine or the volatile anesthetic. However, benzodiazepines in clinical doses do not reliably suppress processing of sensory and, especially, auditory stimuli.[139] When combined with opioids (e.g. alfentanil and midazolam),[140] most patients seem to be in an amnesic–analgesic plane rather than truly unconscious.[141] In a recent study,[142] we found that administration of midazolam 0.03 and 0.05 mg/kg^{-1} to healthy volunteers inhaling 0.2% isoflurane almost completely abolished explicit memory, but there was still some responsiveness in some subjects, particularly with the lower dose of midazolam indicating wakefulness. Other studies in healthy volunteers[143] and in patients using the isolated forearm technique[46,144] demonstrated also responsiveness with no subsequent explicit memory.

Can episodes of intraoperative consciousness without subsequent recall cause harm? There is no direct evidence for this possibility, but there are a few anecdotal reports[23,145] of unfavorable comments voiced during anesthesia and retrieved under hypnosis that caused psychological disorders. Unfortunately, case reports cannot establish a cause and effect relationship, particularly where techniques such as hypnosis, which can sometimes lead to spurious recall, have been used.

Ketamine in subanesthetic doses (0.25 and 0.5 mg/kg intramuscularly and 0.4 mg/kg intravenously) in volunteers impairs immediate and delayed explicit recall.[146–148] Ketamine also produces cardiovascular stimulation due to direct stimulation of sympathetic nervous system outflow from the brain. This effect may be useful in patients who are hypovolemic, but may be absent in the presence of catecholamine depletion. Ketamine also produces positive symptoms of psychosis, such as illusions, disturbances in thought organization and delusions, which may extend into the recovery period. Delirium and recurrent illusions (flashbacks), which may persist for several weeks, may also occur. These psychotogenic and dissociative effects can be ameliorated by premedication with benzodiazepines.[149]

It may be worthwhile to remember using the previously mentioned intravenous agents that they should be given before and not after any expected episode of awareness; e.g. anticipated increase in intensity of surgical stimulus; they should be given in as large doses as can be tolerated by the patient; and supplemental doses or infusion should be considered if a long duration of action is desired. Generally, a continuous administration is preferable to a bolus dosing technique.

Subanesthetic concentrations of inhalation anesthetics and propofol impair explicit memory in a steep dose-response function. MAC awake (the end-tidal concentration preventing voluntary response in 50% of volunteers) is 0.38 MAC for isoflurane, 0.64 MAC for N_2O, and 0.36 MAC for desflurane.[78,83,150] The Cp50-awake for propofol is 2.69 microgram/ml. (Cp50 is the plasma concentration required to prevent a response in 50% of patients.) Explicit memory is prevented by 0.4 MAC isoflurane, but not completely prevented by 0.6 MAC N_2O. Desflurane in a concentration of 0.6 MAC prevents explicit memory to a similar degree to that provided by the same concentration of isoflurane. Propofol is amnestic at concentrations lower than Cp50-awake.[151]

The institution of peripheral nerve blocks, infiltration anesthesia, or low levels of spinal and epidural anesthesia, provided these methods are appropriate for surgery, would reduce the dose of general anesthetic needed to abolish awareness by suppressing the surgical stimulus through deafferentation.[152] (See also Chapter 7 for a study of the incidence of consciousness in patients with and without supplemental epidural anesthesia.)

Finally, physicians administering anesthesia to severely ill patients and major trauma patients are best served by heeding the advice of Hug:[131] 'Unless patient survival is critically dependent on avoiding even momentary hypotension, my first priority is to assure unconsciousness.' Aldrete and Wright[153] have expressed a similar sentiment, suggesting that the anesthesiologist's armamentarium includes drugs that can be used in small doses under circumstances of hemodynamic instability to produce at least amnesia. It is amazing that some patients retain the abilities of learning and recall under adverse physiological states.[66] The inability to identify retrospectively in patients with major traumas, patients who suffered from postoperative recall and those who did not, based on conditions known to reduce anesthetic requirement,[66] probably extends to other patients with hemodynamic instability caused by other factors. It is, therefore, necessary that all patients who receive reduced doses of anesthetics should be considered liable to become aware during surgery and the above mentioned prevention measures instituted.

7 *Periodic maintenance of the anesthesia machine and its vaporizers and meticulous checking of the machine and its ventilator before administration of anesthesia.* Regular checking of the settings of the flow meters and the vaporizer, and the level of the anesthetic in the vaporizing chamber; continuous monitoring of the concentrations of inspired and expired gases, and inhalation agents; and vigilance during the course of anesthesia should eliminate cases due to inadequate anesthetic delivery. Infusion pumps for intravenous anesthetics must have volume and pressure alarms, and the anesthetic infusion should preferably be administered via a dedicated intravenous line. The flow in the chosen vein should not be interrupted, e.g. by a frequently inflated blood pressure cuff, or be susceptible to leakage at a more central site because of surgery. The anesthesiologist should regularly confirm delivery of the anesthetic to the patient by visual inspection of the volume of the drug in the syringe.

8 *Discussion of the potential for awareness and auditory masking.* It has been suggested that in some cases, the anesthesiologist should talk to the patient about the potential for awareness and/or use measures, like earplugs and audiocassette earphones playing music or positive therapeutic suggestions.[154] Informing the patient about the possibility of awareness should be restricted to cases where such a risk is relatively high, e.g. a high risk obstetric or cardiac case. It would add another burden of worry to the patient who is facing the ordeals of anesthesia and surgery, although it may help in protecting the physician from a lawsuit.

The most distressing feature of awareness is pain. In addition to the ability to hear, other frequent complaints of patients are the sensation of paralysis, helplessness, anxiety and panic. It is, therefore, apparent that measures to prevent the patient from hearing operating room sounds fall short of alleviating most patient's complaints. Nevertheless, because patients are most likely to recall emotionally threatening remarks,[105] it is prudent for the operating room team to avoid voicing negative or derogatory remarks about the patients or their prognosis.

9 *Teaching and research.* Cobcroft and Forsdick[104] after reviewing a series of cases of awareness concluded that in most cases understanding of the phenomenon and its management by medical personnel were poor or entirely lacking. In Moerman et al.'s[105] series of cases of awareness, half of the patients had not informed their anesthesiologists because they had not seen him or her since the operation, despite the importance of a postoperative interview that allows the anesthesiologist to deal with this traumatic experience at an appropriate early time.[117] Many cases reported in the literature could have been prevented if there had been better knowledge about the pharmacokinetics, pharmacodynamics and drug delivery system of the anesthetics used.[62,155] It is possible that the incidence of awareness during anesthesia has reached a plateau and that further significant decreases depend on disseminating information to anesthesiologists about the subject through scientific journals and meetings, gaining more knowledge about anesthetic requirements of patients and developing methods to detect consciousness during anesthesia. There is some evidence that reminding anesthesiologists of the potential for awareness and giving them educational material

related to the problem may reduce its incidence through avoidance of 'overly' light anesthesia and decrease in the dose of muscle relaxants used.[64]

10 *Monitor for awareness*. There is current interest in the development and use of a monitor of anesthetic depth. New technological advances and keen interest of the news media in reporting and commenting on cases of awareness have been some of the underlying factors. (The subject of measuring the depth of anesthesia is fully covered in Chapter 3.) We will confine ourselves here to some comments relating to the use of an 'awareness monitor', which would track patients' arousal level and warn of impending wakefulness. Such a monitor should be a rapidly responding 'on-line' instrument, which differentiates reliably wakefulness and unconsciousness at their interface as during induction of anesthesia, when light anesthesia becomes too light and during emergence from anesthesia. However, it should be remembered that because the incidence of awareness is low, it will be difficult to prove that the use of a certain monitor can prevent awareness. Currently, the mid-latency auditory evoked response[59] and the bispectral index of the electroencephalograph[156] are being investigated. At present, the determination of mid-latency auditory evoked responses requires more technical expertise, effort and money than the bispectral index monitoring.

Conclusions

Patients' waking up during their anesthetic is an uncommon complication, though alarming to both patients and anesthesiologists alike. When we consider that approximately 20 million general anesthetics are administered each year in the United States, one case in each 500 anesthetics incidence corresponds to 40,000 cases of awareness annually, an unacceptable number in terms of human suffering. There is a higher incidence in obstetrics, cardiac and trauma surgery. There has also been an increased public concern and consequently more patients seem to harbor some apprehension about being adequately anesthetized during surgery.

Awareness appears to be a dose-related phenomenon and the risk is greatest when muscle relaxants are used. Machine malfunction or misuse may also be another cause. Auditory perception, the sensation of paralysis, panic and pain are frequent complaints. The most feared consequence of awareness is post-traumatic stress disorder. It is not clear how many or why only some patients develop the disorder, the possible measures to prevent it, and the best methods for its treatment. There are also medicolegal consequences for the anesthesia providers, which seem to be increasing, specifically in the USA. Management of a case of awareness should be precise, detailed and documented, but compassionate. Currently, there is no reliable way to detect intraoperative awareness. Observation of patients' movements is the best clinical measure short of a reliable sophisticated monitor. Measures to prevent awareness include avoidance of 'overly' light anesthesia, premedicating patients with amnesic drugs, checking the delivery of anesthetic agents to the patients, teaching of anesthesia practitioners, gaining more knowledge about anesthetic requirements of patients and development of methods to detect consciousness during anesthesia.

References

1. Tulving E. Episodic and semantic memory. In Tulving E, Donaldson W (eds). *Organization of Memory*. New York: Academic Press, 1972, 381–403.
2. Schacter DL, Tulving E. What are the memory systems of 1994? In Schacter DL, Tulving E (eds). *Memory Systems 1994*. Cambridge: MIT Press, 1994, 1–38.
3. Graf P, Schacter DL. Implicit and explicit memory for new associates in normal subjects and amnesic patients. *J Exp Psychol (Learn Mem Cogn)* 1985; **11**:501–518.
4. Schacter DL. Implicit memory: History and current status. *J Exp Psychol (Learn Mem Cogn)* 1987; **13**:501–518.
5. Schacter DL. Implicit knowledge: New perspectives on unconscious processes. *Proc Natl Acad Sci USA* 1992; **89**:11113–11117.
6. Squire LR. Memory and the hippocampus: A synthesis from findings with rats, monkeys and humans. *Psychol Rev* 1992; **99**:195–231.
7. Squire LR. Declarative and nondeclarative memory: Multiple brain systems supporting learning and memory. In Schacter DL, Tulving E (eds). *Memory Systems 1994*. Cambridge: MIT Press, 1994, 203–232.

8. Richardson-Klavehn A, Bjork RA. Measures of memory. *Ann Rev Psychol* 1988; **36**:475–543.

9. Ghoneim MM, Block RI. The word 'awareness': Its ambiguous and confusing use in anesthesia literature on memory (correspondence). *Anesthesiology* 1990; **73**:193.

10. *The Oxford English Dictionary*, 2nd edition, Oxford: Clarendon Press, 1989.

11. Payne JP. Awareness and its medicolegal implications. *Br J Anaesth* 1994; **73**:38–45.

12. Hinrichs JV. Human learning. In Levin IP, Hinrichs JV (eds) *Experimental Psychology: Contemporary Methods and Applications*. Madison: Brown & Benchmark, 1995, 165–204.

13. Andrade J. Consciousness: Current views. In Jones JG (ed). *Depth of Anesthesia. Intern Anesth Clin* 1993; **31**:13–25.

14. Pöppel E, Schwender D. Temporal mechanisms of consciousness. In Jones JG (ed). *Depth of Anesthesia. Intern Anesth Clin* 1993; **31**:27–38.

15. Plourde G, Picton TW. Long-latency auditory evoked potentials during general anesthesia: N1 and P3 components. *Anesth Analg* 1991; **72**:342–350.

16. Vandam LD. History of anesthetic practice. In Miller RD (ed). *Anesthesia* (4th edn). New York: Churchill Livingstone, 1994, 9–19.

17. Calverley RK. Anesthesia as a specialty: Past, present and future. In Barash PG, Cullen BF, Stoelting RK (eds) *Clinical Anesthesia*. Philadelphia: JB Lippincott 1989, 3–33.

18. Pierson AL. Surgical operation with the aid of the 'new gas'. *Bost Med Surg J* 1846; **35**:362–364.

19. Richardson J. Personal experiences under nitrous oxide. *Br J Dent Sci* 1873; **16**:102–106.

20. Crile G. *George Crile: An Autobiography*. Philadelphia: Lippincott, 1947, 197.

21. Jacobson E. Consciousness under anaesthetics. *Am J Psychol* 1911; **22**:333–345.

22. Griffith HR, Johnson GE. Use of curare in general anesthesia. *Anesthesiology* 1942; **3**:418–420.

23. Blacher RS. General surgery and anesthesia: The emotional experiences. In Blacher RS (ed). *The Psychological Experience of Surgery*. New York: John Wiley, 1987; 1–25.

24. Harroun P, Beckert FE, Fisher CW. The physiologic effects of curare and its use as an adjunct to anesthesia. *Surg Gynecol Obstet* 1947; **84**:491–498.

25. Winterbottom EH. Insufficient anaesthesia. *Br Med J* 1950; **1**:247–248.

26. Hutchinson R. Awareness during surgery: A study of its incidence. *Br J Anaesth* 1960; **33**:463–469.

27. Wilson SL, Vaughan RW, Stephen CR. Awareness, dreams and hallucinations associated with general anesthesia. *Anesth Analg* 1975; **54**:609–616.

28. Steinberg H. *Some effects of depressant drugs on behavior*. Ph.D. Thesis, London University, 1953.

29. Steinberg H. Selective effects of an anaesthetic drug on cognitive behavior. *QJ Exp Psychol (A)* 1954; **6**:170–180.

30. Steinberg H. Changes in time perception induced by an anaesthetic drug. *Br J Psychol* 1955; **46**:273–279.

31. James W. *The Varieties of Religious Experience*. New York: Longmans Green, 1905.

32. Parkhouse JD, Henrie JR, Duncan GM, Rome HP. Nitrous oxide analgesia in relation to mental performance. *J Pharmacol Exp Ther* 1960; **128**:44–54.

33. Bruce DL, Bach MJ, Arbit J. Trace anesthetic effects on perceptual, cognitive, and motor skills. *Anesthesiology* 1974; **40**:453–458.

34. Cook TL, Smith M, Starkweather JA, Winter PM, Eger EI II. Behavioral effects of trace and subanesthetic halothane and nitrous oxide in man. *Anesthesiology* 1978; **49**:419–424.

35. Cook TL, Smith M, Starkweather JA, Eger EI II. Effects of subanesthetic concentrations of enflurane and halothane on human behavior. *Anesth Analg* 1978; **57**:434–440.

36. Chenoweth MB. Abuse of inhalational anesthetics. In Sharp CW, Brehm ML (eds). *Review of Inhalants: Euphoria to Dysfunction*. NIDA Research Monogr, DHEW Publication No. (ADM)80-553, Washington DC, US Government Printing Office, 1977, 102–111.

37. Layzer RB. Myeloneuropathy after prolonged exposure to nitrous oxide. *Lancet* 1978; **2**:1227–1230.

38. Rosenberg H, Orkin FK, Springstead J. Abuse of nitrous oxide. *Anesth Analg* 1979; **58**:104–106.

39. Artusio JF. Diethyl ether analgesia: A detailed description of the first stage of ether anesthesia in man. *J Pharmacol Exp Ther* 1954; **111**:343–348.

40. Artusio JF. Ether analgesia during major surgery. *JAMA* 1955; **157**:33–36.

41. Ghoneim MM, Block RI. Learning and memory during anesthesia: An update. *Anesthesiology* 1997; **87**:387–410.

42. Snow J. *On the Inhalation of the Vapour of Ether in Surgical Operations*. London: John Churchill, 1847.

43. Guedel AE. *Inhalation Anaesthesia: A Fundamental Guide*. New York: Macmillan 1937.

44. Eger EI II, Saidman LJ, Brandstater B. Minimum alveolar anesthetic concentration: A standard of anesthetic potency. *Anesthesiology* 1965; **26**:756–763.

45. Tunstall ME. Detecting wakefulness during general anaesthesia for caesarean section. *Br Med J* 1977; **1**:1321.

46. Russell IF. Comparison of wakefulness with two anaesthetic regimens: Total iv v. balanced anaesthesia. *Br J Anaesth* 1986; **58**:965–968.

47. Faulconer A Jr, Bickford RG. *Electroencephalography in Anesthesiology*. Springfield: Charles C. Thomas, 1960.

48. Thornton C, Catley DM, Jordan C, Royston D, Lehane JR, Jones JG. Enflurane increases the latency of early components of the auditory evoked response in man. *Br J Anaesth* 1981; **53**:1102–1103.

49. Private Company interview – Aspect medical systems, Inc. *The Wall Street transcript*, April 19, 1999.

50. Liu J, Singh H, Wu G, Gaines GY, White PF. Use of EEG bispectral index to predict awakening from general anesthesia. *Anesth Analg* 1994; **78**:S254.

51. Rosen M, Lunn JN (eds). *Consciousness, Awareness and Pain in General Anaesthesia*. Boston: Butterworths, 1987.

52. Bonke B, Fitch W, Millar K (eds). *Memory and Awareness in Anaesthesia*. Amsterdam: Swets & Zeitlinger, 1990.

53. Sebel PS, Bonke B, Winograd E (eds). *Memory and Awareness in Anesthesia*. Englewood Cliffs: Prentice Hall, 1993.

54. Bonke B, Bovill JG, Moerman N (eds). *Memory and Awareness in Anesthesia*. Assen: Van Gorcum, 1996.

55. Jordan C, Vaughan DJA, Newton DEF (eds). *Memory and Awareness in Anaesthesia IV*. London: Imperial College Press, 2000.

56. Brice DD, Hetherington RR, Utting JE. A simple study of awareness and dreaming during anaesthesia. *Br J Anaesth* 1970; **42**:535–541.

57. Liu WHD, Thorp TAS, Graham SG, Aitkenhead AR. Incidence of awareness with recall during general anaesthesia. *Anaesthesia* 1991; **46**:435–437.

58. McPherson R. A book review. *Anesthesiology* 1994; **80**:1419.

59. Jones JG. Perception and memory during general anaesthesia. *Br J Anaesth* 1994; **73**:31–37.

60. Blacher RS. On awakening paralyzed during surgery: A syndrome of traumatic neurosis. *JAMA* 1975; **234**:67–68.

61. Ranta SOV, Laurila R, Saario J, Ali-Melkkilä T, Hynynen M. Awareness with recall during general anesthesia: Incidence and risk factors. *Anesth Analg* 1998; **86**:1084–1089.

62. Sandin R, Nordström O. Awareness during total i.v. anaesthesia. *Br J Anaesth* 1993; **71**:782–787.

63. Phillips AA, McLean RF, Devitt JH, Harrington EM. Recall of intraoperative events after general anaesthesia and cardiopulmonary bypass. *Can J Anaesth* 1993; **40**:922–926.

64. Ranta S, Jussila J, Hynynen M. Recall of awareness during cardiac anaesthesia: Influence of feedback information to the anaesthesiologist. *Acta Anaesthesiol Scand* 1996; **40**:554–560.

65. Lyons G, Macdonald R. Awareness during caesarean section. *Anaesthesia* 1991; **46**:62–64.

66. Bogetz MS, Katz JA. Recall of surgery for major trauma. *Anesthesiology* 1984; **61**:6–9.

67. Lubke GH, Kerssens C, Phaf H, Sebel PS. Dependence of explicit and implicit memory on hypnotic state in trauma patients. *Anesthesiology* 1999; **90**:670–680.

68. Utting JE. Awareness: Clinical aspects. In Rosen M, Lunn JN (eds) *Consciousness, Awareness and Pain in General Anaesthesia*. London: Butterworths 1987, 171–179.

69. Ghoneim MM, Block RI, Dhanaraj VJ, Todd MM, Choi WW, Brown CK. The auditory evoked responses and learning and awareness during general anesthesia. *Acta Anaesthesiol Scand* 2000; **44**:133–143.

70. Bennett HL. Awareness, learning, memory and recall. In Russell GB (ed). *Alternate-Site Anesthesia: Clinical Practice Outside the Operating Room*. Boston: Butterworth-Heinemann, 1997; 425–439.

71. Macleod AD, Maycock E. Awareness during anaesthesia and post-traumatic stress disorder. *Anaesth Intensive Care* 1992; **20**:378–382.

72. Russell IF, Wang M. Absence of memory for intraoperative information during surgery under adequate general anaesthesia. *Br J Anaesth* 1997; **78**:3–9.

73. Nordström O, Engström AM, Persson S, Sandin R. Incidence of awareness in total i.v. anaesthesia based on propofol, alfentanil and neuromuscular blockade. *Acta Anaesthesiol Scand* 1997; **41**:978–984.

74. Shalev AY, Peri T, Canetti L, Schreiber S. Predictors of PTSD in injured trauma survivors: A prospective study. *Am J Psychiatry* 1996; **153**:219–225.

75. van der Kolk BA, van der Hart O. Pierre Janet and the breakdown of adaptation in psychological trauma. *Am J Psychiatry* 1989; **146**:1530–1540.

76. Osterman JE, van der Kolk BA. Awareness during anesthesia and post-traumatic stress disorder. *Gen Hosp Psychiat* 1998; **20**:274–281.

77. Eger EI II, Lampe GH, Wauk LZ, Whitendale P, Cahalan MK, Donegan JH. Clinical pharmacology of nitrous oxide: An argument for its continued use. *Anesth Analg* 1990; **71**:575–585.

78. Dwyer R, Bennett HL, Eger EI II, Heilbron D. Effects of isoflurane and nitrous oxide in subanesthetic concentrations on memory and responsiveness in volunteers. *Anesthesiology* 1992; **77**:888–898.

79. Rampil IJ. Anesthetic potency (MAC) is not altered following hypothermic spinal cord transection in rats. *Anesthesiology* 1994; **80**:606–610.

80. Antognini JF, Schwartz K. Exaggerated anesthetic requirements in the preferentially anesthetized brain. *Anesthesiology* 1993; **79**:1244–1249.

81. Gabrieli JDE. Cognitive neuroscience of human memory. *Ann Rev Psychol* 1998; **49**:87–115.

82. Schacter DL. The cognitive neuroscience of memory: Perspectives from neuroimaging research. *Phil Trans R Soc Lond B* 1997; **352**:1689–1695.

83. Chortkoff BS, Eger EI II, Crankshaw DP, Gonsowski CT, Dutton RC, Ionescu P. Concentrations of desflurane and propofol that suppress response to command in humans. *Anesth Analg* 1995; **81**:737–743.

84. Heier T, Steen PA. Awareness in anaesthesia: Incidence, consequences and prevention. *Acta Anaesthesiol Scand* 1996; **40**:1073–1086.

85. Glass PSA, Doherty M, Jacobs JR, Goodman D, Smith LR. Plasma concentration of fentanyl, with 70% nitrous oxide, to prevent movement at skin incision. *Anesthesiology* 1993; **78**:842–843.

86. Ausems ME, Hug CC, Stanski DR, Burm AGL. Plasma concentrations of alfentanil required to supplement nitrous oxide anesthesia for general surgery. *Anesthesiology* 1986; **65**:362–373.

87. Vuyk J, Lim T, Engbers FHM, Burm AGL, Vletter AA, Bovill JG. Pharmacodynamics of alfentanil as a supplement to propofol or nitrous oxide for lower abdominal surgery in female patients. *Anesthesiology* 1993; **78**:1036–1045.

88. Philbin DM, Rosow CE, Schneider RC, Koski G, D'Ambra MN. Fentanyl and sufentanil anesthesia revisited: How much is enough? *Anesthesiology* 1990; **73**:5–11.

89. Spelina KR, Coates DP, Monk CR, Prys-Roberts C, Norley I, Turtle MJ. Dose requirements of propofol by infusion during nitrous oxide anaesthesia in man. *Br J Anaesth* 1986; **58**:1080–1084.

90. Sear JW. Continuous infusions of hypnotic agents for maintenance of anaesthesia. In Kay B (ed). *Total Intravenous Anaesthesia*. Amsterdam: Elsevier 1991; 15–56.

91. Ausems ME, Vuyk J, Hug CC, Stanski DR. Comparison of a computer-assisted infusion *versus* intermittent bolus administration of alfentanil as a supplement to nitrous oxide for lower abdominal surgery. *Anesthesiology* 1988; **68**:851–861.

92. Tammisto T, Takki S. Nitrous oxide–oxygen–relaxant anaesthesia in alcoholics: A retrospective study. *Acta Anaesthesiol Scand (Suppl)* 1973; **53**:68–75.

93. Tammisto T, Tigerstedt I. The need for halothane supplementation of N_2O–O_2 relaxant anesthesia in chronic alcoholics. *Acta Anaesthesiol Scand* 1977; **21**:17–23.

94. Lemmens HJM, Bovill JG, Hennis PJ, Gladines MPRR, Burm AGL. Alcohol consumption alters the pharmacodynamics of alfentanil. *Anesthesiology* 1989; **71**:669–674.

95. Swerdlow BN, Holley FO, Maitre PO, Stanski DR. Chronic alcohol intake does not change thiopental anesthetic requirement, pharmacokinetics, or pharmacodynamics. *Anesthesiology* 1990; **72**:455–461.

96. Bailey PL, Stanley TH. Are opioids anesthetics? Intravenous opioid anesthetics. In Miller RD (ed). *Anesthesia*. New York: Churchill Livingstone, 1994; 290–293.

97. Bailey PL, Wilbrink J, Zwanikken P, Pace NL, Stanley TH. Anesthetic induction with fentanyl. *Anesth Analg* 1985; **64**:48–53.

98. Stanley TH, deLange S. The effect of population habits on side effects and narcotic requirements during high-dose fentanyl anaesthesia. *Can Anaesth Soc J* 1984; **31**:368–376.

99. Shafer A, White PF, Schuettler J, Rosenthal MH. Use of fentanyl infusion in the intensive care unit: Tolerance to its anesthetic effects? *Anesthesiology* 1983; **59**:245–248.

100. Bovill JG, Sebel PS, Wauquier A, Rog P, Schuyt HC. Influence of high-dose alfentanil anesthesia on the electroencephalogram: Correlation with plasma concentrations. *Br J Anaesth* 1983; **55**:199S–209S.

101. Sia RL. Consciousness during general anaesthesia. *Anesth Analg* 1969; **48**:363–366.

102. Guerra F. Awareness and recall. In Hindman BT (ed). *Neurological and Psychological Complications of Surgery and Anesthesia. Intern Anesthesiol Clin* 1986; **24**:75–99.

103. Anonymous. On being aware (editorial). *Br J Anaesth* 1979; **51**:711–712.

104. Cobcroft MD, Forsdick C. Awareness under anaesthesia: The patient's point of view. *Anaesth Intensive Care* 1993; **21**:837–843.

105. Moerman N, Bonke B, Oosting J. Awareness and recall during general anesthesia. Facts and feelings. *Anesthesiology* 1993; **79**:454–464.

106. Guerra F. Awareness during anesthesia (letter). *Can Anaesth Soc J* 1980; **27**:178.

107. Brahms D. Anaesthesia and the law. Awareness and pain during anaesthesia. *Anaesthesia* 1989; **44**:352.

108. Grunshaw N. Anaesthetic awareness. *Br Med J* 1990; **300**:821.

109. Saucier N, Walts LF, Moreland JR. Patient awareness during nitrous oxide, oxygen and halothane anesthesia. *Anesth Analg* 1983; **62**:239–240.

110. Evans JM. Patients' experiences of awareness during general anaesthesia. In Rosen M, Lunn JN (eds). *Consciousness, Awareness and Pain in General Anesthesia.* London: Butterworths, 1987; 184–192.

111. Tracy J. Awareness in the operating room: A patient's view. In Sebel PS, Bonke B, Winograd E (eds). *Memory and Awareness in Anesthesia.* Englewood Cliffs: Prentice-Hall, 1993, 349–353.

112. Domino KB, Posner KL, Caplan RA, Cheney FW. Awareness during anesthesia: A closed claims analysis. *Anesthesiology* 1999; **90**:1053–1061.

113. Heneghan C. Clinical and medicolegal aspects of conscious awareness during anesthesia. In Jones JG (ed.) *Depth of Anesthesia. Intern Anesthesiol Clin* 1993; **31**:1–11.

114. Aitkenhead AR. Awareness during anaesthesia: What should the patient be told? (editorial). *Anaesthesia* 1990; **45**:351–352.

115. Bailey AR, Jones JG. Patients' memories of events during general anaesthesia. *Anaesthesia* 1997; **52**:460–476.

116. Cundy JM. Early intervention in treatment of post-anaesthetic awareness stress disorders. In Sebel PS, Bonke B, Winograd E (eds). *Memory and Awareness in Anesthesia.* Englewood Cliffs: Prentice-Hall, 1993; 343–348.

117. Bennett HL. Treating psychological sequelae of awareness. *Am Soc Anesthes Newsletter* 1994; **58**:12–15.

118. Ghoneim MM, Mewaldt SP. Benzodiazepines and human memory: A review. *Anesthesiology* 1990; **72**:926–938.

119. Ghoneim MM, Mewaldt SP. Effects of diazepam and scopolamine on storage, retrieval and organizational processes in memory. *Psychopharmacologia* 1975; **44**:257–262.

120. Tröster AI, Beatty WW, Staton RD, Rorabaugh AG. Effects of scopolamine on anterograde and remote memory in humans. *Psychobiology* 1989; **17**:12–18.

121. Molchan SE, Martinez RA, Hill JL, *et al.* Increased cognitive sensitivity to scopolamine with age and a perspective on the scopolamine model. *Brain Res Rev* 1992; **17**:215–226.

122. Ghoneim MM, Hinrichs JV, Mewaldt SP. Dose-response analysis of the behavioral effects of diazepam: I. Learning and memory. *Psychopharmacology* 1984; **82**:291–295.

123. McKenna T, Wilton TNP. Awareness during endotracheal intubation. *Anaesthesia* 1973; **28**:599–602.

124. Ghoneim MM, Block RI. Learning and consciousness during general anesthesia. *Anesthesiology* 1992; **76**:279–305.

125. Schwender D, Faber-Zullig E, Klasing S, Pöppel E, Peter K. Motor signs of wakefulness during general anesthesia with propofol, isoflurane and flunitrazepam/fentanyl and midlatency auditory evoked potentials. *Anaesthesia* 1994; **49**:476–484.

126. Russell IF. Conscious awareness during general anesthesia: Relevance of autonomic signs and isolated forearm movements as guides to depth of anaesthesia. In Jones JG, ed. *Depth of Anaesthesia. Clinical Anaesthesiology.* London: Balliere Tindall 1989; 511–532.

127. Ogilvy AJ. Awareness during total intravenous anaesthesia with propofol and remifentanil (correspondence). *Anaesthesia* 1998; **53**:308.

128. Hargrove RL. Awareness: A medicolegal problem. In Rosen M, Lunn JN (eds) *Consciousness, Awareness and Pain in General Anaesthesia.* London: Butterworth 1987, 149–154.

129. Lunn JN, Rosen M. Anaesthetic awareness (correspondence). *Br Med J* 1990; **300**:938.

130. Ghoneim MM, Mewaldt SP, Thatcher JW. The effect of diazepam and fentanyl on mental, psychomotor and electroencephalographic functions and their rate of recovery. *Psychopharmacologia (Berl)* 1975; **44**:61–66.

131. Scamman FL, Ghoneim MM, Korttila K. Ventilatory and mental effects of alfentanil and fentanyl. *Acta Anaesthesiol Scand* 1984; **28**:63–67.

132. Hug CC Jr. Does opioids 'anesthesia' exist? (editorial). *Anesthesiology* 1990; **73**:1–4.

133. McMenemin IM, Parbrook GD. Comparison of the effects of subanaesthetic concentrations of isoflurane or nitrous oxide in volunteers. *Br J Anaesth* 1988; **60**:56–63.

134. Stoelting RK, Miller RD. *Basics of Anesthesia.* New York: Churchill Livingstone 1994, 355–379.

135. Moir DD. Anaesthesia for caesarean section. An evaluation of a method using low concentrations of halothane and 50 per cent of oxygen. *Br J Anaesth* 1970; **42**:136–142.

136. Reves JG, Fragen RJ, Vinik HR, Greenblatt DJ. Midazolam: Pharmacology and uses. *Anesthesiology* 1985; **62**:310–324.

137. Perisho JA, Buechel DR, Miller RD. The effect of diazepam (Valium) on minimum alveolar anaesthetic requirement (MAC) in man. *Can J Anaesth* 1971; **18**:536–540.

138. Melvin MA, Johnson BH, Quasha AL, Eger EI II. Induction of anesthesia with midazolam decreases halothane MAC in humans. *Anesthesiology* 1982; **57**:238–241.

139. Schwender D, Klasing S, Madler C, Pöppel E, Peter K. Effects of benzodiazepines on mid-latency auditory evoked potentials. *Can J Anaesth* 1993; **40**:1148–1154.

140. Desidero D, Thorne AC, Shah NK. Alfentanil-midazolam anaesthesia: Protection against awareness. In Bronk B, Fitch W, Millar K (eds).

Memory and Awareness in Anaesthesia. Amesterdam: Swets and Zeitlinger 1990, 281–285.

141. Russell IF. Midazolam-alfentanil: An anaesthetic? An investigation using the isolated forearm technique. *Br J Anaesth* 1993; **70**:42–46.

142. Ghoneim MM, Block RI, Dhanaraj VJ. Interaction of a subanesthetic concentration of isoflurane with midazolam: Effects on responsiveness, learning and memory. *Br J Anaesth* 1998; **80**:581–587.

143. Andrade J, Munglani R, Jones JG, Baddeley AD. Cognitive performance during anesthesia. *Consciousness Cogn* 1994; **3**:148–165.

144. Schultetus RR, Hill CR, Dharamraj CM, Banner TE, Berman LS. Wakefulness during cesarean section after anesthetic induction with ketamine, thiopental, or ketamine and thiopental combined. *Anesth Analg* 1986; **65**:723–728.

145. Howard JF. Incidents of auditory perception during general anesthesia with traumatic sequelae. *Med J Aust* 1987; **146**:44–46.

146. Harris AJ, Biersner RJ, Edwards D, Bailey LW. Attention, learning and personality during ketamine emergence: A pilot study. *Anesth Analg* 1975; **54**:169–172.

147. Ghoneim MM, Hinrichs JV, Mewaldt SP, Petersen RC. Ketamine: Behavioral effects of subanesthetic doses. *J Clin Psychopharmacol* 1985; **5**:70–77.

148. Krystal JH, Karper LP, Bennett A, *et al.* Interactive effects of subanesthetic ketamine and subhypnotic lorazepam in humans. *Psychopharmacology* 1998; **135**:213–229.

149. White PF, Way WL, Trevor AJ. Ketamine – its pharmacology and therapeutic uses. *Anesthesiology* 1982; **56**:119–136.

150. Gonsowski CT, Chortkoff BS, Eger EI II, Bennett HL, Weiskopf RB. Subanesthetic concentrations of desflurane and isoflurane suppress explicit and implicit learning. *Anesth Analg* 1995; **80**:568–572.

151. Veselis RA, Reinsel RA, Wronski M, Marino P, Tong WP, Bedford RF. EEG and memory effects of low-dose infusions of propofol. *Br J Anaesth* 1992; 246–254.

152. Inagaki Y, Mashimo T, Kuzukawa A, Tsuda Y, Yoshiya I. Epidural lidocaine delays arousal from isoflurane anesthesia. *Anesth Analg* 1994; **79**: 368–372.

153. Aldrete JA, Wright AJ. Concerning the acceptability of awareness during surgery (correspondence). *Anesthesiology* 1985; **63**:460–461.

154. Cork RC, Couture LJ, Kihlstrom JF. Memory and recall. In Yaksh TL, Lynch C III, Zapol WM, Maze M, Biebuyck JF, Saidman LJ (eds). *Anesthesia Biologic Foundations.* Philadelphia: Lippincott-Raven 1998; 451–467.

155. Glass PSA. Prevention of awareness during total intravenous anesthesia (correspondence). *Anesthesiology* 1993; **78**:399–400.

156. Glass P, Gan TJ, Sebel PS, *et al.* Comparison of the bispectral index (BIS) and measured drug concentrations for the monitoring effects of propofol, midazolam, alfentanil and isoflurane. *Anesthesiology* 1995; **83**:A374.

157. Ghoneim MM. Awareness during anesthesia. *Anesthesiology* 2000; **92**:597–602.

Chapter 2

Implicit memory for events during anesthesia

M. M. Ghoneim

Contents

Historical perspective

Early reports by clinical hypnotists

Cheek,[1,2] a gynecologist and an eminent hypnotist, was probably the first to suggest that some patients during general anesthesia may have some form of perception outside awareness (Table 2.1). He reported patients who postoperatively showed signs of anxiety or depression or recovered poorly, without an obvious cause. None of the patients had any explicit memory of surgical events. But, when hypnotized, they repeated offending or threatening remarks made by members of the surgical team. Cheek suggested that these memories unconsciously influenced the patients' postoperative course and reported that recall under hypnosis was followed by a remission of the patients' symptoms. Levinson, a psychiatrist and experienced hypnotist, in an often-quoted work,[3] made statements concerning a

spurious crisis during dental surgery in ten patients receiving ether anesthesia: 'Just a moment! I don't like the patient's colour. Much too blue. Her lips are very blue. I am going to give a little more oxygen .... There, that's better now. You can carry on with the operation.' None of these patients had any recall of the incident in the postoperative period. However, when they were interviewed under hypnosis, four patients were reported to give verbatim or near-verbatim recall of the bogus incident. Four others became anxious and emerged from hypnosis. Wolfe and Millett,[4] and Hutchings[5] administered positive suggestions to patients under anesthesia and claimed highly therapeutic benefits for the patients. Pearson[6] was the first to attempt a controlled and double blind study. He found that patients who received therapeutic suggestions during surgery were discharged sooner from the hospital than those who were played only music or a blank tape, but the experimental and control groups were not matched for the types of surgeries that were performed.

Table 2.1. Mileposts on the history of implicit memory after anesthesia

1959	Cheek[1] suggested that anesthetized patients may have perception without awareness
1960	Wolfe and Millett[4] administered therapeutic suggestions during anesthesia.
1965	Levinson[3] reported a study in which he created a spurious crisis during anesthesia that was only recalled by the patients under hypnosis.
1968	Warrington and Weiskrantz[8] reported on retention without awareness in amnesic patients.
	Milner et al.[12] reported on an amnesic patient who could learn new motor skills.
1983	Millar and Watkinson[15] reported recognition memory for words presented during surgery.
1985	Graf and Schacter[14] introduced the distinction between implicit and explicit memory.
	Bennett et al.[16] investigated the effects of behavioral suggestions presented during surgery.
1986	Bonke et al.[17] studied the efficacy of therapeutic suggestions administered during anesthesia.
1989	The First International Symposium on Memory and Awareness in Anaesthesia was held in Glasgow, Scotland.

Early reports by psychologists and distinction between implicit and explicit memory

The above-mentioned reports by clinical hypnotists languished in the literature for two decades until implicit memory became a major issue in psychology.[7] Although implicit memory had been noted occasionally since the nineteenth century in clinical and experimental reports, systematic research on the subject was fueled by interest in reports by Warrington and Weiskrantz,[8,9] on retention without awareness in amnesic patients, by Weiskrantz[10,11] on perception without awareness in blindsight, and by Milner et al.[12] on reports on patient H.M. When amnesics[8,9] were presented with a list of words, they had great difficulty a few minutes later in recognizing the words. However, when they were given another kind of memory test – they were provided the first three letters of a word, e.g. PEN... or GAR... and asked to supply the remaining letters – they wrote as many words from the previously presented list as normal volunteers. Weiskrantz studies with blindsight[10,11] involved patients with damage to the occipital lobes of their brains. When a light was flashed in the part of visual space affected by the brain damage, the patients claimed to see nothing. But when asked to 'guess' the location of the flash, they performed accurately. Milner and her colleagues[12] described the famous patient H.M., who developed profound amnesia for recent events following bilateral medial temporal lobe resection for the relief of intractable epilepsy. Although he had no ability to retain new information of any kind, he could learn new motor skills in a relatively normal manner. Tulving *et al.*[13] carried out the experiments of Warrington and Weiskrantz[8,9] with word completion test in healthy volunteers and concluded that priming – seeing the words on the list primed the ability of subjects to come up with the correct solution when they tried to complete a word fragment – occurs independent of conscious memory. Graf and Schacter[14] introduced the initial distinction between implicit and explicit memory. Research into priming and implicit memory exploded since then and remains a major theme with wide interest in the area of learning and memory.

Early works in the anesthesia literature and international symposia on memory and awareness in anesthesia

The recent interest in implicit memory after general anesthesia can be traced to the initial works of several authors, including Millar and Watkinson's[15] finding of recognition memory for words presented during surgery, Bennett *et al.*'s[16] work with behavioral suggestions presented during surgery, and Bonke *et al.*'s[17] work with the influence of therapeutic suggestions administered during anesthesia. As we mentioned in the previous chapter, the International Symposium on Memory and Awareness in Anesthesia, which has been held every three years since 1989, has been important for the advancement of research in both explicit and implicit memory during anesthesia.

The two worlds of memory

Memory is composed of different forms and systems.[18,19] Figure 2.1 represents a taxonomy of long-term memory systems. A key distinction when we remember the past is between explicit or declarative or conscious memory and implicit or nondeclarative or unconscious memory. *Explicit memory* refers to the intentional or conscious recollection of prior experiences as assessed by tests of recall or recognition, which are also called *direct* memory tests. It refers to the everyday uses of such terms as 'remembering' when we invoke a previous conscious awareness of past events (e.g. 'I remember the doctor yelling that the patient needs more anesthetic because he is moving'). *Implicit memory*, by contrast, refers to changes in performance or behavior that are produced by prior experiences on tests that do not require any intentional or conscious recollection of these experiences. It is when people are influenced by a past experience without any awareness that they are 'remembering'.[20] Implicit memory leads to automatic responding or habit. Consider the following research scenario that we reported several years ago.[21] Patients are exposed during anesthesia to a list of words. The list may contain the words: 'Pension, Expand and Afford'. Post-operatively, the patients are visited when they are unable to recall any events during anesthesia. But,

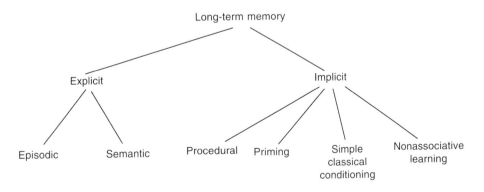

Figure 2.1. A taxonomy of long-term memory systems.

when they are given an incidental test that does not require conscious recollection of the words, e.g. they are presented with a number of three-letter word stems, including PEN..., EXP... and AFF..., and are asked to supply the first words that come to their minds beginning with those letters, they may give the word 'Pension' rather than 'Pencil' or 'Peninsula' or others, which indicates learning and retention of the previously presented word during anesthesia.

This word completion test is called an *indirect* or implicit test. Performance on direct and indirect tests depends critically on the instructions given to the subjects. When amnesic patients were instructed to complete a stem with the first word that comes to mind, they performed as well as control healthy subjects; but when instructed to produce the correct item from the study list, amnesics showed less recall than did controls.[22] Thus, anesthetized patients are asked postoperatively to recall or recognize events that may have occurred during anesthesia in a direct test, while in an indirect test they are asked to give the first word(s) that comes to mind with no mention of events during anesthesia. It should be noted that both types of memories, explicit and implicit, are active all the time during our wakeful life. Every day we acquire information either with or without intention or attention; both processes occurring usually simultaneously.

After this introduction, we are going to discuss the evidence for the existence of implicit memory following anesthesia. Next, we discuss whether it matters if there is implicit memory without postoperative recall. Can it do harm? Finally, we examine whether it is possible to prevent the occurrence of implicit memory after anesthesia.

The search for unconscious learning during anesthesia and implicit memory after anesthesia

The unconscious world of memories following anesthesia has been explored along the following paths:

1 Studies of anesthetized patients using indirect tests of memory
2 Responses to behavioral suggestions administered during anesthesia
3 Studies of the efficacy of administration of therapeutic suggestions during anesthesia
4 Studies of healthy volunteers to whom drugs are administered, usually in subanesthetic concentrations
5 Effects of anesthetics on animal learning and memory
6 Reports of cases of psychosomatic disorders after anesthesia and surgery.

Studies of anesthetized patients using indirect memory tests

Priming

The word completion task, which was mentioned before, probes subjects' memories for a phenomenon known as *priming*: a change in the ability to identify or produce an item as a result of a specific prior encounter with the item. In the above example, the subject produced the word 'pension' because it was presented before. Subjects also perform the task with 'new' stimuli unrelated to those 'old' stimuli that were presented before; i.e. 'Pension, Expand and Afford', that provide a baseline measure of performance. The difference in performance with the old and new stimuli constitutes the measure of priming (Table 2.2). Priming has been the most intensively studied subtype of implicit memory in humans and has been the type used almost exclusively in studies of anesthetics (with the exception of two studies with conditioning (Tables 2.3 and 2.4).

VARIETIES OF PRIMING

Priming can be fractionated into several different subtypes (Figure 2.2). One important distinction is between perceptual priming and conceptual priming. *Perceptual priming* reflects prior processing of stimulus form, while conceptual priming reflects prior processing of stimulus meaning. For obvious reasons, the auditory modality has been used to present the stimuli to the anesthetized patient. Perceptual priming is maximal when study-phase and test-stimuli are perceptually identical, and reduced when there is a study-test change in modality; e.g. the list of words is presented auditorily during anesthesia, but postoperatively the patient is tested by presenting him with written stems of

Table 2.2. Example of the calculation of a priming score

List 1	List 2
PENSION	CLOCK
EXPAND	SEASON
AFFORD	TEACHER

Test

Word beginnings	Target responses by subjects (%)		
	Subjects played list 1	**Subject played list 2**	**Priming (%)**
AFF_____	15	7	8
SEA_____	8	16	8
CLO_____	12	12	0
PEN_____	20	10	10
EXP_____	18	15	3
TEA_____	9	16	7
Mean priming (%)			6

Note: For subjects who were played list 1, the word beginnings corresponding to the list 2 words serve as distractors on the test, and vice-versa (usually, each list consists of more than three items). The priming score for each word beginning is the percentage of subjects who were presented with the list containing the corresponding target word who give that word on the test, minus the percentage of the other subjects who give the word on the test, i.e. the baseline rate of spontaneously giving that word. The bottom row shows the mean priming score for all word beginnings.

words and asking him to write completed words. Even when the same modality is maintained between the presentation phase and the test phase, priming effects will be greater when the same voice is used in the two phases and priming will suffer when the fundamental frequency of a single speaker's voice is changed between the two phases.[23] Perhaps as important for studies in the anesthetized patients, perceptual priming does not depend on semantic or elaborative encoding of an item at the time of the study. Priming has been characterized as perceptual for tasks such as the word completion test. By contrast, *conceptual priming* is maximal when study-phase processing enhances semantic analysis of stimulus meaning and is often unaffected by changes in modalities of the study-test phases. A category generation task, where subjects are presented with a category exemplars (e.g. 'pear', 'tangerine') and then during the test phase are asked to give examples of 'fruits', is considered a conceptual priming task (priming occurs when subjects are biased to produce previously presented category exemplars). Although many priming tasks are well characterized as predominantly perceptual or conceptual in nature, it is likely that most tasks have some elements of each.[24]

Conclusions about preservation of priming in patients with amnesic syndromes are usually based

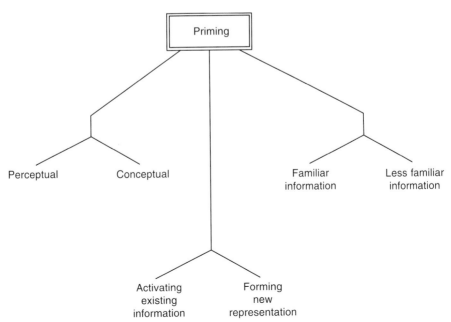

Figure 2.2. Subtypes of priming, which have been used in anesthesia research.

on studies of perceptual priming. Studies of conceptual priming in these patients yielded mixed results.[25] For example, amnesic patients showed impaired priming on a conceptual task that involves answering general knowledge questions (e.g. subjects are played a tape containing statements like 'the blood pressure of an octopus is 80 mmHg', then during the test phase they are asked 'what is the blood pressure of an octopus?'); a task that has been used by several groups of researchers investigating implicit memory after anesthesia. Priming on this task seems also to depend on explicit retrieval processes.[26] It is, therefore, tempting to suggest that anesthetized patients may perform better on perceptual rather than conceptual tasks because of the role of semantic encoding in conceptual priming, however, there is insufficient evidence to confirm this suggestion.

Another distinction pertinent to priming concerns locating and activating information that already exists in memory (e.g. a representation in memory of a word that is already part of a person's vocabulary) *versus* forming a new representation in memory (e.g. learning a new word and storing in memory some kind of cognitive structure that represents that word).[27] There are two important differences between implicit memory for 'old' (already existing) and new representations.[28] First, the creation of new representations in memory may require the participant to engage in some mental activities that are not necessary for locating and activating old representations. Second, priming for new information had been reported initially to be absent in amnesics. Kihlstrom and Schacter[28] have, therefore, hypothesized that implicit memory for events during anesthesia might be confined to the activation of preexisting knowledge. There is now, however, evidence that amnesic patients can show normal priming for novel information.[24] The study of Block et al.[21] using nonsense words, Jelicic et al.[29] using fictitious nonfamous names, and Münte et al.[30] using reading time, suggest that new representations or associations may be formed in memory during anesthesia.

FAMILIARITY OF STIMULI

The issue of familiarity of the material used in the

memory tests is also of interest. So, too, is the material's associative frequency or dominance (i.e. the probability with which a stimulus evokes a response). For example, if participants are asked to name examples of the category 'metal', some examples with high associative frequency or dominance are given frequently (such as iron), whereas other examples with low associative frequency or dominance are given infrequently (such as tungsten). Jelicic et al.[31] and Roorda-Hrdlicková et al.[32] tested patients with a category-generation task using familiar categories and familiar target words. They obtained evidence for learning during anesthesia. However, Bonebakker et al.[33] from the same research group found no such evidence when they used less familiar target words. Bonebakker et al.[34] found that using the word-completion task, patients showed more evidence of priming for words with high associative frequency or dominance compared with words with lesser ratings. Results from studies with conscious persons with and without amnesia show that less familiar words result in larger priming effects.[35,36] This may not be the case in anesthetized patients. Bonebakker et al.[34] suggested that familiarity with the information to which patients are exposed during anesthesia is important for successful priming.

Types of memory tests

Table 2.3 lists the studies that used indirect tests of memory, identifies the anesthetic drugs used for maintenance of anesthesia, specifies whether memory for information that was presented during anesthesia was found, and includes some brief comments. All the tasks, which have been used in more than one study, gave mixed results. Can recognition task measure implicit memory?

The task of recognition is usually construed as a measure of explicit memory, a view based on studies with patients with amnesia, whose performance on the task is usually impaired.[37] An alternative view, based on studies of healthy persons, is that recognition depends on both explicit and implicit memories.[38,39] According to Mandler,[39] two simultaneous processes are involved when a person must decide whether he or she recognizes an item. First, the 'familiarity' of the item is retrieved; secondly, a search process determines whether the item was presented previously. The first process may fall within the domain of implicit memory.

Table 2.3. Studies with indirect tests of memory

Memory test	Parameter measured	Anesthetic (maintenance)	Study	Results	Comments
Category generation	No. of target examples of categories produced	$N_2O:O_2$, isoflurane and sufentanil	Roorda-Hrdličková et al.[32]	+	Used familiar examples
		$N_2O:O_2$ and sufentanil or fentanyl	Jelicic et al.[31]	+	Used familiar examples
		$N_2O:O_2$ and isoflurane or $N_2O:O_2$ with opioids	Block et al.[21]	−	Used examples of difficult categories
		$N_2O:O_2$, isoflurane and fentanyl	Brown et al.[67]	−	Authors suggested without adequate statistical evidence that the results were due to conditioned suppression of material learned during anesthesia
		$N_2O:O_2$, isoflurane and fentanyl	Westmoreland et al.[189]	−	Used familiar examples
		$N_2O:O_2$, isoflurane and sufentanil	Bonebakker et al.[33]	−	Used less frequent examples
		$N_2O:O_2$ and halothane	Russel and Wang[190]	−	Used familiar examples
		$N_2O:O_2$, enflurane and morphine	MacRae et al.[191]	−	Used familiar examples
Conditioning	Electrodermal responses	$N_2O:O_2$ and isoflurane	Ghoneim et al.[192]	−	
Fame judgments	No. of fictitious names presented that were judged as famous	$N_2O:O_2$ and alfentanil	Jelicic et al.[29]	+	
		$N_2O:O_2$ and enflurane	Jelicic et al.[61]	−	Patients, in contrast to previous study, were not paralyzed during anesthesia
		$N_2O:O_2$ and alfentanil	DeRoode et al.[193]	−	Authors attributed the negative results to premedication with midazolam
Free association	No. of targets produced on presentation of cues	Propofol and sufentanil	Donker et al.[194]	−	
		$N_2O:O_2$ and halothane	Lewis et al.[195]	−	
		Isoflurane	Kihlstrom et al.[57]	+	
		$N_2O:O_2$ and sufentanil	Cork et al.[58]	−	
		Fentanyl and propofol or methohexital	Bethune et al.[196]	+	Material was presented during surgery and in the immediate postoperative period
		$N_2O:O_2$ and halothane	Russel and Wang[190]	−	
	Story-related association on presentation of a cue	Fentanyl and flunitrazepam; fentanyl and isoflurane; and fentanyl and propofol	Schwender et al.[59]	+	
		$N_2O:O_2$, fentanyl and isoflurane	van der Laan et al.[89]	+	Subjects in the group that showed priming for a presented

(Contd)

Memory test	Parameter measured	Anesthetic (maintenance)	Study	Results	Comments
					intraoperative story, also heard a story preoperatively; subjects who failed to show priming did not hear a story preoperatively
		$N_2O:O_2$ and bolus doses of fentanyl; $N_2O:O_2$ and alfentanil infusion; and $N_2O:O_2$ and isoflurane	Ghoneim et al.[60]	+	Priming occurred only in the group anesthetized with N_2O and opioid bolus regimen
Forced-choice recognition*	No. of items recognized	$N_2O:O_2$ and halothane or enflurane or thiopental	Dubovsky and Trustman[197]	–	
		$N_2O:O_2$ and halothane	Millar and Watkinson[15]	+	
		$N_2O:O_2$ and halothane or enflurane or isoflurane or opioids	Eich et al.[198]	–	
		$N_2O:O_2$ and halothane or enflurance	Evans and Richardson[85]	+	
		$N_2O:O_2$ and isoflurane or	Block et al.[21]	+	
		$N_2O:O_2$ and opioids			
		$N_2O:O_2$, sufentanil and isoflurane	Caseley-Rondi et al.[53]	+	
		$N_2O:O_2$, isoflurane and sufentanil or propofol and alfentanil	Bonebakker et al.[34]	+	
General knowledge	No. of questions answered correctly	$N_2O:O_2$ and halothane	Goldman[69]	+	
		Isoflurane	Dwyer et al.[199]	–	
		$N_2O:O_2$ and alfentanil	Jelicic et al.[29]	–	
		$N_2O:O_2$ and enflurane	Jelicic et al.[61]	–	
Homophones	Spelling of homophones	Propofol and sufentanil	Donker et al.[194]	–	Patients, in contrast to previous study, were not paralyzed during anesthesia
		$N_2O:O_2$ and halothane or enflurane or isoflurane or opioids	Eich et al.[198]	–	
		$N_2O:O_2$, isoflurane and fentanyl	Brown et al.[67]	–	Authors speculated that the results were due to conditioned suppression of material learned during anesthesia
Preference	No. of items preferred that have been presented before	$N_2O:O_2$, isoflurane and fentanyl	Westmoreland et al.[189]	–	
		$N_2O:O_2$, isoflurane and fentanyl	Winograd et al.[200]	–	Used melodies
		$N_2O:O_2$ and isoflurane or	Block et al.[21]	+	Used nonsense words
		$N_2O:O_2$ with opioids			
		$N_2O:O_2$ and halothane	Bonke et al.[201]	–	Used a coloring task in children

(Contd)

Memory test	Parameter measured	Anesthetic (maintenance)	Study	Results	Comments
		$N_2O{:}O_2$, sufentanil and isoflurane	Caseley-Rondi et al.[53]	−	Used melodies
		$N_2O{:}O_2$ and halothane	Kalff et al.[202]	−	Used a coloring task in children, replicating Bonke et al. Study[201]. Although benzodiazepine premedication was omitted, implicit memory remained undetected
Reading speed	Reading time of previously presented material	$N_2O{:}O_2$, alfentanil and propofol	Münte et al.[30]	+	The authors reported negative results with the word completion task in the first experiment of their study
Word completion	Completion of word stems to targets	$N_2O{:}O_2$ and isoflurane or $N_2O{:}O_2$ with opioids	Block et al.[21]	+	
		$N_2O{:}O_2$, isoflurane and sufentanil or propofol and alfentanil	Bonebakker et al.[34]	+	
		Isoflurane and fentanyl	Lubke et al.[50]	+	Used the bispectral index and the process dissociation procedure. Implicit memory was related to the depth of hypnosis
		$N_2O{:}O_2$, alfentanil and propofol	Münte et al.[30]	−	

+ = positive results; − = negative results.

*Although forced-choice recognition is usually classified as an explicit memory test, there is some basis for considering it an implicit test for material presented during anesthesia.

(Modified from Ghoneim MM, Block RI. Learning and memory during general anesthesia: An update. *Anesthesiology* 1997; **87**:387–410).

The success of some researchers with forced-choice recognition tasks (see Table 2.3), which requires subjects to select the items that have been previously presented – guessing if necessary – may support this contention, assuming that patients are guessing and are guided by feelings of familiarity.

An unforced recognition task, which allows participants not to respond if they are unsure, may be less sensitive to implicit memory than a recognition task in which participants are forced to respond to every test item, even if they believe they are only guessing, because guesses may reflect implicit memory.[40] Several groups of investigators found evidence for memory during anesthesia using forced-choice recognition tasks (see Table 2.3), but not on unforced yes/no procedure.

The above hypothesis, which attempts to explain the success of some studies with a forced recognition task after anesthesia as evidence for implicit memory faces, however, two challenges. First, two methods have been developed that dissociate the roles of conscious recollection and automatic familiarity. The processes dissociation procedure uses inclusion and exclusion tasks that have recollection and familiarity working in concert or in opposition so that separate values for recollection and familiarity can be calculated.[41] The remember/know procedure[42] asks subjects to designate which items in a recognition test they 'remember' from the study list and which items they 'know' were on the list but cannot recollect. Both methods failed to identify familiarity in recognition with the same processes that mediate priming.[43,44] Second, recognition familiarity was found intact in a patient with impaired priming on word-completion and word-identification tasks.[43]

Are learning during anesthesia and memory after anesthesia implicit?

DISTINCTION BETWEEN LEARNING AND MEMORY

In most of the anesthesia literature, the terms implicit learning and implicit memory are used synonymously. In the previous chapter we distinguished and defined learning and memory. Implicit learning refers to subjects who are not aware of what they have learned and implicit memory refers to subjects who cannot consciously remember events. Nevertheless, the relationship between the two during and after anesthesia is far from simple. If learning of auditory information occurs during a period of wakefulness during anesthesia of which the patient is subsequently amnesic, but can be demonstrated by an indirect test of memory during the postoperative period, explicit learning with subsequent implicit memory may be said to have occurred. This would be similar to the case of patients suffering from organic amnesias, where they are aware of experiences around them but cannot consciously recollect them later. Explicit memory can only result from explicit learning. On the other hand, if learning of information has occurred while unconscious, both learning and memory were implicit (Figure 2.3).

ARE THESE LEARNING AND MEMORY CONSCIOUS OR UNCONSCIOUS?

Defining and measuring awareness have presented formidable challenges to both psychologists engaged in memory research[45,46] and anesthesiologists investigating explicit and implicit learning during and memory after anesthesia.[47,48] On a simplistic level, we could argue that any learning during anesthesia is implicit because the patient is rendered unconscious by the general anesthetic drugs, and memory is implicit because the patient in the postoperative period cannot recollect learning anything during anesthesia and has no concept that a relationship exists between material that was presented during anesthesia and performance on an incidental, seemingly 'non-memory' test. If the patient has no concept of such a relationship, he cannot be aware that the presented material influenced his or her performance on the test.

Unfortunately, this may not always be the case for the following reasons. First, memory tests are not process-pure. Performance on both direct and indirect tests may reflect both conscious and unconscious memory processes. For example, the indirect word completion task can be performed using implicit memory, by 'saying the first words that come to mind', or it can be done by explicitly recalling the words that have been presented ('Pension, Expand and Afford' in the example that was mentioned above). Also, an implicit test might show memory while an explicit test does not show memory because the former test is more sensitive than the latter, rather than because it engages a memory system different to the explicit one. Thus, in the same example mentioned above, assessment of implicit memory by performance on the word

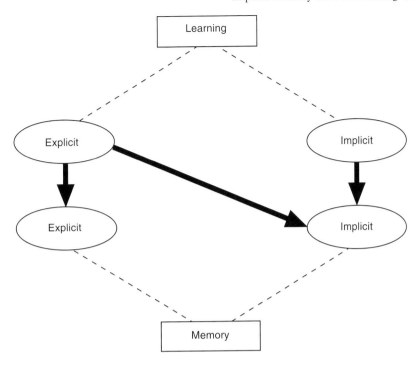

Figure 2.3. The relationship between the two types of learning and memory.

completion task may help cue memory through presentation of the word stems (e.g. 'PEN'), an advantage that is absent in assessment of explicit memory by a free recall task. The latter task is often an insensitive measure of explicit memory. Second, there is no reliable way of ascertaining and proving that patients remain unconscious throughout the surgery, particularly in the paralyzed patient. Explicit recall is abolished before loss of responsiveness, so it is possible for someone to be conscious during surgery and yet not remember being so on recovery. The interaction between the administered anesthetic doses and varying levels of surgical stimulation (Figure 2.4) may lead to 'islands' of awareness.

ASSESSMENT OF CONSCIOUS *VERSUS* UNCONSCIOUS INFLUENCES ON MEMORY AFTER ANESTHESIA

It is therefore important if we are going to answer the previous question to be able to separate explicit from implicit memory and monitor the adequacy of anesthesia. One method to dissociate explicit and implicit influences on memory performance is to use Jacoby's Process Dissociation Procedure (PDP).[38] The PDP consists of two parts, an inclusion and an exclusion part, used in combination with the memory task. As an example for its use with the word completion task, suppose the word 'pension' was used in a list of words that was presented during anesthesia. In the *inclusion* part, patients are asked to complete the word stem 'PEN' with a word presented during surgery, or, otherwise, with the first word that comes to mind. In the *exclusion* part, the patients are asked not to use presented words for stem completion, but to use any other word they could think of (e.g. 'PENCIL'). Implicit memory would result in a higher proportion of completion with the word 'PENSION' in both parts of the test because the subjects cannot recollect the words. On the other hand, explicit memory would enhance performance only in the inclusion part. In the exclusion part, it would result in hit rates (i.e. completion with the word 'PENSION') lower than the baseline rate (see Table 2.2 for explanation of baseline rate) because the subjects can recall the words and therefore use *different* words according to the instructions.

Initially, it was assumed that the method may be too complex for patients in the early part of the recovery phase who may be suffering from drowsiness, nausea, pain and difficulty to concentrate.[49]

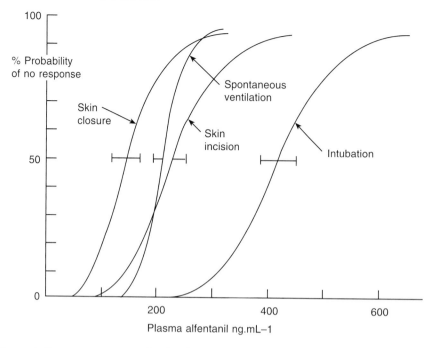

Figure 2.4. Concentration response curves for the plasma concentration of alfentanil with 66% nitrous oxide and the probability of no response after intubation, skin incision, and skin closure for patients undergoing abdominal surgery. – indicates ± SD of the mean Cp50 (Reprinted with permission from Ausems ME, Vuyk J, Hug CC, Stanski DR. Comparison of a computer-assisted infusion versus intermittent bolus administration of alfentanil as a supplement to nitrous oxide for lower abdominal surgery. *Anesthesiology* 1988; **68**:851–861.)

Bonebakker *et al.*[34] used only the exclusion component and found that unconscious influences were dominant in their patients' memory. Lubke *et al.*[50] used both components in trauma patients and found evidence for implicit but not explicit memory. Lubke *et al.*[51] also used both components in patients who underwent cesarean sections. They found a weak form of explicit memory. The authors suggested that the division in explicit and implicit memory provided by PDP may be too crude to describe the underlying processes. The PDP may also be at a disadvantage with low levels of memory. Implicit memory can make words seem familiar even when there is no explicit recollection of having encountered words earlier.[52] If, in the exclusion condition, patients excluded words that seemed familiar as well as words they explicitly recalled, then explicit memory would have been over-estimated and implicit memory underestimated (see Chapter 4).

Another method to separate explicit from implicit memory is to use tests of those types of memory that are equally sensitive and are as comparable as possible in all respects except whether they overtly request recollection of previously presented information. Under these circumstances, if participants show more memory on the implicit test than the explicit test, unconscious learning can be inferred. If the explicit and implicit tests differ in other respects,[53] these other differences might be responsible for any differences in performance and would complicate an interpretation in terms of unconscious learning. Two studies that used the most similar explicit and implicit tests – forced-choice recognition and preference judgments, respectively – did not demonstrate differential performance on these tests.[21,53]

A third method to ascertain unconscious learning and memory is to use a monitor which has a well-defined point for loss of consciousness and can assess the adequacy of anesthesia (see Chapter 3).

OTHER FACTORS AFFECTING IMPLICIT MEMORY IN ANESTHETIZED PATIENTS USING INDIRECT MEMORY TESTS

We wrote above about the type of instructions given before testing with indirect memory tasks; the types of information presented and tested, specifically, perceptual *versus* conceptual priming, old *versus* novel information, and familiar *versus* less familiar stimuli; and the appropriateness of the forced-choice recognition task as a test for implicit memory. Here we will discuss other factors that may determine the outcomes of studies looking for implicit memory after anesthesia, namely, the influence of anesthetic regimens, the time of postoperative testing, the number of stimulus presentations during anesthesia and the sample size.

Influence of anesthetic regimens on outcomes of studies

Because some benzodiazepines impair implicit memory,[54–56] it is prudent to avoid their use in studies of implicit memory during anesthesia. Although it is possible that the probability of learning would vary with the *type of anesthetic* drugs used, a review of the literature (see Table 2.3) does not support such a hypothesis. Kihlstrom *et al.*[57] found evidence for implicit memory during anesthesia with isoflurane, but no implicit memory in a second study[58] in which they used nitrous oxide and sufentanil. Their results are contradictory to many others (see below) and may represent failure of replication of an earlier study rather than a difference caused by the two anesthetic methods.

Perhaps more important for elicitation of implicit memory after anesthesia is the *depth of anesthesia* achieved by the drugs during surgical stimulation. Schwender *et al.*[59] found that in patients with implicit memory after operations, the midlatency auditory-evoked potentials during anesthesia continued to show a pattern similar to the awake state, but in contrast, in the patients without implicit memory, the waveforms were severely attenuated or abolished. Most of the patients in the first group were anesthetized with flunitrazepam and fentanyl, and most of the patients in the second group were anesthetized with isoflurane and fentanyl or propofol, and fentanyl. Ghoneim *et al.*,[60] using the midlatency auditory-evoked potentials, found similar results. Implicit memory occurred only in patients anesthetized with nitrous oxide and bolus fentanyl supplementation but not in patients anesthetized with nitrous oxide and isoflurane or nitrous oxide and alfentanil infusion. Lubke *et al.*[50] also recently found using the bispectral index that the probability of implicit memory was related to the depth of

hypnosis. Their patients were anesthetized with isoflurane and fentanyl. Too light anesthesia is easier to detect and correct in a spontaneously breathing non-paralyzed patient than in a patient who is artificially ventilated because of administration of neuromuscular blockers. In the former case, a change in breathing pattern and/or movement may alert the anesthesia provider to increase the dose of the anesthetic. Jelicic *et al.*[29] found evidence of implicit memory when their patients were anesthetized with nitrous oxide and opioids together with muscle relaxants, but not in patients anesthetized with nitrous oxide and enflurane, and left spontaneously breathing.[61] We therefore suggest that implicit memory may be possible mainly following light anesthesia. As a corollary for investigators, they should monitor the anesthetic depth in their studies or failing this, at least standardize the anesthetic methods used as closely as possible with respect to drugs and their dosages.

Time of postoperative testing

Priming effects were found in anesthetized patients when they were tested very early after operation[31] (3–5 h after surgery) or as late as five days after surgery.[59] The optimal time of testing after operation could be influenced by several factors. Patients should be tested when they have recovered sufficiently from the detrimental effects of anesthetics on cognitive functions that could impair their performance, but before priming effects have dissipated. Durations of the priming effects may vary according to the task used,[27] although they can persist for as long as a year.[62] Andrade[48] suggests that testing should be conducted in the hospital to minimize changes in context between stimulus presentations and the memory test. Extraneous stimuli may also interfere with the specific stimuli administered during anesthesia if the testing is delayed. Merikle and Daneman[40] conducted a meta-analysis of studies investigating memory for events during anesthesia. Memory decreased systematically as the interval between the end of surgery and the administration of the memory test increased, and there seemed to be no memory when testing was delayed more than 36 h after surgery.

In contrast, consolidation of implicit memory, active during sleep, depends strongly on rapid eye movement sleep.[63] Sleep pattern after surgery is severely disturbed with early depression of rapid eye movement and slow wave sleep, and with rebound of rapid eye movement sleep on the second and third nights.[64] Conceivably, this might favor testing on the third postoperative day.

Number of stimulus presentations

In conscious persons, repetition and duration of exposure to the stimulus seem to enhance conceptual, but not perceptual, priming.[65,66] Bonebakker et al.[34] found that memory during anesthesia was apparent after one but not after 30 presentations of a word list. An explanation that has been offered for these results is that patients may unconsciously associate the presented material with an aversion period after surgery. Brown et al.[67] found that performance on indirect memory tests was worse for words that were presented three times during anesthesia than for words that were not presented at all. The investigators suggested that memory may be suppressed by the aversion experience of surgery. However, this somewhat implausible speculation stands in contrast to several studies that showed memory effects after multiple presentations.[21,29,57] Brown et al.'s[67] statistical analyses of their results were also questionable. Because the effect was only marginal in the primary analysis, follow-up analyses were not warranted. The analyses were also based on pooling the results of two entirely separate types of tests.

Sample size

In studies providing evidence of learning during anesthesia, the effects usually have been small.[15,21,57] This is consistent with the possibility that only a minority of persons can learn during anesthesia, perhaps due to a relatively light level of anesthesia. Positive findings seem more likely to be replicated in studies with substantial samples of patients, which provide adequate power to detect relatively small effects. Studies with small samples, such as 20–30 patients, may lead to conflicting results.

Conclusions of the section

Research requires that the results of an experiment can be replicated in another one and if replication fails, plausible reasons for the discrepancy should be considered. Yet, the results of studies of anesthetized patients that used indirect tests of memory, show a quality of 'now-you-see-it-now-you-don't', a confusing pattern of positive and negative outcomes. It is, however, somewhat reassuring that Merikle and Daneman's[40] meta-analysis of the data from 2517 patients in 44 studies, showed evidence of implicit memory for information that was presented during surgery. One hopes that future studies, which either match the level of difficulty of implicit and explicit tasks, or use experimental manipulations to ensure that the implicit task is not contaminated by explicit retrieval and employ measures to monitor the depth of anesthesia, would lead to more consistent results.

Postoperative performance after behavioral suggestions presented during anesthesia

Cheek and Le Cron[68] suggested that nonverbal responses (raising one finger for 'yes' and a different finger for 'no') were more trustworthy than verbal responses for hypnotic recollection of meaningful sounds heard during anesthesia. Patients were often unaware of their nonverbal responses. Bennett et al.[16] following on this suggestion, measured learning during anesthesia using a post-anesthetic motor behavior. In an important departure from previous work, Bennett et al. performed a randomized and double-blind study in which patients were assigned to either suggestions or control groups. The suggestion patients were exposed during anesthesia to a statement about the importance of touching their ear during a postoperative interview. Compared with controls, they touched their ears more frequently, though they were amnesic for the spoken message, both without and under hypnosis. Positive responses to intraoperative instructions are evidence for implicit memory: a change in behavior (touching a certain body part) that is attributable to a past evidence (presentation of the instructions) in the absence of conscious recall of that event. Bennett et al.'s pioneering experiment was followed initially by replication of the positive results by two other groups of investigators,[21,69] although there have been criticisms of the methodologies used and some unexplained discrepancies.[47,70–73] Later reports have been mostly negative both in anesthetized patients and in healthy volunteers treated with subanesthetic concentrations of inhalation anesthetics. Table 2.4 summarizes the literature in this area in patients and Table 2.6 in healthy volunteers.

Table 2.4. Studies with behavioral suggestions presented during anesthesia

Study	Results	Comments
Bennett et al.[16]	+	(1) There was no baseline assessment of 'ear pulling' frequency. (2) The difference between groups was due to the extreme reaction of two patients. If these two 'outliers' were excluded, the difference between groups would not be significant. (3) Using more appropriate statistical tests would have led to negative results. (4) Some patients could have been too lightly anesthetized while receiving the suggestions.
Goldmann et al.[69]	+	(1) Failed to replicate ear touching results but succeeded in increasing chin touching. (2) Absence of baseline assessment. (3) The message was presented during very light anesthesia. (4) The statistical analysis can be criticized.
Block et al.[21]	+	The effect of suggestions was only apparent on the day of surgery but not on the day after.
McLintock et al.[203]	–	There were reduced analgesic requirements in the early postoperative period.
Jansen et al.[204]	–	
Bethune et al.[196]	–	The authors tested the effects of suggestions in two separate studies. In one study, they tested the patients 36 to 48 hours postoperatively and in the other 7 days afterwards.
Dwyer et al.[199]	–	

Responses to therapeutic suggestions administered during anesthesia

If, during anesthesia, one gives a patient information and suggestions to behave in a manner conducive to optimal postoperative recovery, such as 'everything is going well; the operation will be soon over; you soon will wake up calm, relaxed, comfortable and with good appetite; your healing will start immediately and you will leave the hospital very shortly; etc.' And, if such presentation improves the recovery of the patient, this would imply that the information that was presented has been encoded and stored in implicit memory. The reason is that the positive effects of intraoperative suggestions fit the formal definition of implicit memory: a change in behavior, thought, and performance, which is produced by a past event (delivery of the suggestions) in the absence of conscious recollection of that event. In addition to providing evidence of unconscious learning during anesthesia, improvement of the postoperative course of patients through an easy, cost-effective and non-pharmacological method would be an attractive clinical goal for research in this area.

Rationale

There is well-documented evidence that psychological and behavioral preparation prior to surgery can speed postoperative recovery.[74,75] Early reports of positive effects of intraoperative therapeutic suggestions[6] by clinical hypnotists led to modeling of those suggestions on hypnotic suggestions. The efficacy of such suggestions is enhanced when subjects feel at ease and are not distracted; feel they are in a special kind of expectancy situation in which unusual events may occur; and can feel, remember, think, imagine, and experience in new or unusual ways.[76] It has also been claimed that hypnosis produces more profound bodily relaxation than do waking-state interventions, elicits greater clarity of visual imagery, and increases responsiveness to suggestions for therapeutic change.[77] It has been speculated that suggestions administered during anesthesia might incorporate some of the desirable conditions that increase their efficacy. However, although hypnotizability seems to mediate the somatic outcomes of hypnotic suggestion,[78,79] Casely-Rondi et al.,[53] Korunka et al.,[80] and Lebovits et al.[81] found no significant association between hypnotizability and therapeutic outcome after surgery.

IF THERAPEUTIC SUGGESTIONS ARE EFFECTIVE, HOW MIGHT THEY WORK?

Barber,[76] in a review of the literature on physiologic effects of suggestions, concluded that if they are effectively communicated and accepted at a 'deep' level, they could influence cellular (especially vascular and immunologic) functioning to conform to the suggested alterations. Supposedly, by becoming deeply absorbed in the imagined physiologic change as a result of the suggestions, the feelings that accompanied the actual physiologic change would be reinstated, and these feelings would stimulate the cells to produce the actual change. Wadden and Anderton[77] in a review of the clinical use of hypnosis, concluded that hypnosis was more effective in treating non-voluntary disorders, such as pain, than disorders involving self-initiated behavior, such as overeating. The authors suggested this might be because pain, unlike eating, was not affectively rewarding and there would be no conflicting motivation concerning its avoidance, as there might be with food. Consequently, individuals suffering from non-voluntary disorders might be highly motivated to accept therapeutic suggestions. However, the analogy between the hypnotic and anesthetized states is limited. Caseley-Rondi et al.[53] and Korunka et al.[80] raise the issue of what mediates the therapeutic effect of suggestions during anesthesia. They suggest that it is possible that the soothing tones of a voice rather than semantic processing of connected discourse may be important. Soothing tones, by reducing stress, might aid recovery. The beneficial effect of music in the Korunka et al.[80] study may be consistent with such an explanation and suggests that evidence for postoperative benefit does not necessarily imply that memory is involved.

Comments on the contents of the tape and its presentation

Some researchers[82] stress the importance of gaining close rapport with the patients during the preoperative interview to enhance motivation for the study and convince them of its relevance for their well-being. Some researchers believe that the message should use the patient's preferred name; should be presented slowly, but at normal listening volumes; should be phrased in direct, grammatically simple and affirmative statements; and should be repeated continuously during anesthesia. Clinical hypnotists[83] stress the importance of using positive terms (such as 'comfortable' or 'fine') and avoiding the use of negative ones (such as 'no pain' or 'no trouble') to maximize benefits to the patients. This is based on the argument that the unconscious mind may not register sounds and words in the same way as the conscious mind, and inclusion of negative

terms like 'pain' or 'trouble', albeit denied, may influence the patient negatively. The text may contain direct suggestions, e.g. 'You are completely relaxed'; third person suggestions simulating positive comments made by surgeons, e.g. 'Great … That looks excellent, very good indeed'; and suggestions on the best way to cope with postoperative sequelae, e.g. 'You will swallow to clear your throat and everything will go one way, straight down … so that you can get good food to make you strong after the operation, your stomach and intestines will begin churning and gurgling soon after your operation'. Some researchers think that the tape should be recorded by the interviewer or the patient's own anesthesiologist or surgeon. Woo et al.[84] asked patients to record the positive message in their own voices.

The contents of the tape presented to the control group has varied. Some investigators have presented a blank tape (or simply plugged the ears), whereas some have played noise, sea sounds or similar neutral sounds, or sounds of the operating room. The latter may have been the sounds during the patient's own operation or prerecorded operating room sounds. Each option has its merits and disadvantages. For example, recording and playing the patient's actual operating room sounds may be disturbing to some members of the operating room team and may contain pessimistic statements, which if registered by the patient's mind may be detrimental to his or her well-being. Noise might affect the patient negatively.

The tape should be presented through headphones placed over the patient's ears. Usually, the audio cassette player is set on an auto-reverse mode and played continuously. The player should be set at a comfortable listening volume and should only be audible to the patient to avoid bias of members of the health care team.

Current literature

Table 2.5 lists studies that have been done in this area. The following are some comments on some of the more recent studies arranged according to the main outcome measurements that were used. The studies were selected to reflect the general state of the literature in this area.

HOSPITAL STAY

Evans and Richardson[85] reported that patients who

Table 2.5. Therapeutic suggestions studies

Study	Outcome measure(s)	Anesthetic (maintenance)	Surgery	Results	Comments
Wolfe and Millett[4]	Postoperative pain, nausea, and vomiting, and many others	Not stated	Wide variety	No measurement done	Uncontrolled study
Hutchings[5]	Postoperative pain, nausea and vomiting, and many others	Not stated	Wide variety	No measurements done	Uncontrolled study
Pearson[6]	Duration of hospitalization	Not stated	Several types	Shortened	Experimental and control groups not matched Small sample size
Abramson et al.[205]	Postoperative analgesic requirements and duration of hospitalization	Not stated	Abdominal and orthopedic procedures	No effect	
Bonke et al.[17]	Duration of hospitalization, postoperative pain, nausea and vomiting, subjective well-being, and nurses' evaluations	$N_2O:O_2$ and fentanyl; sometimes with dyhydrobenzperiodol	Biliary tract	Shortened the duration of hospitalization in older patients	
Woo et al.[84]	Duration of hospitalization, postoperative analgesic requirements, days until p.o. fluids and solid food, and wound drainage	$N_2O:O_2$ and enflurane	Abdominal hysterectomy	No effect	Small sample size
Boeke et al.[206]	Duration of hospitalization, postoperative pain, nausea and vomiting, subjective well-being, and nurses' evaluations	$N_2O:O_2$ and fentanyl; sometimes enflurane added	Cholecystectomy	No effect	
Evans and Richardson[85]	Duration of hospitalization, pyrexia, pain intensity and distress, nausea and vomiting, urinary difficulties, difficulties with bowels, flatulence, mobilization rating and nurses' assessment of recovery	$N_2O:O_2$ and halothane or enflurane	Abdominal hysterectomy	Shorter hospital stay, shorter period of pyrexia, and better rating by nurses	
McLintock et al.[203]	Postoperative analgesic requirements, pain scores, and nausea and vomiting	$N_2O:O_2$ and enflurane	Abdominal hysterectomy	Reduced analgesic requirements in the early postoperative period	Analgesia was provided through a PCA system
Block et al.[207]	Duration of hospitalization, postoperative analgesic	$N_2O:O_2$ and isoflurane or $N_2O:O_2$	Several types	No effect	Analgesia was provided through a PCA system to

(Contd)

Study	Outcome measure(s)	Anesthetic (maintenance)	Surgery	Results	Comments
Block et al.[207] (continued)	requirements, nausea and vomiting, gastrointestinal and urinary symptoms, and rating of pain, anxiety, and recovery	and opioids			52% of patients
Liu et al.[86]	Duration of hospitalization, postoperative analgesic requirements, nausea, flatulence, pyrexia, ease of mobility, mood states and anxiety level, and nurses' assessments	$N_2O:O_2$ and enflurane	Abdominal hysterectomy	No effect	
Korunka et al.[80]	Duration of hospitalization, postoperative analgesic requirements, and pain ratings	$N_2O:O_2$, fentanyl, and isoflurane or halothane	Hysterectomy; abdominal or vaginal	Relative to presentation of operating room sounds, presentation of therapeutic suggestions reduced time elapsed until the first postoperative analgesic dose and some ratings of pain, whereas presentation of music reduced not only these two measures but total analgesic consumption as well	
Jelicic et al.[88]	Duration of hospitalization and subjective well-being	$N_2O:O_2$ and sufentanil or fentanyl	Cholecystectomy	Patients who received both affirmative and non-affirmative suggestions spent less time in hospital than patients who received affirmative or nonaffirmative suggestions separately, or some irrelevant text	It is difficult to explain why mixed suggestions produced the best results
Caseley-Rondi et al.[53]	Duration of hospitalization, postoperative analgesia requirements, patients and nurses' ratings, and assessments of anxiety, mood and nausea	$N_2O:O_2$, sufentanil, and isoflurane	Abdominal hysterectomy	Reduced analgesic requirements for the first 2 postoperative days	Analgesia was provided through a PCA system

(Contd)

Study	Outcome measure(s)	Anesthetic (maintenance)	Surgery	Results	Comments
Williams et al.[90]	Nausea and vomiting	$N_2O:O_2$ and isoflurane	Major gynecologic surgery	Incidence and severity reduced	
Hughes et al.[93]	Smoking	Not specified	Several types	Stopped or reduced	
Oddby-Muhrbeck et al.[91]	Nausea and vomiting	$N_2O:O_2$, fentanyl, and isoflurane	Breast surgery	No effect	The experiment group had a lower frequency of recall of their nausea and vomiting compared with the control group
van der Laan et al.[89]	Postoperative analgesic requirements	$N_2O:O_2$, fentanyl, and isoflurane	Hysterectomy, myomectomy, or gynecologic laparotomy	No effect	Analgesia was provided through a PCA system
Myles et al.[94]	Smoking	Isoflurane, enflurane and others	Elective or semielective surgery	No effect	
Maroof et al.[92]	Vomiting	$N_2O:O_2$ and halothane	Hysterectomy	Incidence and severity reduced	
Lebovits et al.[81]	Pain, nausea and vomiting, and other side effects	$N_2O:O_2$, propofol, fentanyl and sometimes isoflurane	Outpatient hernia repair	Incidence of nausea and vomiting, and other side effects were reduced	Incomplete report

PCA = patient-controlled analgesia
(Modified from Ghoneim MM, Block RI. Learning and memory during general anesthesia: An update. *Anesthesiology* 1997; **87**:387–410).

received therapeutic suggestions during anesthesia for hysterectomy had shorter postoperative stays than did a non-suggestion control group. In contrast, Liu et al.[86] could not find positive effects. Millar[87] conducted a meta-analysis of the results of Evans and Richardson and Liu et al. He concluded that Evans and Richardson's results may have been caused by chance bias in allocation of patients to the control group as a result of a relatively small sample size (Figure 2.5). Jelicic et al.[88] exposed patients to both affirmative ('you will be comfortable') and non-affirmative ('you will have no pain') suggestions, affirmative or non-affirmative suggestions separately, or some irrelevant text. They obtained somewhat contradictory and confusing findings: patients who received both affirmative and non-affirmative suggestions spent less time in the hospital than did patients in the other three groups. The authors acknowledge the possibility that the outcome might have been due to chance.

POSTOPERATIVE PAIN AND ANALGESIC USE

Korunka et al.[80] found that suggestions or music prolonged the period before patients asked for their first postoperative analgesic, compared with a control tape of operating room sounds, but only the music tape reduced total analgesic consumption. Caseley-Rondi et al.[53] also reported reduction in analgesic requirements in patients who were played therapeutic suggestions during anesthesia. However, differences between the experimental and control groups were only marginally significant in analyses controlling for the greater age of the patients and longer duration of anesthesia (and presumably larger doses of intraoperative opioids) in the experimental group. Furthermore, the significance level in the

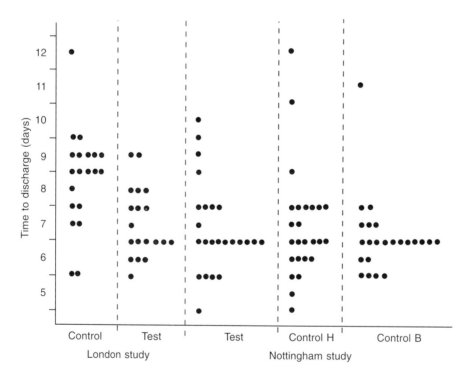

Figure 2.5. Distribution of patient data points (days to discharge) in the two groups of Evans and Richardson[85] in London and three groups of Liu et al.[86] in Nottingham. Test groups were presented with therapeutic suggestions during anesthesia. The suffixes 'B' and 'H' indicate that those control groups received a blank or 'history' tape, respectively, in the Nottingham study. With the presentation of data in scatter plots, it is evident that, although four of the groups were similar in their mean and typical durations of stay in the hospital, the London control group was distinctive, with most patients staying longer in the hospital. (Reprinted with permission from Millar K. Efficacy of therapeutic suggestions presented during anaesthesia: Re-analysis of conflicting results. *Br J Anaesth* 1993; **71**:597–601.)

analysis of morphine use after operation was not adjusted for the number of measures of post-operative recovery that were assessed, increasing the probability of a type 1 error. Van der Laan *et al.*[89] also found that therapeutic suggestions had no effect on postoperative analgesic requirements.

NAUSEA AND VOMITING

Williams *et al.*[90] reported that presentation of positive intraoperative suggestions reduced patients' recalled incidence of vomiting in the first 24 hours after surgery by 37% compared with a control group. Patients who received therapeutic suggestions also required smaller doses of metoclopramide. Oddby-Muhrbeck *et al.*[91] more recently failed to find positive effects on postoperative nausea and vomiting, although therapeutic suggestions did reduce patients' recall of these distressing post-operative symptoms. Maroof *et al.*[92] in a very short correspondence reported that therapeutic suggestions reduced the incidence and severity of post-hysterectomy emetic episodes. Lebovits *et al.*[81] recently reported that therapeutic suggestions reduced the incidence of nausea and vomiting in ambulatory surgery patients over the first 90 minutes post-anesthesia.

SMOKING

Hughes *et al.*[93] presented smokers during surgery with a tape encouraging them to give up smoking or a control tape. Compared with patients who received the control tape, more of those who received the suggestions tape had stopped or reduced their smoking according to self-reports one month after operation. However, Myles *et al.*[94] failed to confirm this finding. The strength of the findings of Hughes *et al.*[93] as evidence of implicit learning during anesthesia is limited, because of several factors. Although no patients recalled the message, their memory was not tested until one month after operation; however, some might have recalled it had their memory been probed earlier. The assessment of postoperative smoking was not based on objective records of cigarette smoking or on self-reports obtained at frequent intervals, but only on a single, delayed self-report covering a one-month period. The validity of such a self-report, especially for patients who reported decreased smoking rather than complete abstention, is uncertain.

Critiques of the studies in this section

STATISTICAL CONCERNS

Andrade and Munglani[95] criticized many studies reporting beneficial effects of presentation of therapeutic suggestions during anesthesia on the grounds that some of these effects might have been due to chance, because the studies assessed multiple measures of recovery without controlling statistically for the number of variables analyzed. When many variables are analyzed and a statistical method, such as Bonferroni's method, is used to control for the number of variables, an effect must be rather large to be deemed statistically significant. Because beneficial effects of presentation of therapeutic suggestions may not be large, judicious selection while planning a study of a smaller set of dependent variables may be preferable.

METHODOLOGIC CONCERNS

Millar[87] made useful suggestions for improving the methods used. The first suggestion concerns the sample size. Considerably larger sample sizes than the usual samples of 20 or fewer are required, considering the likely possibility that only a few patients in a given sample may be in a state to register auditory information during anesthesia. The second suggestion concerns the mode of presentation of the results. Millar suggests that rather than presenting the data exclusively in the summary form of means and standard deviations, better insights into treatment effects may be gained by presenting full data sets in graphic form (see Figure 2.5).

Measures of postoperative well-being and recovery are affected by complex sets of factors that may not be controlled by the experimenter and that may lead to bias when assessing their interactions with presentations of therapeutic suggestions.

HOSPITAL STAY

It appears that the length of hospital stay is not influenced by presentation of therapeutic suggestions to anesthetized patients[47] and there does not seem to be a good reason any more to focus on this measure of postoperative recovery. This measure is likely to be affected by factors that are usually beyond the experimenters' control.

POSTOPERATIVE PAIN AND ANALGESIC USE

Although patient-controlled analgesia provides a better measure of patients' requirements of opioids than drugs prescribed on an as-needed basis by physicians and delivered by nurses, some pitfalls may confound this measure. One issue is that the dose and timing of administration of preoperative and intraoperative opioids may reduce postoperative patient-controlled analgesic consumption.[96,97] Another issue is sample size. A simulation study suggested that detecting a 25% decrease of analgesic use between control and intervention groups (the effect size that has been reported in studies of therapeutic suggestions with positive results) requires a sample size of 116 patients.[98] This suggests that none of the studies of therapeutic suggestions had large enough sample sizes.

NAUSEA AND VOMITING

The cause of nausea and vomiting is also multi-factorial; that is, it is influenced by type of surgery; anesthetic agents and techniques; patient sex, age, and weight; duration of anesthesia; experience of the anesthesiologist; history of postoperative nausea and vomiting, motion sickness, middle ear disease, pain and few other factors.[99–101] Authors should report these factors and specify whether they were equally represented in patients receiving therapeutic suggestions and controls. This has not been the case.

Conclusions of the section

It is, therefore, apparent that therapeutic suggestion tasks are particularly liable to both type I and type II errors. This is probably the reason for inconsistent results in this area. It is usually difficult to explain in many of the studies that used multiple measures of recovery the reasons why some outcome measures improved, although they were not referred to on the tape, while some other measures were not affected, although they were explicitly and repeatedly mentioned. A recent meta-analysis of studies in this area by Merikle and Daneman[40] found little or no effect of therapeutic suggestions on postoperative recovery. However, it should be remembered that negative results do not preclude the existence of implicit memory following anesthesia. Intraoperative therapeutic suggestions

may be encoded in memory, but remain unexpressed because of lack of capacity to execute them (consider the analogy to a person who remembers the details of a dietary regimen but for one reason or another does not comply with it or the person who remembers the telephone number of his mother-in-law but lacks the enthusiasm to call her).

Studies of healthy volunteers

Advantages

Work with healthy volunteers gives investigators the opportunity to use within-subjects experimental designs and controlled conditions without the many possible confounding factors that may be present when studying patients, e.g. varying surgical stimuli, varying doses of anesthetics, varying rates of postoperative recovery, side effects of anesthesia and surgery, and effects of postoperative treatments with analgesics, antiemetics and others. It also allows the investigators to use subanesthetic and very light concentrations of drugs to define the concentrations required for loss of consciousness and amnesia, which would not be ethically possible in the surgical patients. It enables the investigators to construct dose-response curves, which would show the patterns of decrement in explicit and implicit memory. The use of a single drug rather than the usual mixture of drugs used in clinical practice allows better control of the experiments and allows us to determine whether different anesthetics have different effects on memory. Table 2.6 summarizes the literature with healthy volunteers in which indirect memory tests were used. (For review of other studies in which direct memory tests were only used, please see Ghoneim and Block.[73])

Concentration-effect relations

The concentrations of anesthetics that block explicit memory are less than those that prevent voluntary responses to verbal commands.[102–106] Thus, anesthetic concentrations that prevent voluntary responses also prevent conscious memory. At minimum alveolar concentration-awake and Cp50 awake (the plasma concentration required to prevent responsiveness to command in 50% of patients), both explicit and implicit memory may be abolished. These results are inconsistent with reports of implicit

Table 2.6. Studies of healthy volunteers

Study	No. of subjects	Anesthetic agents	Tasks	Design	Results
Block et al.[107]	32	30% N$_2$O	Recall and recognition of word lists and first names, category-example task, free associations, word completion and preference, and recognition of nonsense words	Double-blind and randomized	Recall and recognition were impaired. Impairments were milder in forced choice recognition than in yes/no recognition. Performance in category-example task and word completion showed resistance to memory impairment
Block et al.[208]	32	30% N$_2$O	Classical conditioning of skin conductance responses	Double-blind	Although N$_2$O seemed to prevent conditioning during its inhalation, learning took place because conditioned responses could be elicited after cessation of inhalation
Newton et al.[209]	8	0, 0.1, 0.2, and 0.4 MAC of isoflurane	Recall and recognition of word lists, responses to commands, and auditory evoked response (AER)	Double-blind, randomized, and crossover	Recall and recognition were lost at 0.2 MAC. Half of the subjects recalled a 'shock' word at the same concentration. Responses to command were lost at 0.4 MAC. It was difficult to demonstrate changes in the AER that were specifically related to changes in memory.
Dwyer et al.[106]	17	0.15, 0.3, and 0.45 MAC isoflurane and 0.3, 0.45 and 0.6 MAC N$_2$O	Responses to commands, learning of obscure general knowledge, responses to behavioral suggestions, and EEG	Open, randomized, and crossover; the different concentrations of each drug were given consecutively in a fixed order in one session	Explicit and implicit memory were prevented by 0.45 MAC isoflurane. N$_2$O did not completely prevent either type of memory. EEG showed very limited relationships to response to command and learning
Chortkoff et al.[112]	10	0.15, 0.28 and 0.4 MAC isoflurane	Category-example task and response to behavioral suggestions	Open; the different concentrations were given consecutively in a fixed order in one session	0.4 MAC abolished both explicit and implicit memory

(Contd)

Study	No. of subjects	Anesthetic agents	Tasks	Design	Results
Chortkoff et al.[135]	24	40% N_2O combined with 0.06, 0.22, and 0.38% isoflurane	Category-example task, learning of obscure general knowledge, responses to commands, and responses to behavioral suggestions	Open; the different concentrations were given consecutively in a fixed order in one session	There was a small degree of antagonism between the two anesthetics. There was no evidence of learning during inhalation of the high concentration
Polster et al.[109]	35	Midazolam and propofol in subanesthetic concentrations	Perceptual facilitation on word identification and recognition tasks	Double-blind and randomized	Both drugs had little effect on performance with the implicit memory test. Midazolam had a more profound amnesic effect than propofol on the recognition memory test
Ghoneim et al.[55]	72	0, 0.05 and 0.1 mg/kg midazolam and 0, 1 and 3 mg flumazenil	Free recall, recognition, word completion and other cognitive tasks	Double-blind, randomized and crossover. Subjects participated in three sessions, at least 1 week apart	Midazolam impaired explicit and implicit memory. Flumazenil reversed both the sedative and memory effects of the drug
Munglani et al.[210]	7	0, 0.2, 0.4 and 0.8% isoflurane	Category-example task and measurement of the 'coherent frequency' of the AER	Open; the different concentrations were given consecutively in a fixed order in one session	Increasing concentrations of isoflurane decreased coherent frequencies and performance on the tests. There was no evidence of implicit learning with 0.8% concentration. Dose of anesthetic was a better predictor of cognitive function than coherent frequency.
Zacny et al.[134]	9	0, 0.3 and 0.6% isoflurane and 0, 20 and 40% N_2O	Immediate and delayed free recall	Double-blind, randomized and crossover	Both drugs impaired immediate and delayed recall in a concentration-related fashion. There were no differences between the two drugs
Chortkoff et al.[110]	22	Desflurane and propofol concentrations were increased in stepwise fashion until the subjects stopped following commands	Response to commands	Open; order of administration of the two drugs was randomized over two sessions	MAC-awake for desflurane was 2.6% and the Cp50-awake for propofol was 2.69 microgram/ml

(Contd)

Study	No. of subjects	Anesthetic agents	Tasks	Design	Results
Chortkoff et al.[149]	23	Desflurane and propofol at a concentration 1.5–2 times each individual MAC-awake or its equivalent for propofol	Presentation of emotionally charged information, learning of obscure general knowledge and responses to behavioral suggestions	Subject and interviewers were blinded to the information that was presented; materials and treatments were randomized and balanced	The drugs prevented explicit and implicit learning
Zacny et al.[211]	10	0, 30% N_2O and 0.2 and 0.4% isoflurane, alone, and in combination with 30% N_2O	Immediate and delayed free recall	Single-blind, randomized and crossover; different sessions for each treatment	Drug combinations produced profound impairments. Isoflurane appeared to produce more impairment than N_2O
Gonsowski et al.[111]	12	0.6 MAC desflurane or isoflurane, followed by 1.7 MAC, then 0.6 MAC again	Category-example task, learning of obscure general knowledge, and responses to behavioral suggestions	Open and crossover	0.6 MAC prevented explicit and implicit learning
Andrade et al.[212]	12	Propofol in subanesthetic concentrations. Mean infusion rate of 3.62 mg.kg^{-1} hr^{-1} for 'light' sedation and 4.35 mg.kg^{-1} hr^{-1} for 'deep' sedation	Recognition and fame judgments tasks	Open; propofol concentrations were given consecutively in a fixed order in one session	There was no memory for stimuli presented during light or deeper propofol sedation
Ghoneim et al.[187]	28	0.2% isoflurane and 0.03 or 0.06 mg.kg^{-1} midazolam	Responses to commands, word completion, free recall and forced choice recognition tasks	Double-blind and randomized	After administration of midazolam, recall and, to a lesser degree, implicit memory were absent. Recognition was also absent after administration of midazolam 0.06 mg.kg^{-1} and sometimes after administration of 0.03 mg.kg^{-1}. Responsiveness was more frequent with midazolam 0.03 mg.kg^{-1} than with 0.06 mg.kg^{-1}

(Modified from Ghoneim MM, Block RI. Learning and memory during general anesthesia: An update. Anesthesiology 1997; **87**:387–410).

memory during general anesthesia, and the differences are usually explained by the arousing effects of surgery, which may promote learning and the salience of any stimulus during surgical operations, which may have relevance to survival in patients (see Chapter 4).

Variability of results

There are also inconsistencies in the results of the different volunteer studies. Andrade[49] classified these studies into three main categories:

1 Single dose studies with low doses of anesthetics, e.g. Block *et al.*[107,108] and Polster *et al.*,[109] which showed that light sedation impairs explicit but not implicit memory

2 Single dose studies with larger doses of anesthetics, which prevented motor response to command, e.g. Chortkoff *et al.*[110] and Gonsowski *et al.*,[111] which showed that these doses abolished both explicit and implicit memory

3 Multiple dose studies, e.g. Dwyer *et al.*[106] and Chortkoff *et al.*,[112] which showed that explicit and implicit memory were abolished by doses of anesthetics that prevented subjects from moving their hands in response to commands and impaired equally both explicit and implicit memory.

Methodological issues

The above classification of studies by Andrade,[49] while accurate, is confounded by other differences between the studies, which may explain the discrepancies and necessitate caution in making final conclusions. One important issue is the use of adequate comparison groups. There are two components of value in the design of experiments investigating the effects of drugs on cognition. The first is comparison of the behavior of the patient before and after administration of the drug, allowing unambiguous attribution of behavioral changes to the influence of the drug in question. The second design component is the use of a non-drug (placebo) control in which the same or other persons receive identical treatment except for administration of the drug. Pre-post comparisons alone are imperfect because practice on experimental tasks (Figure 2.6), environmental influences, fatigue, and other factors (Figure 2.7) can change behavior over time and

affect the comparison of performance before and after drug administration. Comparison of separate treatment and control groups alone does not provide evidence that the groups were equivalent before treatment, so the possibilities that observed differences could have been present regardless of treatment or true differences could have been masked by different baseline levels between groups cannot be excluded. It is unfortunate that some studies have omitted one or the other of these design components.

In the multiple dose studies, investigators rather than testing different concentrations of an anesthetic in separate sessions or with separate participants, have used a series of increasing and then decreasing concentrations of the drug within a single session. Practice effects, fatigue effects, cumulative effects of the anesthetic agent, tolerance development, proactive or retroactive interference, and other potential confounders are inherent risks of this type of design. Some investigators administered the indirect test(s) of memory only during the inhalation of the highest concentration of the anesthetic. In the absence of testing in a control group, during inhalation of lower concentrations of the anesthetic, or both, it is difficult to determine whether the absence of learning was due to the effect of the drug, insensitivity of the task, or both.

Other concerns are use of different lists of words with no evidence that they were comparable in their normative characteristics or had been equated in pilot studies; absence of counterbalancing of lists over treatments, which may confound differences among lists with differences among treatments; and use of tasks that have not been adequately validated, which may result in studying one unknown with another.

There are two additional concerns that apply specifically to the elucidation of unconscious memory under the influence of anesthetics. The first is the failure to use comparable tests of explicit and implicit memory. For example, Block *et al.*[107] assessed explicit memory by asking subjects to recall the study words and implicit memory by asking them to complete word stems, which may help cue memory, but this support is not available in the free recall task. Thus, the observed failure to recall words presented during anesthetic administration may reflect the difficulty of the recall task rather than a genuine loss of explicit memory.[49] Investigators should ensure that tests of these types

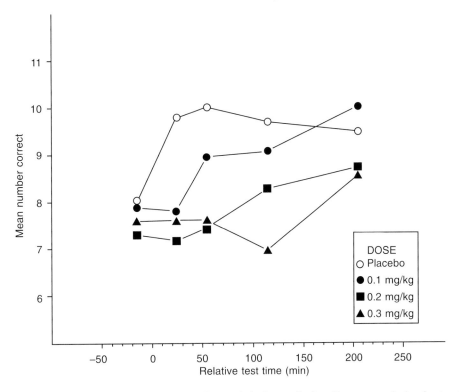

Figure 2.6. The mean number of digits recalled at intervals before and after diazepam and placebo treatments. Zero was the time of drug administration. Different random 15-digit numbers were presented each time. The score represents the mean of three trials. A delayed practice effect caused by varying doses of diazepam is apparent. (Reprinted with permission from Ghoneim MM, Hinrichs JV, Mewaldt SP. Dose-response analysis of the behavioral effects of diazepam: I. Learning and memory. *Psychopharmacology* 1984; **82**:291–5.)

of memory are equally sensitive.[113] The second concern is the use of relatively complex type of stimuli in the implicit memory tests by some investigators, e.g. answers to Trivial Pursuit-type questions, which need more cognitive processing *versus* use of simpler stimuli by others, e.g. single words which can perceptually be processed at a more superficial level as in the word stem completion task. Again, the presence or absence of implicit memory may be a function of different sensitivities of the tasks used. Investigators should pay considerable attention to the literature on indirect memory tests before making their choices. Table 2.7 provides a checklist, which may be useful for the design of studies or evaluation of the literature.

Conclusions of the section

One can conclude: first, explicit memory is blocked by concentrations of anesthetics that may allow conscious awareness. Second, there may be a pharmacological window during which explicit memory is blocked while implicit memory is retained. Third, the precise concentrations of anesthetics that guarantee absence of recall, both conscious and unconscious, may differ in surgical patients from the healthy volunteers. These results have been of interest but those of us who have hoped for concrete and robust conclusions on implicit memory during anesthesia to match the results of studies of implicit memory in healthy volunteers in the psychology laboratories have not yet been rewarded. There is a lot still to be done, e.g. assessments of the degrees of memory impairments with different anesthetics and different types of memory tasks, effects of gender and aging, interactions of anesthetics with one another and with arousing stimulation and correlations between electroencephalographic changes and consciousness and memory.

Studies of the effects of anesthetics on memory need to take advantage of functional neuroimaging

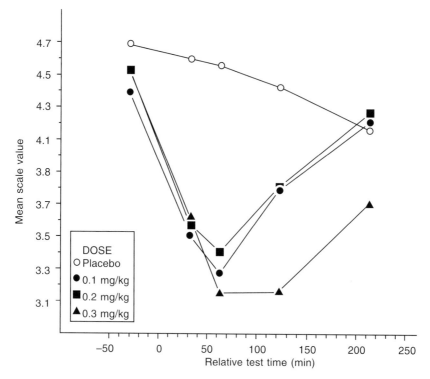

Figure 2.7. Composite mood evaluation scores on visual analog scales before and after administration of diazepam and placebo. The vertical axis represents the mean value of seven scales. A decreasing score is associated with increasing sedation. The figure illustrates changes in subjective mood evaluations over time with or without active drug treatment. (Reprinted with permission from Ghoneim MM, Mewaldt SP, Hinrichs JV. Dose-response analysis of the behavioral effects of diazepam:II. Psychomotor performance, cognition and mood. *Psychopharmacology* 1984; **82**:296–300.)

techniques using positron emission tomography (PET) or functional magnetic resonance imaging (fMRI). These technologies permit the visualization of memory processes in the brain. Functional neuroimaging studies allow for the design of

Table 2.7. A checklist for the design of studies of memory effects of anesthetics in volunteers

1 Use adequate comparison groups:
   (a) Pretreatment *vs* post-treatment
   (b) Treatment *vs* control group.
2 Use separate sessions or separate participants in multiple dose studies.
3 Use adequately validated tasks.
4 Word lists should be comparable in their normative characteristics or had been equated in pilot studies.
5 Counterbalance word lists over treatments.
6 Use comparable tests of explicit and implicit memory.
7 Use the most sensitive tasks, if the aim is to demonstrate the existence of memory.

experiments targeted at specific memory processes. Studies have identified specific roles of hippocampal and parahippocampal regions, the amygdala, the basal ganglia, and various neocortical areas in explicit memory. Priming is mediated by neocortical areas, reflecting experience-induced decrements in activity in the same neural networks that subserved initial processing. Separate cortical areas mediate perceptual and conceptual priming. As examples, priming on visual word stem completion tasks is associated with reduced activity, relative to baseline, in bilateral occipitotemporal regions. Priming on conceptual tasks as in generation of verbs to nouns or of semantically related words is associated with reduced activity in left frontal neocortex.[24]

Electroencephalography records electric activity of the brain from the scalp and hence does not accurately localize the source of neuronal activity. It records the signals associated with neuronal activity over a much shorter time period than PET and fMRI. Functional neuroimaging techniques are also unlikely to resolve directly the flow of information processing that occurs over very brief time scales, such as on the order of 10s of milliseconds. A combination of brain imaging and electric recording may complement each other and define the anatomy of the circuits and the time course of events in these circuits that are involved in a particular behavior. Thus, more recently developed methods, such as event-related functional MRI, will provide additional new avenues for memory research.[114] Studies of healthy volunteers in the awake state and during anesthesia using well-defined cognitive tasks may provide answers to questions difficult to obtain in other ways.

Effects of anesthetics on animal learning and memory

Advantages

Studies in anesthetized patients having surgery who were subjected to multitudes of extraneous influences, which constitute most of the current literature, may not produce conclusive and convincing results for implicit memory during anesthesia. Conclusive and convincing evidence can be taken to mean appropriately analyzed and statistically significant data that have been obtained from experiments employing suitable control conditions and that have not proved difficult to replicate, even by researchers holding different presuppositions. By such criteria, there may not be yet conclusive evidence for implicit memory during anesthesia. Animals offer the opportunity to gather information that is not obtainable in any other way and allow tight control of the experimental procedures. The situation is similar to the literature on the effects of volatile anesthetics on various physiologic functions, where data from animals and healthy volunteers breathing equipotent concentrations of these drugs established their actions. The effects of other variables associated with disease and surgery were then studied.

Methods of study

THE HUMAN AND NON-HUMAN SPECIES

Animals are capable of different types of learning (e.g. habituation, classical conditioning, operant conditioning, and imprinting). Different tasks have been used to evaluate learning and memory in experimental animals. The study of animal memory usually involves associative learning of some sort. Basic associative learning is the way organisms learn about causal relationships in the world. Classical conditioning and operant conditioning probably are responsible for a majority of an animal's learned responses.[115] Compared to humans, animal subjects often require elaborate training programs and possess a much more restricted repertoire of behavior. Because of the absence of highly developed language in animals, there is no easily measurable phenomenon of 'free recall'. Typical animal studies of amnesia involve a failure of recognition.

DIFFICULTIES OF FINDING A MODEL TO STUDY MEMORY WITH AND WITHOUT AWARENESS

Although there is evidence for different memory systems in animals, it is not clear whether the memories produced by these systems are analogous to implicit and explicit memory as defined in the human literature.[116] It is difficult to dissociate the latter two memory systems in animals and determine whether a particular task taps into one of these systems or the other. No one knows any method that would allow one to identify 'conscious recollection' in nonverbal animals.

ASSOCIATIVE LEARNING

The classical or Pavlovian conditioning paradigm includes different procedures that can be used to study various aspects of the conditioned response. All of these procedures have in common the association of a neutral conditioned stimulus (CS), such as a tone or white noise, with an unconditioned stimulus (US), such as an electric shock or air puff. Initially, the conditioned stimulus does not elicit a response but the unconditioned stimulus elicits an unconditioned response (UR). With repeated pairings, however, the conditioned stimulus alone also elicits a response – the conditioned response (CR) (Figure 2.8). Although there are many types of conditioning, only three forms have been used during anesthesia: the conditioned nictitating membrane/eye lid response, an example of a discrete skeletal muscle response; conditioned fear, mostly in the form of conditioned lick suppression, a

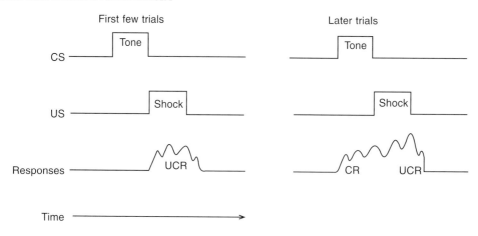

Figure 2.8. The events of a classical or Pavlovian conditioning trial before a conditioned response (CR) is established and after. The upward deflection of the trace indicates stimulus or response onset. The downward deflection indicates offset. A tone (the CS or conditioned stimulus) is paired with shock (the US or unconditioned stimulus). The latter elicits the unconditioned response (UCR). Responses may be salivation, eyelid closure, increased skin conductance, and so on. During later conditioning trials, repeated pairings of the tone and shock elicits a response to the tone (the CR) and to the shock.

conditioned emotional response; and conditioned food aversion. When an animal consumes a flavored fluid and becomes nauseated afterwards, it will acquire a conditioned flavor aversion associating the flavor with sickness.

DELAY *VERSUS* TRACE CONDITIONING

One of the important conditions for the formation of an association between CS and US is temporal contiguity. CR is sensitive to variation in the temporal interval between CS and US, being best established when the CS precedes the US by a short (but not too short) interval, and declining rapidly as this interval increases.[117] In the standard basic delay conditioning, the CS and US overlap in time. In trace conditioning, the CS terminates and there is a period of no stimulation between CS offset and US onset (Figure 2.9). In trace conditioning, as Pavlov proposed years ago,[118] the organism must maintain a 'trace' of the CS in the brain in order for the CS and the US to become associated. The standard simple delay conditioning represents processing of the CS–US relationship in an automatic reflexive way where the CS serves as an adaptive, defensive response to the US; features that are characteristic of nondeclarative or implicit memory. By contrast, trace conditioning represents acquiring conscious knowledge of the CS–US relationship and remembering it across many trials;

features that are characteristic of declarative or explicit memory.[119]

The classification of associative learning using the standard delay procedure as involving the implicit memory system and the trace procedure as involving the explicit memory system is supported by some persuasive evidence. Amnesic patients show relatively normal classical conditioning using the delay procedure accompanied by complete failure to recollect the conditioning episode.[120–123] Evidence from eye-blink conditioning of healthy human subjects also suggests that even if they were aware of the CS–US contingency during learning they blink to the tone CS after associative learning has taken place reflexively, rather than by explicitly recollecting the training episodes.[123] In animals, the cerebellum and its associated brain stem tracts contain the necessary circuitry for the acquisition, storage and expression of the CR.[124] Transection of the brain stem just rostral to the pons spares both the acquisition and retention of the CR.[125] If the entire forebrain is not needed for conditioning, then conscious knowledge of the CS–US associations seems less likely to play an essential role in learning.[18]

On the other hand, trace classical conditioning seems to be more dependent on the declarative or explicit memory system. This is supported by studies in animals in which large bilateral lesions of the hippocampus made before training markedly

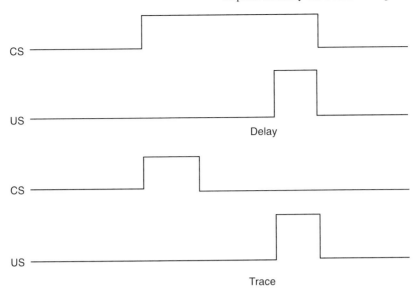

Figure 2.9. The temporal relationship between the conditioned stimulus (CS) and unconditioned stimulus (US) for the delay and trace conditioning procedures.

impaired this type of conditioning, while the same lesions had no effect on the delay CRs.[126] The hippocampus and related structures of the medial temporal lobe support declarative memory.[19] Amnesic patients acquired delay conditioning at a normal rate, but failed to acquire trace conditioning. For normal volunteers, awareness was unrelated to successful delay conditioning, but was a prerequisite for successful trace conditioning.[119] Thus, the above discussion raises the possibility that delay and trace conditioning can be used to study implicit and explicit memory in animals.

A NEED FOR A MODEL OF PRIMING

There is a notable absence of a well-developed animal model of priming to compare with the vast literature on the subject in humans, particularly anesthetized patients and to extend our understanding of the phenomenon. A possible recent exception is the use of single-unit recording techniques in primates.[127] Animals were made to fixate on a series of visual objects, while the activity of population of cells in inferior temporal (IT) cortex was recorded. Repeated exposure to the same stimulus yielded reduced responses in IT cells. These findings resemble the priming-related activation reductions observed in neuroimaging studies in humans.[25]

Current literature

The literature on the effects of anesthetics on learning and memory in animals is limited (Table 2.8). Weinberger *et al.*[128] demonstrated that epinephrine enabled the learning of a Pavlovian conditioned fear response during pentobarbital and chloral hydrate anesthesia. Gold *et al.*,[129] from the same group of investigators, using the same anesthetic and Dariola *et al.*,[130] using thiopental have replicated these findings. El-Zahaby *et al.*[131] tested the effect of epinephrine in rabbits treated with subanesthetic concentrations of isoflurane. Learning and retention were tested using Pavlovian conditioning of the nictitating membrane response (NMR). Epinephrine did not improve retention. Isoflurane showed a dose-dependent effect on acquisition. The results were similar to those obtained by Chortkoff *et al.*[112] in human volunteers. There was no learning during treatment with a 0.8% (0.4 MAC in rabbits) concentration. Even a 0.4% (0.2 MAC in rabbits) concentration, which allowed some learning, abolished retention. Moon *et al.*[132] in a series of experiments with the rabbit NMR examined the effects of nitrous oxide on associative learning. The gas in concentrations of 0%, 33% and 67% impaired acquisition of CRs. This was attributable to its attenuation of the intensity of tone CSs and shock USs and/or UR amplitude, which affected their ability

Table 2.8. Studies of animal learning and memory during anesthesia

Study	Animals used	Anesthetic agents	Types of classical conditioning used	Result	Comments
Weinberger et al.[128]	Rats	Pentobarbital and chloral hydrate	Conditioned fear (lick suppression)	+	Learning only occurred in rats that were treated with epinephrine
Gold et al.[129]	Rats	Pentobarbital and chloral hydrate	Conditioned fear (lick suppression)	+	Learning only occurred in rats that were treated with epinephrine
Edeline and Neuensch-wander-El Massioui[139]	Rats	Ketamine	Conditioned fear (suppression of instrumental responses)	+	
Bermudez-Rattoni et al.[141]	Rats	Pentobarbital	Conditioned food aversion	+	Uncertainties
Dariola et al.[130]	Rats	Thiopental	Conditioned fear (lick suppression)	+	Learning only occurred in rats that were treated with epinephrine
Ghoneim et al.[140]	Rabbits	Ketamine	Conditioned nictitating membrane response	+	Marginal results
El-Zahaby et al.[131]	Rabbits	Isoflurane	Conditioned nictitating membrane response	−	Epinephrine did not enhance retention
Moon et al.[132]	Rabbits	Nitrous oxide	Conditioned nictitating membrane response	−	Nitrous oxide, in subanesthetic concentrations produced an appreciable impairment of learning
Ghoneim et al.[138]	Rabbits	Nitrous oxide	Conditioned nictitating membrane response	±	Nitrous oxide, in subanesthetic concentrations impaired explicit memory more than implicit memory
El-Zahaby et al.[133]	Rabbits	Nitrous oxide and isoflurane	Conditioned nictitating membrane response	±	The two drugs interacted additively on suppression of learning
Pang et al.[136]	Mice	Halothane	Conditioned fear (lick suppression)	+	Halothane was not measured in the experimental chamber
Kandel et al.[137]	Rats	Desflurane and two nonanesthetics	Conditioned fear (fear-potentiated startle)	−	Desflurane, perfluoropentane, and 1,2-dichloro-perfluorocyclobutane abolished learning at subanesthetic concentrations or their equivalents.

(Modified from Ghoneim MM, Block, RI. Learning and memory during general anesthesia: An update. *Anesthesiology* 1997; **87**:387–410.)

to enter into the establishment of CS–CR connections and, therefore, the development of associative learning. El-Zahaby et al.[133] used the same preparation to study the interaction between nitrous oxide and isoflurane on suppression of learning. Both drugs interacted additively. This supported the results of Zacny et al.[134] in humans, but was contradictory to those of Chortkoff et al.[135] who reported a slight antagonism between the two drugs.

Pang et al.[136] examined the effects of halothane anesthesia on the acquisition and retention of Pavlovian fear conditioning in mice. Animals trained under anesthesia exhibited significant suppression of drinking relative to the control group. Then, Kandel et al.[137] came with another different result using conditioned fear in rats. Desflurane and two nonanesthetics abolished learning at subanesthetic concentrations or their equivalents. These results were similar to those obtained during nitrous oxide or isoflurane treatments using the conditioned NMR.[131,132,138]

Edeline and Neuenschwander-El Massioui[139] treated rats with ketamine and trained them during anesthesia. Seven days after the acquisition phase, a tone presentation elicited a significant conditioned suppression of instrumental response only in the groups in which the tone was paired with shock during training. Ghoneim et al.[140] administered ketamine to rabbits and determined its effect on the acquisition and retention of the classically conditioned NMR. Ketamine blocked the display of CRs during acquisition. However, the animals learned faster during retention than naive saline-treated rabbits that had received no acquisition training. This 'savings' may suggest that learning has occurred during ketamine treatment; however, the results were rather marginal. Lastly, Ghoneim et al.[138] used the NMR preparation to examine trace and delay classical conditioning during nitrous oxide treatment. Trace conditioning was more impaired than delay conditioning. This suggests that the drug impairs explicit memory more than implicit memory.

Several studies examined the acquisition of conditioned flavor aversion during anesthesia. Food aversions can be conditioned with very long interstimulus intervals of several hours between CS and US. An example of such studies is the study by Bermudez-Rattoni et al.,[141] in which rats drank water associated with a taste (saccharin) and odor (almond extract) cues. The animals were then anesthetized with pentobarbital. Lithium was

administered 10 minutes after the pentobarbital administration. The rats demonstrated retention of a conditioned flavor aversion after they recovered from the anesthetic, although they were anesthetized during lithium treatment.

Critiques and conclusions of the section

The results of the studies cover a wide spectrum, including findings of no learning during anesthesia, learning only when epinephrine is administered, learning during ketamine anesthesia in which there is sympathetic nerve stimulation, and learning without epinephrine or apparent sympathetic nerve stimulation. The development of flavor aversions when the nauseating agent is administered during anesthesia can provide evidence for learning during anesthesia. However, none of the available reports[141–145] provides a compelling result. The depth and duration of anesthesia produced by bolus doses of pentobarbital or urethane are difficult to determine, as are the durations of actions of nauseating agents such as lithium chloride or apomorphine. It is possible that the effects of the latter may linger during recovery from anesthesia.

Classical conditioning may be the best method available to investigate learning and memory during anesthesia in animals. Fear conditioning has been more successful in providing evidence of learning during anesthesia than conditioning of a skeletal muscle response, such as eye-blink conditioning. The application of a strong, painful, potentially life-threatening and anesthesia-lightening unconditioned stimulus compared with a slight electrotactile one might account for the different results. The question of the possibility of learning during 'adequate' anesthesia in animals has yet to be answered.

Reports of cases of psychosomatic disorders after anesthesia and surgery

The evidence

There is the case of a patient who had an uneventful surgery but postoperatively suffered from a severe sleeping disorder. She was afraid of going to sleep and when she did, she was awakened by nightmares. Under hypnosis she remembered that during anesthesia she heard the words 'she will sleep the sleep of death'. The anesthesiologist confirmed that he did say such a phrase. Subsequent psychotherapy cured the patient. Another patient became depressed and suicidal after a minor operation. Under hypnosis she recalled the surgeon exclaiming, 'she is fat, isn't she?'[146] Goldmann[147] reported the case of a patient who suffered high postoperative anxiety and had no recall of intraoperative experience. Under hypnosis, he described his leg being cut, hearing voices, and feeling as if he 'wasn't going to pull through it'. He became flushed and uncomfortable and spontaneously terminated hypnosis, restoring his intraoperative amnesia.

These anecdotal reports suggest the presence of implicit memory because the patient had no explicit memory for the negative remarks, which were voiced during surgery. They fit the formal definition of implicit memory, which I cited earlier: changes in behavior that are produced by past experiences, in the absence of conscious recollection of those experiences.

Levinson in 1965[3] made statements concerning a spurious crisis during surgery to 10 patients receiving ether anesthesia. None of the patients had any recall of the incident in the postoperative period. However, when they were interviewed under hypnosis, four patients recalled the bogus incident. Four others became anxious and emerged from hypnosis. Blacher[148] claimed that his group could replicate the results of Levinson[3] by creating a similar fake crisis during anesthesia. However, a more recent study in healthy subjects could not replicate these results.[149]

Related to these cases are studies with the isolated forearm technique during light anesthesia. A forearm is isolated from the circulation before injection of muscle relaxants by inflating a tourniquet and then the patient is verbally instructed to move the non-paralyzed arm.[150] Patients may comprehend and respond to the commands, but are usually amnesic postoperatively for these events.[104] (For more details, see Chapter 7.) This conscious perception with subsequent amnesia may be analogous to patients suffering from amnesias whose learning is conscious or explicit, but most of their memories are implicit rather than explicit.

Potential clinical significance of implicit memory after anesthesia

Does it matter if there is implicit memory without postoperative recall? Can it do harm? And why? We will try to answer these questions now. (For more information, see Chapter 8.) Figure 2.10 is a schematic illustration of the hypothesis by which negative information about the anesthetized patient voiced during surgery may impair post-operative recovery and the role of hypnosis in eliciting recall.

Rationale

Implicit effects of past experiences may shape our emotional reactions. Therefore, the possibility that affective stimuli, like unfavorable comments about the patient or his disease, voiced during anesthesia may cause harm is a matter of potential great significance, in addition to its support of the existence of implicit memory during anesthesia.

Information that is acquired during anesthesia may not be retrieved from explicit memory

There are three reasons why this conceivably may occur:

1 Adequate anesthesia may interfere with retrieval of previously acquired information. Ghoneim et al.[151] observed in studies with healthy volunteers using 30% nitrous oxide that the drug may affect memory retrieval as well as acquisition. However, anesthesia usually produces anterograde rather than retrograde amnesia.

2 State-dependent retrieval, i.e. the phenomenon in which retrieval of information is easiest if the drug state remains the same between presentation and testing or learning and retrieval; any change makes retrieval more difficult.[152] For example, consider the alcoholic who, while intoxicated one evening, placed his wallet somewhere and the next morning when he recovered could not remember its place. However, when he started drinking that evening he could remember its place. That is, information learned while under the influence of alcohol is better recalled when the subject is intoxicated than when he or she is sober, and vice versa. For the anesthetized patient, this means that information learned during anesthesia might be remembered better during the same state than while awake. However, state-dependent memory

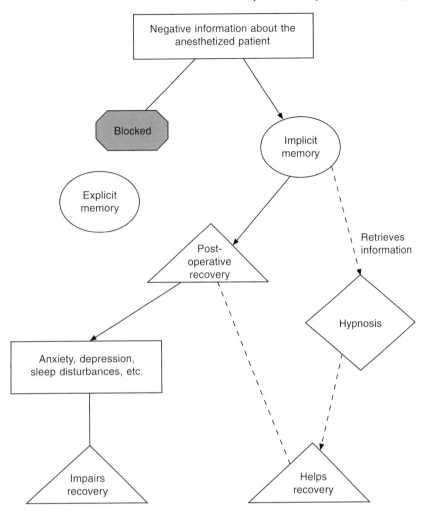

Figure 2.10. Illustration of the hypothesis of the method by which negative information about the patient voiced during anesthesia may impair postoperative recovery and the role of hypnosis in eliciting recall.

in general has been better observed in animals than in humans. Mewaldt *et al.*[153] working with a subanesthetic concentration of nitrous oxide in healthy volunteers found an unusual form of asymmetrical state-dependent memory. Material which was learned while breathing placebo (100% oxygen), was poorly recalled during nitrous oxide inhalation, but material learned while receiving nitrous oxide could be recalled in either the placebo or drug state.

3 The information, which was acquired during anesthesia, was particularly traumatic and its recall was therefore blocked. Psychogenic amnesia has been well documented[154] and some patients may show implicit memory for the traumatic events.[155]

Information that is acquired during anesthesia may be retrieved through implicit memory

There are several reasons why this conceivably may occur:

1 Affective or emotional priming can be elicited with minimal access to content. Independent systems may encode and process affect and content and physiological and behavioral effects may occur with too short an exposure to reveal any content.[156] As an example, Murphy and Zajonc[157] presented subjects for very brief periods with photographs of faces with either angry or happy expressions before showing them Chinese ideographs. Subjects were asked to guess

the meaning of the Chinese ideographs and to rate them on a scale of 'good/bad'. Although the subjects could not recognize the faces that were presented, the expression of the face strongly influenced the attractiveness of the Chinese characters. Happy faces primed good ratings and angry faces bad ratings. When pictures of the faces were presented for a longer period to allow conscious perception, they had no effect on the ideograph ratings. Thus, consciousness may inhibit the processing of stimuli with an 'emotional' meaning.

2 Affective priming, measured by changes in emotional responses, has been demonstrated to be stronger in unconscious than conscious states.[157-159]

3 The work of Damasio group in patients with brain damage,[160] LeDoux[161,162] in animals, and others may provide a biological basis for understanding why someone might experience emotions and affects that result from incidents that are not recollected explicitly. The amygdala is a critical structure in the brain network that regulates emotions, including emotional aspects of memory. The amygdala plays a vital role in emotionally charged memories, while the hippocampus is essential for explicit memory. As an example, Damasio group conducted a conditioning experiment in patients.[160] The unconditioned stimulus was the startling sound of a loud horn, which produced an increase in skin conductance response, the unconditioned response. They presented a slide with a specific color as the conditioned stimulus, which was accompanied by the jarring noise. After the slide had been presented several times with the sound, presentation of the slide alone to healthy subjects produced an increase in skin conductance – a conditioned response – evidence that emotional conditioning had occurred. (See Figure 2.8 for explanation of the events of conditioning. A slide replaced the tone and a loud noise replaced the shock in Damasio group experiment.) Patients with selective hippocampal damage showed normal emotional conditioning to the slide, but remembered little of what had occurred during the trials. In striking contrast, patients with amygdala damage remembered what had happened, but failed to show any effects of conditioning. Thus, the effects of emotional conditioning depend on the amygdala and are

processed separately from explicit knowledge about what happened during the conditioning episode, which depends on the hippocampus.

4 Some patients with psychogenic amnesia may show implicit memory for the traumatic events.[155] This largely anecdotal evidence has been mentioned before.

5 It is possible that emotional learning and responsivity may be relatively preserved at levels of anesthesia that are sufficient to obliterate cognitive processing. There is a persistent tradition in the literature that unfavorable comments about patients voiced during anesthesia are particularly likely to be recalled. The evidence is anecdotal.[3] Can structures like the amygdala and hippocampus with their neural networks have different sensitivities to the effects of anesthetics? This remains to be tested.

Recovery from surgery depends partially upon psychosomatic processes

Surgery has been widely regarded as a stressor or stressful life event that requires coping and adaptation for a successful outcome.[163-165] The psychological consequences of surgery have been of interest to health care providers and stress researchers for many years.[166-169] Not only may the patient's psychological state affect postoperative morbidity and mortality, it is also an important index of recovery.[170-172] There is some evidence that patients who are psychologically prepared for surgery suffer less depression and anxiety after surgery relative to controls.[75]

Anesthetized patients may be vulnerable to psychosomatic influences

It is theoretically possible that if memories of intraoperative events cannot be consciously recollected, they may exert a stronger influence on emotions than in the normal waking state for three reasons:

1 Anesthetized patients are less able to defend themselves against the implications of what they have 'heard'; that is, to use normal, conscious cognitive processes to rationalize or cope with 'bad news'.

2 Information that bypasses consciousness may activate complexes (repressed systems of emo-

tionally charged ideas), with unfortunate psychological consequences, such as post-operative anxiety or depression.[157,159,173,174]

3 Weak physical condition, which may be present during or after surgery may contribute to psychosomatic deterioration.

The role of hypnosis

The reports that memories of pessimistic or derogatory operating room conversations may sometimes only be apparent with the aid of hypnosis could be explained as:

1 Hypnosis may induce a state of altered consciousness similar to that of anesthesia to facilitate state-dependent retrieval.

2 If the information that was acquired during anesthesia was particularly traumatic, and its recall was therefore blocked, hypnosis may disinhibit the patient and thereby encourages recollection of previously repressed information. (It should be remembered that hypnosis has failed in aiding recall of neutral verbal stimuli that were presented during anesthesia.)[16,147,175,176]

Critiques and conclusions about the clinical significance of implicit memory after anesthesia

How accurate are these reports of psychosomatic disorders as evidence for implicit memory of intraoperative events?

To invoke implicit memory for a past experience, it is essential to demonstrate that a behavior or symptoms are specifically related to that experience. With general symptoms like sleep disturbances, anxiety and depression following surgery, it is difficult to ascertain that implicit memory for intraoperative events is the source of these symptoms. As we mentioned before, emotional distress following surgery is relatively common and there are strong predictors of such reactions, e.g. patient's personality, disease, surgery, rate of recovery, etc.[177] In the laboratory, experimenters can control the events that give rise to implicit memories. In case reports where patients do not explicitly remember, it is impossible to make controlled comparisons. The therapist may engage

in unwarranted interpretations of insomnia, anxiety, depression and other symptoms as signs of implicit memory. This is particularly troublesome in cases where hypnosis was used. It is possible that much of the material 'recalled' under hypnosis may be incorrect.[178,179] A panel of the council on Scientific Affairs of the American Medical Association[180] reviewed the evidence concerning the effect of hypnosis on memory and concluded that 'recollections obtained during hypnosis can involve confabulations and pseudomemories, and not only fail to be more accurate, but actually appear to be less reliable than non-hypnotic recall'. It is, therefore, worrisome that most of the reports following anesthesia did not use techniques that would exclude confabulation as the basis for 'memories' that were hypnotically retrieved. Also, details concerning the interview between hypnotist and patient were usually insufficient to establish if leading questions were asked and if the patient's recall was accurate. It is hard to distinguish accurate from spurious recall without specific stimuli to score. Lastly, remission of the patient's symptoms through hypnosis or psychoanalysis may be due to causes other than the bringing of intraoperative events into consciousness.

Are we using the optimal tests?

Unfortunately, controlled studies, for ethical and legal reasons, use neutral stimuli. Some investigators[148,181,182] claim that meaningfulness of the material to be learned is of paramount importance, and it is difficult in controlled studies to use personally meaningful or emotional materials comparable to those mentioned in some case reports. Blacher[148] claimed that his group could replicate the results of Levinson[3] by creating a similar fake crisis during anesthesia, but were unsuccessful when they administered 'benign' stimuli (he supplied no details). Memories of traumatic experiences are qualitatively different from memories of everyday events and are characterized by having a substantial sensorimotor or affective quality with sometimes little or no narrative component.[183,184] Unlike smells, colors, sounds or other sensory stimuli that trigger memories, verbal tests, such as the word completion task, a free association task or others developed in the laboratory may not be the optimal tests for implicit memory of intraoperative events.[184] Osterman and van der Kolk[185] suggest that such memories are more likely to be recalled with one sensory element stimulating recall of other emotional memories. They cite as an example a woman with only a few isolated memories of her painful awareness experience who visited a hospital several weeks postoperatively. She was flooded with previously unrecalled memories and flashbacks of her trauma when she was approached by a hospital employee wearing an operating room scrub suit. She was overcome with feelings of terror and re-experienced feelings of paralysis and helplessness. Levinson[181] described the difference between meaningful and neutral stimuli in a colorful way: 'The brain has a censoring mechanism that carefully monitors all input. For example, a mother is sleeping. A bus passes, shaking the wall. She remains asleep. Her baby makes an odd noise and she immediately wakens'. His analogy for the controlled studies using neutral stimuli during anesthesia is: 'I am walking across a suspension bridge. It is only ropes and a few slats of wood. Thousands of feet below me is a raging, rock strewn river.... My whole being is focused on getting to the other side. Behind me, someone is saying … orange … pigeon … what is the blood pressure of the octopus …? The only way to transfix the censoring apparatus is to present it with a life-threatening or life-preserving stimulus'.

Therein lies a dilemma

Case reports cannot establish a cause-and-effect relation between unconscious learning during anesthesia and a patient's psychological disorder or determine the frequency of such occurrences. But neither should they be dismissed, particularly if there is corroborating evidence from persons other than the patient and the therapist concerning the remembered intraoperative events. For several years there have been few new reports linking unconscious learning during anesthesia and postoperative psychosomatic disorders. Are there no new cases to report? Or is there a lack of interest to report on the part of clinicians or to publish on the part of journal editors? Andrade and Jones[186] recently suggested that future research should be directed at the emotional impact of light anesthesia in well-controlled studies to see if it would do any harm (assuming that affective priming would be likely during light rather than adequate anesthesia). Although such studies may be difficult because psychological complications following surgery are caused by many factors and ethical concerns about the use of light anesthesia may be raised, the subject is too important to be lightly dismissed. In the meantime, even with the present level of knowledge, it is reasonable to caution operating room personnel to exercise restraint in their conversations and assume that some of these conversations may be retained by the unconscious and vulnerable patient with adverse consequences.

Prevention of implicit memory following anesthesia

If there is a possibility that implicit memory following anesthesia may cause harm to the patients, we need to consider how to prevent unconscious information processing during surgery. There are at least three methods. First, as we mentioned before, there is recent evidence of a correlation between implicit memory and the level of hypnosis. Thus, *deepening the level of the anesthetic* should obliterate this memory. How deep? Lubke *et al.*'s recent study[50] suggests a bispectral index of 40 and below. We look forward to future confirmation of these interesting results. Second, *prevention of auditory perception of operating room sounds*. This could be done by playing music, neutral sounds or therapeutic suggestions to the patients through head phones; using ear plugs; and prevention of voicing negative or derogatory remarks about the patients or their diseases during anesthesia. Third, administration of benzodiazepines, specifically *midazolam*. In healthy volunteers, administration of 0.1 mg/kg or 0.06 mg.kg^{-1} together with 0.2% isoflurane obliterates implicit memory as tested by the word completion task for at least the next 30 to 45 minutes following its administration.[187] There is no available information about the adequacy of the drug in patients during surgery.

General comments and conclusions

Implicit memory after anesthesia has often proved to be an elusive phenomenon. Studies that search for implicit learning and memory during and after anesthesia continue to generate a bewildering array of positive and negative results. The use of procedures that dissociate explicit and implicit influences on memory performance; or match the level of difficulty of explicit and implicit tasks; and use of a monitor that has a well-defined point for loss of consciousness and can assess the adequacy of anesthesia may elucidate the nature of learning and memory during anesthesia. This may also lead to more consistent outcomes for the studies that can be replicated. Then, it would be much easier to study the influence of experimental variables that may affect unconscious learning and memory.

Current state of knowledge suggests that implicit memory occurs in few patients, only some of the time, and particularly after light levels of anesthesia. Learning may be more perceptual than engaging in elaborate processing of complex information and may be limited to single, relatively familiar words. Memory may be more evident if tested as soon as possible after surgery.

The study of implicit memory after anesthesia is important for two main reasons. First and foremost, it may have important clinical implications. Preferences, feelings and biases can be shaped by experiences that people do not remember consciously. Implicit influences may be especially traumatic because they operate outside our awareness and affect the potentially vulnerable surgical patient. We need to study the emotional as well as the cognitive consequences of implicit memories on the postoperative outcomes of patients. Our knowledge could promote recovery and prevent debilitating psychosomatic complications. The proposition is difficult to prove, but it needs to be addressed.

The second reason for studying implicit memory after anesthesia is theoretical and concerns the use of general anesthesia as a tool for memory research. A voluminous literature in human learning and cognition has addressed the question of whether it is possible to learn without awareness.[46] However, the existence of this so-called implicit learning remains contentious, partly because of the problem of ensuring that all subjects are unaware of all the information to be learned.[49] Experimental psychologists have tried to induce conscious subjects to perceive unconsciously by presenting stimuli under suboptimal conditions. For example, in a subliminal learning study, visual or auditory stimuli may be presented for a very short duration (e.g. 50 ms) and in a divided attention study, subjects are asked to perform secondary distracting tasks (e.g. subjects wear earphones. One message is played through

one ear and a different message is played through the other. Subjects are asked to pay attention to one of the messages and to repeat it back aloud as it is being played. Then, they are stopped unexpectedly in the middle of the task and asked to recall the 'unattended' message). Anesthetics provide an attractive alternative approach to these methods. Unconsciousness is directly induced and any demonstration of memory afterwards constitutes evidence for implicit learning, provided that we can monitor the level of awareness to ascertain its absence.[40,188] One can also study the effects of varying the level of consciousness by varying the dose of the anesthetic. Anesthetics, therefore, have the potential to reveal not only whether implicit learning is possible, but also the ways in which awareness during learning affects later memory and the distinction between its types.

References

1. Cheek DB. Unconscious perception of meaningful sounds during surgical anesthesia as revealed under hypnosis. *Am J Clin Hypn* 1959; **1**:101–113.
2. Cheek DB. Surgical memory and reaction to careless conversation. *Am J Clin Hypn* 1964; **6**: 237–240.
3. Levinson BW. States of awareness during general anesthesia. *Br J Anaesth* 1965; **37**:544–546.
4. Wolfe LS, Millett JB. Control of post-operative pain by suggestion under general anesthesia. *Am J Clin Hypn* 1960; **3**:109–112.
5. Hutchings DD. The value of suggestions given under general anesthesia: A report and evaluation of 200 consecutive cases. *Am J Clin Hypn* 1961; **4**:26–29.
6. Pearson RE. Response to suggestions given under general anesthesia. *Am J Clin Hypn* 1961; **4**: 106–114.
7. Cork RC, Couture LJ, Kihlstrom JF. Memory and recall. In Yaksh TL, Lynch C III, Zapol WM, Maze M, Biebuyck JF, Saidman LJ (eds).*Anesthesia Biologic Foundations*. Philadelphia: Lippincott-Raven 1998; 451–467.
8. Warrington EK, Weiskrantz L. New method for testing long-term retention with special reference to amnesic patients. *Nature* 1968; **217**:972–974.
9. Warrington EK, Weiskrantz L. The effect of prior learning on subsequent retention in amnesic patients. *Neuropsyhologia* 1974; **12**:419–428.
10. Weiskrantz L. Some aspects of visual capacity in monkeys and man following striate cortex lesions. *Arch Italiennes de biologie* 1978; **116**:318–323.

11. Weiskrantz L. *Blindsight. A Case Study and Implications.* Oxford: Clarendon Press, 1986.

12. Milner B, Corkin S, Teuber HL. Further analysis of the hippocampal amnesic syndrome: Fourteen year follow-up study of H.M. *Neuropsychologia* 1968; **6**:215–234.

13. Tulving E, Schacter DL, Stark H. Priming effects in word-fragment completion are independent of recognition memory. *J Exp Psychol (Learn Mem Cogn)* 1982; **8**:336–342.

14. Graf P, Schacter DL. Implicit and explicit memory for new associations in normal subjects and amnesic patients. *J Exp Psychol (Learn Mem Cogn)* 1985; **11**:501–518.

15. Millar K, Watkinson N. Recognition of words presented during general anesthesia. *Ergonomics* 1983; **26**:585–594.

16. Bennett HL, Davis HS, Giannini AJ. Non-verbal response to intraoperative conversation. *Br J Anaesth* 1985; **57**:174–179.

17. Bonke B, Schmitz PIM, Verhage F, Zwaveling A. Clinical study of so-called unconscious perception during general anesthesia. *Br J Anaesth* 1986; **58**:957–964.

18. Squire LR, Hamann S, Knowlton B. Dissociable learning and memory systems of the brain. *Behav Brain Sci* 1994; **17**:422–430.

19. Squire LR, Zola SM. Structure and function of declarative and nondeclarative memory systems. *Proc Natl Acad Sci USA* 1996; **93**:13515–13522.

20. Schacter D. Implicit knowledge: New perspectives on unconscious processes. *Proc Natl Acad Sci USA* 1992; **89**:11113–11117.

21. Block RI, Ghoneim MM, Sum Ping ST, Ali MA. Human learning during general anesthesia and surgery. *Br J Anaesth* 1991; **66**:170–178.

22. Graf P, Squire LR, Mandler G. The information that amnesic patients do not forget. *J Exp Psychol (Learn Mem Cogn)* 1984; **10**:164–178.

23. Church BA, Schacter DL. Perceptual specificity of auditory priming: Implicit memory for voice intonation and fundamental frequency. *J Exp Psychol (Learn Mem Cogn)* 1994; **20**:521–533.

24. Gabrieli JDE. Cognitive neuroscience of human memory. *Annu Rev Psychol* 1998; **49**:87–115.

25. Schacter DL, Buckner RL. Priming and the brain. *Neuron* 1998; **20**:185–195.

26. Vaidya CJ, Gabrieli JDE, Demb JB, Keane MM, Wetzel LC. Impaired priming on the general knowledge task in amnesia. *Neuropsychology* 1996; **10**:529–537.

27. Schacter DL. Implicit memory. History and current status. *J Exp Psychol (Learn Mem Cogn)* 1987; **134**:501–518.

28. Kihlstrom JF, Schacter DL. Anaesthesia, amnesia, and the cognitive unconscious. In Bonke B, Fitch W, Millar K (eds). *Memory and Awareness in Anesthesia.* Amsterdam: Swets & Zeitlinger, 1990, 21–44.

29. Jelicic M, De Roode A, Bovill JG, Bonke B. Unconscious learning during anaesthesia. *Anaesthesia* 1992; **47**:835–837.

30. Münte S, Kobbe I, Demertzis A, *et al.* Increased reading speed for stories presented during general anesthesia. *Anesthesiology* 1999; **90**:662–669.

31. Jelicic M, Bonke B, Appelboom DK. Indirect memory for words presented during anaesthesia. *Lancet* 1990; **2**:249.

32. Roorda-Hrdlicková V, Wolters G, Bonke B, Phaf RH. Unconscious perception during general anesthesia demonstrated by an implicit memory task. In Bonke B, Fitch W, Millar K (eds). *Memory and Awareness in Anaesthesia.* Amsterdam: Swets & Zeitlinger, 1990, 150–155.

33. Bonebakker AE, Bonke B, Klein J, Wolters G, Hop WCJ. Implicit memory during balanced anaesthesia: Lack of evidence. *Anaesthesia* 1993; **48**:657–660.

34. Bonebakker AE, Bonke B, Klein J, *et al.* Information-processing during balanced anaesthesia: Evidence for unconscious memory. *Mem Cogn* 1996; **24**:766–776.

35. Foster KI, Davies C. Repetition priming and frequency attention in lexical access. *J Exp Psychol (Learn Mem Cogn)* 1984; **10**:680–698.

36. McLeod CM. Word context during initial exposure influences degree of priming in word-fragment completion. *J Exp Psychol (Learn Mem Cogn)* 1989; **15**:398–406.

37. Squire LR. Declarative and nondeclarative memory: Multiple brain systems supporting learning and memory. *J Cognitive Neuroscience* 1992; **4**:232–243.

38. Jacoby LL, Toth J, Yonelinas A. Separating conscious and unconscious influences of memory: Measuring recollection. *J Exp Psychol (Gen)* 1993; **122**:139–154.

39. Mandler G. Recognizing: The judgment of previous occurrence. *Psychol Rev* 1980; **87**:252–271.

40. Merikle PM, Daneman M. Memory for unconsciously perceived events: Evidence from anesthetized patients. *Consciousness Cogn* 1996; **5**:525–541.

41. Jacoby LL. A process dissociation framework: Separating automatic from intentional uses of memory. *J Mem Lang* 1991; **30**:513–541.

42. Gardiner JM. Functional aspects of recollective experience. *Mem Cogn* 1988; **16**:309–313.

43. Wagner AD, Gabrieli JDE, Verfaellie M. Dissociations between familiarity processes in explicit-recognition and implicit-perceptual memory. *J Exp Psychol (Learn Mem Cogn)* 1997; **23**:305–323.

44. Knowlton BJ, Squire LR. Remembering and

knowing: Two different expressions of declarative memory. *J Exp Psychol (Learn Mem Cogn)* 1995; **21**:699–710.

45. Merikle PM, Reingold EM. Comparing direct (explicit) and indirect (implicit) measures to study unconscious memory. *J Exp Psychol (Learn Mem Cogn)* 1991; **17**:224–233.

46. Shanks DR, St. John MF. Characteristics of dissociable human learning systems. *Behav Brain Sci* 1994; **17**:367–395.

47. Ghoneim MM, Block RI. Learning and memory during general anesthesia: An update. *Anesthesiology* 1997; **87**:387–410.

48. Andrade J. Learning during anaesthesia: A review. *Br J Psychol* 1995; **86**:479–506.

49. Andrade J. Investigations of hypesthesia: Using anesthetics to explore relationships between consciousness, learning and memory. *Conscious Cogn* 1996; **5**:562–580.

50. Lubke GH, Kerssens C, Phaf H, Sebel PS. Dependence of explicit and implicit memory on hypnotic state in trauma patients. *Anesthesiology* 1999; **90**:670–680.

51. Lubke GH, Kerssens C, Gershon RY, Sebel PS. Memory formation during general anesthesia for emergency cesarean section. *Anesthesiology*, 2000;**92**:1029–1034.

52. Jacoby LL, Kelley CM. Becoming famous without being recognised. Unconscious influences of memory produced by divided attention. *J Exp Psychol (Gen)* 1989; **118**:115–125.

53. Caseley-Rondi G, Merikle PM, Bowers KS. Unconscious cognition in the context of general anesthesia. *Conscious Cogn* 1994; **3**:166–195.

54. Ghoneim MM, Mewaldt SP. Benzodiazepines and human memory: A review. *Anesthesiology* 1990; **72**:926–938.

55. Ghoneim MM, Block RI, Sum Ping ST, El-Zahaby HM, Hinrichs JV. The interactions of midazolam and flumazenil on human memory and cognition. *Anesthesiology* 1993; **79**:1183–1192.

56. Brown MW, Brown J, Bowes JB. Absence of priming coupled with substantially preserved recognition in lorazepam-induced amnesia. *Q J Exp Psychol* 1989; **41A**: 599–617.

57. Kihlstrom JF, Schacter DL, Cork RC, Hurt CA, Behr SE. Implicit and explicit memory following surgical anesthesia. *Psychol Sci* 1990; **1**:303–306.

58. Cork RC, Kihlstrom JF, Schacter DL. Absence of explicit and implicit memory in patients anesthetized with sufentanil/nitrous oxide. *Anesthesiology* 1992; **76**:892–898.

59. Schwender D, Kaiser A, Klasing S, Peter K, Pöppel E. Midlatency auditory evoked potentials and explicit and implicit memory in patients undergoing cardiac surgery. *Anesthesiology* 1994; **80**:493–501.

60. Ghoneim MM, Block RI, Dhanaraj VJ, Todd MM, Choi WW, Brown CK. The auditory evoked responses and learning and awareness during general anesthesia. *Acta Anesthesiol Scand* 2000; **44**:133–143.

61. Jelicic M, Asbury AJ, Millar K, Bonke B. Implicit learning during enflurane anaesthesia in spontaneously breathing patients? *Anesthesia* 1993; **48**:766–768.

62. Cave CB. Very long-lasting priming in picture naming. *Psychol Sci* 1997; **8**:322–325.

63. Karni A, Tanne D, Rubenstein BS, Askenasy JJM, Sagi D. Dependence on REM sleep of overnight improvement of a perceptual skill. *Science* 1994; **265**:679–682.

64. Rosenberg J, Wildschiøsdtz G, Pedersen MH, von Jessen F, Kehlet H. Late postoperative nocturnal episodic hypoxaemia and associated sleep pattern. *Br J Anaesth* 1994; **72**:145–150.

65. Challis BH, Sidhu R. Dissociative effect of massed repetition on implicit and explicit measures of memory. *J Exp Psychol (Learn Mem Cogn)* 1993; **19**:115–127.

66. Musen G. Effects of verbal labeling and exposure duration on implicit memory for visual patterns. *J Exp Psychol (Learn Mem Cogn)* 1991; **17**: 954–962.

67. Brown AS, Best MR, Mitchell DB, Haggard LC. Memory under anesthesia: Evidence for response suppression. *Bull Psychonom Soc* 1992; **30**: 244–246.

68. Cheek DB, Le Cron JM. *Clinical Hypnotherapy*: New York: Grune and Stratton, 1968.

69. Goldmann L, Shah MV, Hebden MW. Memory of cardiac anaesthesia. *Anaesthesia* 1987; **42**: 596–603.

70. Millar K. Unconscious perception during general anaesthesia (letter). *Br J Anaesth* 1987; **59**:1334.

71. Wilson ME, Spiegelhalter D. Unconscious perception during anesthesia (letter). *Br J Anaesth* 1987; **59**:1333.

72. Merikle PM, Rondi G. Memory for events during anesthesia has not been demonstrated: A psychologist's view point. In Sebel PS, Bonke B, Winograd E (eds). *Memory and Awareness in Anesthesia*. Englewood Cliffs: Prentice-Hall 1993, 476–497.

73. Ghoneim MM, Block RI. Learning and consciousness during general anesthesia. *Anesthesiology* 1992; **76**:279–305.

74. Mumford E, Schlesinger HJ, Glass G. The effect of psychological intervention on recovery from surgery and heart attacks: An analysis of the literature. *Am J Public Health* 1982; **72**:141–151.

75. Rogers M, Reich P. Psychological intervention with surgical patients: Evaluation outcome. In Guggenheim FG (ed). *Psychological Aspects of Surgery*. Basel: Karger, 1986, 23–50.

76. Barber TX. Changing 'unchangeable' bodily processes by (hypnotic) suggestions: A new look at hypnosis, cognitions, imagining, and the mind-body problem. In Sheikh AA (ed.) *Imagery and Healing (Imagery and Human Development Series)*. Farmingdale: Baywood Publ Co, 1984, 69–127.

77. Wadden TA, Anderton CH. The clinical use of hypnosis. *Psychol Bull* 1982; **91**:215–243.

78. Bowers KS. Hypnosis: An informational approach. *Ann NY Acad Sci* 1977; **296**:222–237.

79. Bowers KS, Kelly P. Stress, disease, psychotherapy, and hypnosis. *J Abnorm Psychol* 1979; **88**:490–505.

80. Korunka C, Guttmann G, Schleinitz D, Hilpert M, Haas R, Ritzal S. Die auswirkung von suggestionen und musik wahren vollnarkose auf postoperative befindlichkeit (The effect of suggestions and music during general anesthesia on postoperative well-being). *Zeitschrift fur Klinische Psychologie* 1992; **21**:272–285.

81. Lebovits SH, Twersky R, McEwan B. Intra-operative therapeutic suggestions in day-case surgery: Are there benefits for postoperative outcome? *Br J Anaesth* 1999; **82**:861–866.

82. Bennett HL. Influencing the brain with information during general anaesthesia: A theory of 'unconscious hearing'. In Bonke B, Fitch W, Millar K (eds). *Memory and Awareness in Anaesthesia*. Amsterdam: Swets and Zeitlinger, 1990, 50–56.

83. Münch F, Zug H-D. Do intraoperative suggestions prevent nausea and vomiting in thyroidectomy patients? An experimental study. In Bonke B, Fitch W, Millar K (eds). *Memory and Awareness in Anaesthesia*. Amsterdam: Swets and Zeitlinger, 1990, 185–188.

84. Woo R, Seltzer JL, Marr A. The lack of response to suggestion under controlled surgical anesthesia. *Acta Anaesthesiol Scand* 1987; **31**:567–571.

85. Evans C, Richardson PH. Improved recovery and reduced postoperative stay after therapeutic suggestions during general anaesthesia. *Lancet* 1988; **2**:491–493.

86. Liu WHD, Standen PJ, Aitkenhead AR. Therapeutic suggestions during general anaesthesia in patients undergoing hysterectomy. *Br J Anaesth* 1992; **68**:277–281.

87. Millar K. Efficacy of therapeutic suggestions presented during anaesthesia: Re-analysis of conflicting results. *Br J Anaesth* 1993; **71**: 597–601.

88. Jelicic M, Bonke B, Millar K. Effect of different therapeutic suggestions presented during anaesthesia on post-operative course. *Eur J Anaesthesiol* 1993; **10**:343–347.

89. van der Laan WH, van Leeuwen BL, Sebel PS, Winograd E, Baumann PL, Bonke B. Therapeutic suggestion has no effect on postoperative morphine requirements. *Anesth Analg* 1996; **82**:148–152.

90. Williams AR, Hind M, Sweeney BP. The incidence and severity of postoperative nausea and vomiting in patients exposed to positive intraoperative suggestions. *Anaesthesia* 1994; **49**:340–342.

91. Oddby-Muhrbeck E, Jakobsson J, Enqvist B. Implicit processing and therapeutic suggestion during balanced anesthesia. *Acta Anaesthesiol Scand* 1995; **39**:333–337.

92. Maroof M, Ahmed SM, Khan RM, Bano S, Haque AW. Positive suggestions during surgery reduces post-hysterectomy emesis (correspondence). *Can J Anaesth* 1997; **44**:227–230.

93. Hughes JA, Sanders LD, Dunne JA, Tarpey J, Vickers MD. Reducing smoking: The effect of suggestion during general anaesthesia on post-operative smoking habits. *Anaesthesia* 1994; **49**:126–128.

94. Myles PS, Hendrata M, Layher Y, *et al.*. Double-blind, randomized trial of cessation of smoking after audiotape suggestion during anaesthesia. *Br J Anaesth* 1996; **76**:694–698.

95. Andrade J, Munglani R. Therapeutic suggestions during general anaesthesia (letter). *Br J Anaesth* 1994; **72**:730.

96. Richmond CE, Bromley LM, Woolf CJ. Pre-operative morphine pre-empts postoperative pain. *Lancet* 1993; **342**:73–75.

97. Mansfield MD, James KS, Kinsella J. Influence of dose and timing of administration of morphine on postoperative pain and analgesic requirements. *Br J Anaesth* 1996; **76**:358–361.

98. d'Amours RH, Kramer TH, Mannes AJ. A Monte Carlo simulation of iv PCA use to examine its sensitivity as an analgesic assay. *Anesthesiology* 1995; **83**:A790.

99. Muir JJ, Warner MN, Offord KP, Buck CF, Harper JV, Kunkel SE. Role of nitrous oxide and other factors in postoperative nausea and vomiting: A randomized and blinded prospective study. *Anesthesiology* 1987; **66**:513–518.

100. Anonymous. Nausea and vomiting after general anesthesia (editorial). *Lancet* 1989; **1**:651–652.

101. Wachta MF, White PF. Postoperative nausea and vomiting. Its etiology, treatment and prevention. *Anesthesiology* 1992; **77**:162–184.

102. Russell IF. Comparison of wakefulness with two anaesthetic regimens: Total iv v. balanced anaesthesia. *Br J Anaesth* 1986; **58**:965–968.

103. Russell IF. Conscious awareness during general anaesthesia: Relevance of autonomic signs and isolated arm movements as guides to depth of anesthesia. In Jones JG (ed.) *Depth of Anaesthesia. Clinical Anesthesiology*, Vol. 3. London: Baillière Tindall, 1989, 511–532.

104. Russell IF. Midazolam-alfentanil: An anaesthetic?

An investigation using the isolated forearm technique. *Br J Anaesth* 1993; **70**:42–46.

105. King H-K, Ashley S, Brathwaite D, Decayette J, Wooten DJ. Adequacy of general anesthesia for cesarean section. *Anesth Analg* 1993; **77**:84–88.

106. Dwyer R, Bennett HL, Eger EI II, Heilbron D. Effects of isoflurane and nitrous oxide in subanesthetic concentrations on memory and responsiveness in volunteers. *Anesthesiology* 1992; **77**:888–898.

107. Block RI, Ghoneim MM, Pathak D, Kumar V, Hinrichs JV. Effects of a subanesthetic concentration of nitrous oxide on overt and covert assessments of memory and associative processes. *Psychopharmacology* 1988; **96**:324–331.

108. Block RI, Ghoneim MM, Hinrichs JV, Kumar V, Pathak D. Effects of a subanesthetic concentration of nitrous oxide on memory and subjective experience. Influence of assessment procedures and types of stimuli. *Hum Psychopharmacol* 1988; **3**:257–265.

109. Polster MR, Gray PA, O'Sullivan G, McCarthy RA, Park GR. Comparison of the sedative and amnesic effects of midazolam and propofol. *Br J Anaesth* 1993; **70**:612–616.

110. Chortkoff BS, Eger II EI, Crankshaw DP, Gonsowski CT, Dutton RC, Ionescu P. Concentrations of desflurane and propofol that suppress response to command in humans. *Anesth Analg* 1995; **81**:737–743.

111. Gonsowski CT, Chortkoff BS, Eger EI II, Bennett HL, Weiskopf RB. Subanesthetic concentrations of desflurane and isoflurane suppress explicit and implicit learning. *Anesth Analg* 1995; **80**:568–572.

112. Chortkoff BS, Bennett HL, Eger EI II. Subanesthetic concentrations of isoflurane suppress learning as defined by the category-example task. *Anesthesiology* 1993; **79**:16–22.

113. Reingold EM, Merikle PM. Using direct and indirect measures to study perception without awareness. *Perception & Psychophysics* 1988; **44**:563–575.

114. Buckner RL, Koutstaal W. Functional neuroimaging studies of encoding, priming and explicit memory retrieval. *Proc Natl Acad Sci USA* 1998; **95**:891–898.

115. Mackintosh NJ. *The Psychology of Animal Learning*. New York: Academic Press, 1974.

116. Polster MR. Drug-induced amnesia: Implications for cognitive neuropsychological investigations of memory. *Psychol Bull* 1993; **114**:477–493.

117. Smith MC, Coleman SR, Gormezano I. Classical conditioning of the rabbit's nictitating membrane response at backward, simultaneous and forward CS-US intervals. *J Comp Physiol Psychol* 1969; **69**:226–231.

118. Pavlov IP. *Conditioned reflexes* (translated by Anrep GV). London: Oxford University Press, 1927.

119. Clark RE, Squire LR. Classical conditioning and brain systems: The role of awareness. *Science* 1998; **280**:77–81.

120. Daum I, Channon S, Canavar A. Classical conditioning in patients with severe memory problems. *J Neurol Neurosurg Psychiatry* 1989; **52**:47–51.

121. Daum I, Channon S, Polkey CE, Gray JA. Classical conditioning after temporal lobe lesions in man: Impairment in conditional discrimination. *Behav Neurosci* 1991; **105**:396–408.

122. Warrington EK, Weiskrantz L. Conditioning in amnesic patients. *Neuropsychologia* 1979; **17**:187–194.

123. Woodruff-Pak DS. Eyeblink classical conditioning in H. M: Delay and trace paradigms. *Behav Neurosci* 1993; **107**:911–925.

124. Thompson RF. Neural mechanisms of classical conditioning in mammals. *Philos Trans R Soc Lond (B)* 1990; **329**:161–170.

125. Mauk MD, Thompson RF. Retention of classically conditioned eyelid responses following acute decerebration. *Brain Res* 1987; **403**:89–95.

126. Thompson RF, Jeansok JK. Memory systems in the brain and localization of a memory. *Proc Natl Acad Sci USA* 1996; **93**:13438–13444.

127. Desimone R, Miller EK, Chelazzi L, Lueschow A. Multiple memory systems in the visual cortex. In Gazzaniga MS (ed.) *The Cognitive Neurosciences*. Cambridge, MA: MIT Press, 1995, 475–486.

128. Weinberger NM, Gold PE, Sternberg DB. Epinephrine enables Pavlovian fear conditioning under anesthesia. *Science* 1984; **233**:605–607.

129. Gold PE, Weinberger NM, Sternberg DB. Epinephrine-induced learning under anesthesia: Retention performance at several training-testing intervals. *Behav Neurosci* 1985; **99**:1019–1022.

130. Dariola MK, Yadava A, Malhotra S. Effects of epinephrine on learning under anaesthesia. *J Indian Acad Appl Psychol* 1993; **19**:47–51.

131. El-Zahaby HM, Ghoneim MM, Johnson GM, Gormezano I. Effects of subanesthetic concentrations of isoflurane and their interactions with epinephrine on acquisition and retention of the rabbit nictitating membrane response. *Anesthesiology* 1994; **81**:229–237.

132. Moon Y, Ghoneim MM, Gormezano I. Nitrous oxide: Sensory, motor, associative and behavioral tolerance effects in classical conditioning of the rabbit nictitating membrane response. *Pharmacol Biochem Behav* 1994; **47**:523–529.

133. El-Zahaby HM, Ghoneim MM, Block RI. The interaction between nitrous oxide and isoflurane on suppression of learning: A study using classical

conditioning in rabbits. *Acta Anaesthesiol Scand* 1996; **40**:798–803.

134. Zacny JP, Sparacino G, Hoffmann PM, Martin R, Lichtor JL. The subjective, behavioral and cognitive effects of subanesthetic concentrations of isoflurane and nitrous oxide in healthy volunteers. *Psychopharmacology* 1994; **114**:409–416.

135. Chortkoff BS, Bennett HL, Eger EI II. Does nitrous oxide antagonize isoflurane-induced suppression of learning? *Anesthesiology* 1993; **79**:724–732.

136. Pang R, Turndorf H, Quartermain D. Pavlovian fear conditioning in mice anesthetized with halothane. *Physiol Behav* 1996; **59**:873–875.

137. Kandel L, Chortkoff BS, Sonner J, Laster MJ, Eger El II. Nonanesthetics can suppress learning. *Anesth Analg* 1996; **82**:321–326.

138. Ghoneim MM, El-Zahaby HM, Block RI. Classical conditioning during nitrous oxide treatment: Influence of varying the interstimulus interval. *Pharmacol Biochem Behav* 1999; **62**:449–455.

139. Edeline J-M, Massioui N. Retention of CS–US association learned under ketamine anesthesia. *Brain Res* 1988; **457**:274–280.

140. Ghoneim MM, Chen P, El-Zahaby HM, Block RI. Ketamine: acquisition and retention of classically conditioned responses during treatment with large doses. *Pharmacol Biochem Behav* 1994; **49**: 1061–1066.

141. Bermudez-Rattoni F, Forthman DL, Sanchez MA, Perez JL, Garcia J. Odor and taste aversions conditioned in anesthetized rats. *Behav Neurosci* 1988; **102**:726–732.

142. Roll DL, Smith JC. Conditioned taste aversion in anesthetized rats. *Biological Boundaries of Learning.* Seligman MEP, Hager JL (eds). New York, Appleton-Century-Crofts, 1972, 98–102.

143. Rozin P, Ree P. Long extension of effective CS–US interval by anesthesia between CS and US. *J Comp Physiol Psychol* 1972; **80**:43.

144. Millner JR, Palfai T. Metrazol impairs conditioned aversion produced by Li Cl: A time dependent effect. *Pharmacol Biochem Behav* 1975; **3**: 201–204.

145. Buresová O, Bures J. The effect of anesthesia on acquisition and extinction of conditioned taste aversion. *Behav Biol* 1977; **20**:41–50.

146. Howard JF. Incidents of auditory perception during general anesthesia with traumatic sequelae. *Med J Aust* 1987; **146**:44–46.

147. Goldmann L. Information-processing under general anaesthesia: A review. *J Roy Soc Med* 1988; **81**:224–227.

148. Blacher RS. General surgery and anesthesia: The emotional experience. In Blacher RS (ed.) *The Psychological Experience of Surgery.* New York: Wiley, 1987, 1–25.

149. Chortkoff BS, Gonsowski CT, Bennett HL, *et al.* Subanesthetic concentrations of desflurane and propofol suppress recall of emotionally charged information. *Anesth Analg* 1995; **81**:728–736.

150. Tunstall ME. Detecting wakefulness during general anaesthesia for Caesarean section. *Br Med J* 1977; **1**:1321.

151. Ghoneim MM, Mewaldt SP, Petersen RC. Subanesthetic concentration of nitrous oxide and human memory. *Prog Neuro-psychopharmacol* 1981; **5**:395–402.

152. Overton DA. Historical context of state dependent learning and discriminative drug effects. *Behav Pharmacol* 1991; **2**:253–264.

153. Mewaldt SP, Ghoneim MM, Choi WW, Korttila K, Petersen RC. Nitrous oxide and human state-dependent memory. *Pharmacol Biochem Behav* 1988; **30**:83–87.

154. Schacter DL. *Searching for Memory: The Brain, the Mind, and the Past.* New York: Basic Books, 1996, 218–247.

155. Tobias BA, Kihlstrom JF, Schacter DL. Emotion and implicit memory. In Christianson S-Å (ed.) *The Handbook of Emotion and Memory: Research and Theory.* Hillsdale: Erlbaum, 1992, 67–92.

156. Kunst-Wilson WR, Zajonc RB. Affective discrimination of stimuli that cannot be recognized. *Science* 1980; **207**:557–558.

157. Murphy ST, Zajonc RB. Affect, cognition and awareness: Affective priming with optimal and suboptimal stimulus exposures. *J Pers Soc Psychol* 1993; **65**:723–739.

158. Lewicki P, Hill T, Czyewska M. Nonconscious acquisition of information. *Amer Psychologist* 1992; **47**:796–801.

159. Bornstein RF. Subliminal mere exposure effects. In Bornstein RF, Pittman TS (eds). *Clinical and Social Perspectives.* New York: Guilford Press, 1992, 191–210.

160. Bechara A, Tranel D, Damasio H, Adolphs R, Rockland C, Damasio AR. Double dissociation of conditioned and declarative knowledge relative to the amygdala and hippocampus in humans. *Science* 1995; **269**:1115–1118.

161. LeDoux JE. Emotion as memory: Anatomical systems underlying indelible neural traces. In Christianson S-Å (ed.) *The Handbook of Emotion and Memory: Research and Theory.* Hillsdale: Erlbaum, 1992, 269–288.

162. LeDoux JE. Emotion, memory and the brain. *Scientific American* 1994; **270**:32–39.

163. Bradley C. Psychological factors affecting recovery from surgery. In Watkins J, Salo M (eds). *Trauma, Stress and Immunity in Anesthesia and Surgery.* Woburn, MA: Butterworth, 1982, 335–361.

164. Cohen F, Lazarus RS. Active coping processes, coping dispositions, and recovery from surgery. *Psychosom Med* 1973; **35**:375–389.

165. Sime AM. Relationship of preoperative fear, type of coping, and information received about surgery to recovery from surgery. *J Pers Soc Psychol* 1976; **34**:717–724.

166. Janis IL. *Psychological Stress: Psychoanalytic and Behavioral Studies of Surgical Patients.* New York: Academic Press, 1958.

167. Titchener JL, Levine M. *Surgery as a Human Experience: The Psychodynamics of Surgical Practice.* New York: Oxford University Press, 1960.

168. Blacher RS (ed.) *The Psychological Experience of Surgery.* New York: Wiley, 1987.

169. Guggenheim FG (ed.) *Psychological Aspects of Surgery.* New York: S. Karger, 1986.

170. Johnston M. Dimensions of recovery from surgery. *Int Rev Appl Psychol* 1984; **33**:505–520.

171. Johnston M. Preoperative emotional states and postoperative recovery. In Guggenheim FG (ed.) *Psychological Aspects of Surgery.* New York: S Karger, 1986, 1–22.

172. Mayou R. The psychiatric and social consequences of coronary artery surgery. *J Psychosom Res* 1986; **30**:255–271.

173. Dixon NF. Unconscious perception and general anesthesia. *Baillieres Clin Anesthesiol* 1989; **3**: 473–485.

174. LeDoux JE. Cognitive-emotional interactions in the brain. *Cognition and Emotion* 1989; **3**: 267–289.

175. Terrell RK, Sweet WO, Gladfelter JH, Stephen CR. Study of recall during anesthesia. *Anesth Analg* 1969; **48**:86–90.

176. Goldmann L, Levy AB. Orienting responses under general anaesthesia. *Anaesthesia* 1986; **41**: 1056–1057.

177. O'Hara MW, Ghoneim MM, Hinrichs JV, Mehta MP, Wright EJ. Psychological consequences of surgery. *Psychosom Med* 1989; **51**:356–370.

178. Dywan J, Bowers K. The use of hypnosis to enhance recall. *Science* 1983; **222**:184–185.

179. Laurence J-R, Perry C. Hypnotically created memory among highly hypnotizable subjects. *Science* 1983; **222**:523–524.

180. Council on Scientific Affairs. Council report: Scientific status of refreshing recollection by the use of hypnosis. *JAMA* 1985; **253**:1918–1923.

181. Levinson BW. Quo Vadis. In Sebel PS, Bonke B, Winograd E (eds). *Memory and Awareness in Anesthesia.* Englewood Cliffs: Prentice-Hall, 1993, 498–500.

182. Bennett HL. Memory for events during anesthesia does occur: A psychologist's viewpoint. In Sebel PS, Bonke B, Winograd E (eds). *Memory and Awareness in Anesthesia.* Englewood Cliffs: Prentice-Hall, 1993, 459–466.

183. van der Kolk BA, Fisher R. Dissociation and the fragmentary nature of traumatic memories: Overview and exploratory study. *J Traumatic Stress* 1995; **8**:505–525.

184. Christianson S, Engelberg E. Remembering and forgetting traumatic experiences: A matter of survival. In Conway MA (ed.) *Recovered Memories and False Memories.* Oxford: Oxford University Press, 1997, 231–250.

185. Osterman JE, van der Kolk BA. Awareness during anesthesia and post-traumatic stress disorder. *Gen Hosp Psychiatry* 1998; **20**:274–281.

186. Andrade J, Jones JG. Is amnesia for intraoperative events good enough? (editorial). *Br J Anesth* 1998; **80**:575–576.

187. Ghoneim MM, Block RI, Dhanaraj VJ. Interaction of a subanesthetic concentration of isoflurane with midazolam: Effects on responsiveness, learning and memory. *Br J Anaesth* 1998; **80**:581–587.

188. Andrade J. Is learning during anaesthesia implicit? *Behav Brain Sci* 1994; **17**:396.

189. Westmoreland CL, Sebel PS, Winograd E, Goldman WP. Indirect memory during anesthesia. *Anesthesiology* 1993; **78**:237–241.

190. Russell IF, Wang M. Absence of memory for intraoperative information during surgery under adequate general anesthesia. *Br J Anaesth* 1997; **78**:3–9.

191. MacRae WJ, Thorp JM, Millar K. Category generation testing in the search for implicit memory during general anaesthesia. *Br J Anaesth* 1998; **80**:588–593.

192. Ghoneim MM, Block RI, Fowles DC. No evidence of classical conditioning of electrodermal responses during anesthesia. *Anesthesiology* 1992; **76**: 682–688.

193. DeRoode A, Jelicic M, Bonke B, Bovill JG. The effect of midazolam premedication on implicit memory activation during alfentanil-nitrous oxide anaesthesia. *Anaesthesia* 1995; **50**:191–194.

194. Donker AG, Phaf RH, Porcelijn T, Bonke B. Processing familiar and unfamiliar auditory stimuli during general anesthesia. *Anesth Analg* 1996; **82**:452–455.

195. Lewis SA, Jenkinson J, Wilson J. An EEG investigation of awareness during anaesthesia. *Br J Psychol* 1973; **64**:413–415.

196. Bethune DW, Ghosh S, Gray L, *et al.* Learning during general anaesthesia: Implicit recall after methohexitone or propofol infusion. *Br J Anaesth* 1992; **69**:197–199.

197. Dubovsky SL, Trustman R. Absence of recall after general anesthesia: Implications for theory and practice. *Anesth Analg* 1976; **55**:696–701.

198. Eich E, Reeves JL, Katz RL. Anesthesia, amnesia, and the memory/awareness distinction. *Anesth Analg* 1985; **64**:1143–1148.

199. Dwyer R, Bennett HL, Eger EI II, Peterson N.

Isoflurane anesthesia prevents unconscious learning. *Anesth Analg* 1992; **75**:107–112.

200. Winograd E, Sebel PS, Goldman WP, Clifton CL, Lowden JD. Indirect assessment of memory for music during anaesthesia. *J Clin Anesth* 1991; **3**:276–279.

201. Bonke B, Van Dam ME, VanKleef JW, Slijper FME. Implicit memory tested in children during inhalation anaesthesia. *Anaesthesia* 1992; **47**: 747–749.

202. Kalff AC, Bonke B, Wolters G, Manger FW. Implicit memory for stimuli present during inhalation anesthesia in children. *Psychological Reports* 1995; **77**:371–375.

203. McLintock TTC, Aitken H, Downie CFA, Kenny GNC. Postoperative analgesic requirements in patients exposed to positive intraoperative suggestions. *BMJ* 1990; **301**:788–790.

204. Jansen CK, Bonke B, Klein J, van Dasselaar N, Hop WCJ. Failure to demonstrate unconscious perception during balanced anaesthesia by postoperative motor response. *Acta Anaesthesiol Scand* 1991; **35**:407–410.

205. Abramson M, Greenfield I, Heron WT. Response to or perception of auditory stimuli under deep surgical anesthesia. *Am J Obstet Gynecol* 1966; **96**:584–585.

206. Boeke S, Bonke B, Bouwhuis-Hoogerwerf MI, Bovill JG, Zwaveling A. Effects of sounds presented during general anesthesia on post-operative course. *Br J Anaesth* 1988; **60**:697–702.

207. Block RI, Ghoneim MM, Sum Ping ST, Ali MA. Efficacy of therapeutic suggestions for improved postoperative recovery presented during general anesthesia. *Anesthesiology* 1991; **75**:746–755.

208. Block RI, Ghoneim MM, Fowles DC, Kumar V, Pathak D. Effects of a subanesthetic concentration of nitrous oxide on establishment, elicitation and semantic and phonemic generalization of classically conditioned skin conductance responses. *Pharmacol Biochem Behav* 1987; **28**:7–14.

209. Newton DEF, Thornton C, Konieczko KM, *et al.* Levels of consciousness in volunteers breathing sub-MAC concentrations of isoflurane. *Br J Anaesth* 1990; **65**:609–615.

210. Munglani R, Andrade J. Sapsford DJ, Baddeley A, Jones JG. A measure of consciousness and memory during isoflurane administration: The coherent frequency. *Br J Anaesth* 1993; **71**: 633–641.

211. Zacny JP, Yajnik S, Lichtor JL, *et al.* The acute and residual effects of subanesthetic concentrations of isoflurane/nitrous oxide combinations on cognitive and psychomotor performance in healthy volunteers. *Anesth Analg* 1996; **82**:153–157.

212. Andrade J, Jeevaratnum D, Sapsford D. Explicit and implicit memory for names presented during propofol sedation. In Bonke B, Bovill JG, Moerman N (eds). *Memory and Awareness in Anaesthesia III*. Assen: Van Gorcum, 1996, 10–16.

213. Ausems ME, Vuyk J, Hug CC, Stanski DR. Comparison of a computer-assisted infusion versus intermittent bolus administration of alfentanil as a supplement to nitrous oxide for lower abdominal surgery. *Anesthesiology* 1988; **68**:851–861.

214. Ghoneim MM, Hinrichs JV, Mewaldt SP. Dose-response analysis of the behavioral effects of diazepam: I. Learning and memory. *Psychopharmacology* 1984; **82**:291–295.

215. Ghoneim MM, Mewaldt SP, Hinrichs JV. Dose-response analysis of the behavioral effects of diazepam: II. Psychomotor performance, cognition and mood. *Psychopharmacology* 1984; **82**: 296–300.

Chapter 3

Monitoring the depth of anesthesia

J. G. Jones and Sanjay Aggarwal

Contents

Introduction to depth of anesthesia

A gradual increase in anesthetic dose produces a progressive impairment of working memory until events occurring only 1–2 seconds before cannot be remembered explicitly. A small further increase in anesthetic dose is associated with a loss of conscious awareness and this may be followed by a stage of hyperexcitability. A further gradual increase in anesthetic dose (deepening anesthesia) stops this excitable state and produces a progressive impairment of the reflex activity of both the upper airway and the somatic muscles. For the first 100 years of anesthetic practice the basic principles were to ablate conscious awareness and produce a deep stage of anesthesia to facilitate surgery by profound relaxation of skeletal muscle. This deep stage could be achieved only with a relatively high concentration of general anesthetic and it was difficult to avoid 'too deep' anesthesia with the risk of fatal cardiorespiratory depression. The introduction of curare into anesthetic practice in the 1940s produced neuromuscular paralysis without the need for a high concentration of anesthetic; the problem of 'too deep' anesthesia gave way to 'too light' anesthesia with the danger of conscious awareness. In the decade following the introduction of curare the incidence of conscious awareness was about 1% in the UK because N_2O/O_2 was used without supplemention by either opioid or volatile anesthetic agent. With the increased use of volatile or intravenous agent supplementation the incidence may have fallen to less than 0.01[1] in the 1990s. Now, with the realization that we do not need to give doses of anesthetic sufficient to abolish movement, we are tending to give even lighter anesthetics and to adjust the depth of anesthetic sedation so as to ablate memory.[2]

This chapter discusses depth of anesthesia in terms of its effect on memory and consciousness and relates monitoring methods to these entities. It is divided into three parts: What is awareness? What is the incidence of this condition? and How can it be monitored?

What is awareness during 'general anesthesia'?

The possibility of awareness under 'anesthesia' is frightening to both patients and anesthesiologists, yet awareness remains a rather nebulous concept. Awareness suggests 'consciousness' that must incorporate elements of perception, attention, introspection, volition and explicit memory. We use the term 'conscious awareness' to summarize these elements and we distinguish this state from other states of awareness (subconscious awareness) where information is registered by the brain but it does not enter consciousness (e.g. implicit memories). If a patient has conscious awareness during an operation, but subsequently has no explicit memory of these events, then this falls into the category of 'conscious awareness' but this is qualified by having 'no explicit memory of the event'. To assess conscious awareness in anesthetized patients, it is necessary to seek evidence of phenomena that might imply consciousness.

Does movement in response to a noxious stimulus imply conscious awareness?

Movement in response to stimulation does not indicate consciousness nor does the lack of organized movement on stimulation imply unconsciousness. An example of this is the use of the term MAC, a standard of anesthetic potency. MAC is the Minimum Alveolar Concentration of a volatile anesthetic, which prevents movement in response to surgical stimulation in 50% of patients. The concentration needed to impair consciousness (MAC awake) is usually about half of the concentration required to prevent movement (Table 3.1). Antognini and Schwartz[3] and Rampil[4] confirmed that it was subcortical, rather than cortical, structures, that determined movement in response to painful stimulation during anesthesia.

Another difficulty is the use of neuromuscular blockade to facilitate surgery. This obviously prevents voluntary movement if the 'anesthetized' patient becomes conscious. We then have to rely on the patient's memories of intraoperative events based on postoperative interviews. This is unreliable because of the powerful effects of general anesthetics on memory. Alternatively it is possible to use the isolated forearm technique (IFT) where the arm remains non-paralyzed and is used for communicating with the patient during surgery. Although a

Table 3.1. The general anesthetic dose needed to abolish consciousness (MAC awake) is compared with the concentration required to abolish movement (MAC)

	MAC awake %	MAC %	MAC awake % MAC
Halothane	0.4	0.7	57
Isoflurane	0.5	1.3	38
Desflurane	2.5	5.0	50
Sevoflurane	0.7	1.7	41
Propofol (equiv. dose, [gm]g/ml)	3–4	8–12	38

NB Propofol is an intravenous anesthetic. The plasma levels are those needed to achieve the equivalent MAC awake and MAC end-points.

well-known technique, it is very rarely used in routine anesthetic practice.

Memories of intraoperative events

Can depth of anesthesia be deduced by examining patients' memories of intraoperative events? Here we consider explicit memories of intraoperative events, the likelihood of sequelae, under reporting of conscious awareness and the important subject of vague memories of intraoperative events. The latter may include implicit memories of intraoperative events.

Explicit memories of intraoperative events

There are many well-documented cases of patients waking up during surgery when they are supposedly anesthetized. However, because they are paralyzed with curare-like drugs the anesthesiologist does not realize, at the time, that the patient is awake. A full explicit memory of the event may be retained. Thus one patient reported that: 'The feeling of helplessness was terrifying. I tried to let the staff know I was conscious but I couldn't move even a finger or eyelid. I began to feel that breathing was impossible and I just resigned myself to dying.'[5] Similar disturbing cases involving medically qualified patients have also been reported.[6] 'I was lying there, covered in green towels, my abdomen slit open, strange people delving inside me … My first reaction to this was an irrational surge of fear and panic …. The closest parallel I can think of is being in a coffin, having been buried alive'. The latter experience reminds us of Edgar Alan Poe's terrifying classic entitled 'Premature Burial'.

Three studies have analysed patient's explicit memories and responses to intraoperative awareness. Schwender et al.[7] described 45 patients' experiences of awareness (Table 3.2). Moerman et al.[8] studied 26 patients with conscious awareness referred by colleagues from a large university hospital. Before that Evans[5] had studied 27 patients after advertising in four British newspapers.

Not every patient with intraoperative conscious awareness develops sequelae

While many patients who experience conscious awareness during anesthesia go on to develop a post-traumatic stress disorder, it is remarkable that

Table 3.2. Summary of memories and sequelae in 45 patients awake during 'anesthesia'

Auditory perceptions	45 (All)
No pain	34
Recall of conversations	33
No after-effects	32
Localization of touch	28
Helpless	28
Feeling paralyzed	27
Anxious/fearful	22
Severe panic	18
Saw silhouettes	11
Clear vision	10
Severe pain	8
PTSD	3

PTSD = Post-traumatic stress disorder
(After Schwender D, Kunze-Kronawitter H, Dietrich P, Klasing S, Forst H, Madler C. Conscious awareness during general anesthesia: Patients perceptions, emotions, cognition and reactions. Br J Anaesth 1998; **80**:133–139.)

32 out of 45 awake patients had no sequelae in Schwender's study.[7] In Moerman et al.'s[8] study 8 out of 26 awake patients had no sequelae. Half of the patients with after-effects had experienced pain during the episode of conscious awareness but only one of the patients without after-effects had a painful experience. The latter patient explained that his happiness at having survived a car accident had eclipsed the sensations he recalled from the period of awareness during his operation.

Under-reporting of conscious awareness

Moerman et al.[8] were surprised by the low percentage of patients who had informed their anesthesiologists about being aware; 17 out of the 26 aware patients had not informed the anesthesiologist. Six others were greeted with disbelief. There are three reasons why conscious awareness during general anesthesia may be under-reported.

1 Patients may have conscious awareness during the 'anesthetic' but subsequently they have no explicit memory of this experience. The isolated forearm technique may be used to elucidate cognitive function in apparently anesthetized and paralyzed patients who subsequently have no memory of waking during anesthesia. In outline, one of the patient's arms is isolated by an inflated blood pressure cuff from the effects of neuromuscular blocking drugs injected into a vein in

the patient's other arm. If the patient wakes up they can respond to verbal commands by squeezing the anesthesiologist's hand using the non-paralyzed (isolated) arm. With some anesthetic techniques more than 40% of patients responded intraoperatively to a verbal command[9,10] but had no subsequent memory of the event (see Chapter 7 for more details).

2 Patients may have conscious awareness but be completely free of pain because of high dose opioid administration and although they may recall the experience afterwards they do not mention it to anyone.

3 Patients may have conscious awareness but they are either afraid to mention it afterwards, or they mention it but nobody believes them. Blacher[11] described six patients who woke up during anesthesia and who later suffered from nightmares, anxiety and a preoccupation with death. These patients were reluctant to discuss both their symptoms and the fact that they were awake during anesthesia lest they were thought to be insane. Today, because of wide publicity in the press and TV, there has been a considerable change in attitude of both the public and of the medical profession to the problem of conscious awareness during anesthesia. Nowadays patients are more likely to complain and to be believed. However, with such wide publicity it is difficult to refute the proposal that the individual adds to their experience from the barrage of press and TV reports of intraoperative events. Consequently their memories may be inaccurate.

Vague memories of intraoperative events

A distinction should be made between conscious awareness with vivid, explicit memories of events during 'general anesthesia', which is probably rare, and a more common group who may have some vague recollection of intraoperative events, these coming to light only when they are prompted afterwards. Lyons and Macdonald[12] described an important prospective study of conscious awareness during anesthesia for cesarean section. Their study lasted from 1982 to 1989 and subsequently Lyons and Macdonald reported (personal communication to J.G. Jones) their subsequent unpublished results until 1993. The average number of anesthetics in their study was 375 per year during the first 8 years. During these 8 years 3076 general anesthetics were given for cesarean section. All patients were asked in a postoperative interview 'Do you remember anything about your operation?' If the answer was 'no', they were asked, 'Did you dream during your operation?' Twenty-eight patients (0.9%) recalled something about their operation and 189 (6%) had dreams. If the context of the dream represented an unequivocal recall of an intraoperative event they were deemed to have been awake at some time. No patient out of the 3076 was able, at the time of the postoperative interview, to recall the operation or the experience of pain. One patient, 3 years after the event, claimed that she remembered tracheal intubation, surgical manipulations, crying babies and operating room noises, although she made no mention of this at the postoperative interview. Four case histories were given, three of which illustrated some vague memory of intraoperative events and the other patient remembered her leg slipping off the operating table when she was moved into the operating room.

Implicit memories of intraoperative events require sophisticated psychological testing techniques. Because they may depend on depth of anesthesia they will be mentioned later in this chapter but will be discussed in more detail by Ghoneim and by Andrade in Chapters 2 and 4.

Incidence of conscious awareness during 'general anesthesia'

To define the incidence of awareness during anesthesia we must distinguish between two situations outlined in above.

1 The patient has conscious awareness, has a clear explicit memory of events, may be distressed and may seek legal redress

2 The patient has only the vaguest recollections of intraoperative discomfort, which is discovered only by postoperative prompting and are unlikely to be distressed.

Unfortunately, because of the poor quality or absence of critical incident recording, we have to rely on legal claims to determine the incidence of conscious awareness. Consequently, the actual incidence of conscious awareness during 'general anesthesia' is not known with any certainty. A recent paper[7] quoted an incidence of 0.5–2% whereas another paper[1] states that patients with a full explicit memory of the intraoperative events are probably very rare, less than 0.01% general anesthetics (1/10 000). The former figure is more relevant to cases of vague intraoperative awareness and the latter to conscious awareness with explicit memory of intraoperative events.

Conscious awareness with explicit memories is very rare

Pederson and Johansen[13] found two patients out of 7306 who were awake and in pain during 'general anesthesia', that is 1 in 3653. In the Lyons and Macdonald[12] study, only 1 in 3000 patients consulted a lawyer. The authors concluded that the remainder of their patients, who had vague memories of awareness, did not regard their experiences as being other than trivial complications. I have previously argued[1] that if 1 in 3000 were a reasonable estimate of the incidence of conscious awareness of sufficient severity to take legal action, then we would expect about 800 cases per year in the UK. But Hargrove[14] described only about four cases per year reported to the UK Medical Defence Union. *This is a huge discrepancy, which suggests that 1 in 3000 is a considerable overestimate.* If we assume, instead, an incidence of conscious awareness of 1 in 10,000 anesthetics[1] we would expect three cases of awareness in our Cambridge hospital per year. On this basis over the 6-year period since April 1993, for which we have good medical negligence records, we would have expected 18 cases of conscious awareness in our hospital. In fact the hospital legal department has dealt with only two claims for awareness in that time. This gives an even lower incidence of 1 in 90,000 general anesthetics, which is based on 30,000 general anesthetics administered per year. I carried out a further investigation in 11 hospitals in my region in the UK. Between June 1996 and June 1999 there were 558,000 general anesthetics given but only seven cases of anesthetic awareness were reported by the legal department; an incidence of 1 in 80,000.

Vague memories of intraoperative events are more common

In the first part of their study Lyons and Macdonald[12] reported the incidence of vague awareness as 14 per 1000. The anesthetic technique was changed half way through the study and the incidence of awareness fell to 4 per 1000. In a further 5-year period from 1989 to 1993 there was only one case of awareness, giving an incidence of about 0.7 per 1000 (personal communication). Liu *et al.*[15] described a prospective study on 1000 patients who were interviewed postoperatively. Two patients had memory of intraoperative events, one remembered tracheal intubation, the other remembered being wheeled into the operating room. Neither recalled any part of the operation nor were they distressed by the experience. From these two studies it is suggested that some vague, non-distressing recollection of part of the intraoperative procedure is mentioned on interview by about 0.7–2 in 1000 patients.

Methods for assessing depth of anesthesia

When anesthetic sedation is gradually increased there are major changes in working memory before loss of consciousness occurs. Studying this effect on memory is the most sensitive method for assessing depth of anesthesia.

Examining the effect of anesthetics on memory

The effect of general anesthetics on memory may be the key to conscious awareness. Baddeley[16] has replaced the old concept of short-term memory and instead has formulated a model of working memory, which is characterized by low capacity, short duration and large processing potential. These processes are very sensitive to sedative doses of general anesthetics. Unlike working memory, which is very sensitive to the effects of anesthetics, the registration of new implicit memories may be more resistant to the effects of anesthetics than the registration of new explicit memories.[17,18] Implicit memories are not accessible to the conscious mind but are evident in their subsequent effect on behaviour. Functional neuroimaging techniques reveal the anatomical correlates of implicit memory.[19–24] For example, Dehaene *et al.*[24] showed that words presented to non-sedated subjects so briefly (43 ms) that they cannot be seen (i.e. they do not enter consciousness) do, in fact, facilitate the subsequent processing of related words. This unconscious processing was accompanied by measurable modifications of brain electrical activity and of cerebral blood flow measured by functional magnetic resonance imaging. This concurs with the observation of a modulation of the activity of the amygdala by very briefly presented pictures of faces.[22,25,26]

Memory as a measure of depth of anesthesia

Artusio,[27] more than 40 years ago, showed that sedative doses of ether had powerful adverse effects on recent memory. Several recent studies have investigated the effect of gradually increasing anesthetic doses on cognitive function. Newton *et al.*[28] showed that at 0.2–0.4% end tidal isoflurane, *memory is lost before loss of response to commands.* These changes were reflected by changes in the auditory evoked potential (AEP).[29] To add to Newton's work, Block *et al.*[30] suggested that at levels of anesthetic sufficient to suppress explicit memory, implicit memories could still be laid down.

We have shown in our laboratory in Cambridge, using low doses of either isoflurane[31] or propofol,[32] that there are powerful effects of these anesthetics on working memory using the Within-list Recognition (WLR) and Category Recognition tests. For example, a number of word-lists, like those in Table 3.3, are read to the subject; a word is read out every 2 seconds. Some words in the list are repeated at different intervals and the subject has to identify the repeated words *as soon as they are recognized.* Some words are easy to remember, e.g. favor, because there are no (0 in Table 3.3) intervening words so there is only a 2-second interval between repeats. Others are much more difficult, e.g. dignity, with 16 intervening words (16 in Table 3.3) or 32 seconds between repeats.

An example from our work using isoflurane sedation[31] is shown in Figure 3.1.

The percent correct response to words with either no (INT 0), 4 or 16 intervening words is shown at different stages of the study.

- Stage 1 is without isoflurane.
- Stage 2 with 0.2% end tidal isoflurane. Working memory for words repeated with 16 intervening words is profoundly impaired whereas those with no intervening words are normally remembered.

Table 3.3. Word list used for the Within-list Recognition test (WLR). Some words are repeated at different intervals. For these words that are repeated, the number of intervening words is shown on the list (see text).

ABILITY
FAVOR
FAVOR 0
DIGNITY
DEMONSTRATION
MEMBER
SUGGESTION
CHARACTER
SUGGESTION 1
SEGMENT
EXPEDITION
QUANTITY
OVERTONE
EXPEDITION 2
SEGMENT 4
BAYONET
CHARACTER 8
LIBERTY
LIBERTY 0
ATTEMPT
DIGNITY 16
SOLUTION
SALVATION

- Stage 3 with 0.4% end tidal isoflurane. All words repeated with 16 intervening words were not recognized and 60% of words repeated after only 2 seconds were not recognized. Subjects are able to respond normally to commands at this stage.
- Stage 4 with 0.4% end tidal isoflurane and a painful stimulation.
  The severe impairment of working memory at 0.4% isoflurane is partially compensated for by the arousal effect of a painful stimulation.
- *During recovery*, memory improves in stage 5, (0.2% end tidal isoflurane) and in stage 6, (zero end tidal isoflurane). Whereas the memory of words repeated with 0 interval returns to normal, memory of words repeated with 4 and 16 intervening words is severely impaired.

Similar results were found with sedative doses of propofol.[32] In Figure 3.2 we compare the results using the WLR in two groups of subjects, one with isoflurane as in Figure 3.1 and the other with propofol. The mean percent correct responses are

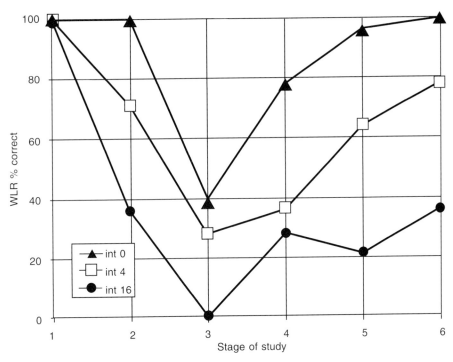

Figure 3.1. Mean WLR score at different end-tidal isoflurane values. (Stage 1 = 0%, stage 2 = 0.2%, stage 3 = 0.4%, stage 4 = 0.4% + painful stimulation, stage 5 = 0.2% (recovery), stage 6 = 0). Results of WLR for three different word intervals (Int) are shown: Int 0, Int 4, and Int 16 are the number of intervening words. (See text.)

shown for each group for all word intervals. The stages of propofol study are similar to those shown in Figure 3.1.

- Stage 1 is no propofol.
- Stage 2 is low dose propofol. This causes a 40% reduction in WLR score.
- Stage 3 is high dose propofol adjusted to just abolish the response to words repeated with no intervening word (0), i.e. within 2 seconds, although subjects were still obeying commands.
- Stage 4 is the same dose as stage 3 but with a painful stimulus.
- *On recovery,* stage 5 shows the result with low dose.
- Stage 6 is when the subjects were fully alert.

Thus with sedative doses of these anesthetics, a word presented within 2 seconds of a previous presentation was not recognized even when subjects appeared fully conscious and were obeying commands. On recovery the easier memory task recovers before the more difficult task. As we shall see towards the end of this chapter, in both of these

studies the auditory steady state potential in the EEG reflected the reduction in performance. *However, unlike the study of Block et al.[30] we found that the implicit memory of new events tested with category recognition was abolished by low doses of anesthetics even in subjects who were still conscious and responding normally to verbal commands.*

Stages of anesthesia based on memory and consciousness

Four stages of general anesthesia have been proposed based on the effect of increasing or decreasing depth of anesthesia on memory:

1 Conscious awareness with explicit memory of contemporary events.
2 Conscious awareness without explicit memory of contemporary events.
3 Subconscious awareness with implicit, but no explicit, memory of contemporary events.
4 No awareness (after Jones and Konieczko[33]).

Stage 1 includes implicit memory of contemporary

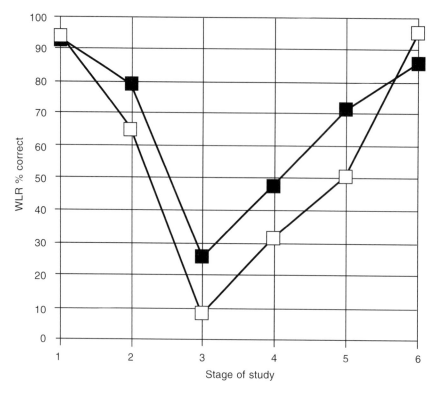

Figure 3.2. Mean WLR score for all word intervals for different study stages for isoflurane (■) or propofol (□) sedation. (See also Figure 3.7.) Isoflurane stages are those shown in Figure 3.1. For propofol doses, stage 1 is zero, stage 2 is low, stage 3 is high, stage 4 is high +painful stimulation, stage 5 is low (recovery) and stage 6 is 20 min post-propofol. (See text.)

events in normal, awake, non-sedated subjects. It is controversial whether anesthetic sedation also impairs implicit learning in this stage.

Stage 2 is associated with very light anesthesia and, in patients with neuromuscular blockade, it is demonstrated using the isolated forearm technique. Increasing anesthetic concentration moves the subject down through these stages to stages 3 and 4. This is referred to as increasing 'depth of anesthesia'. Increasing painful stimulation at a constant anesthetic concentration may precipitate conscious awareness in a previously unconscious anesthetized patient by moving subjects up from deeper stages to stage 2.[34] This concept represents depth of anesthesia as a balance between the depressive effects of anesthetics and the increased arousal brought about by surgical stimulation.

Stage 3, subconscious perception with implicit memory of intra-anesthetic events, concerns learning under anesthesia. Implicit memory is revealed when a previous event facilitates performance on a task

that does not require conscious recollection of this experience.

Stage 4 is assumed at about 1 MAC when implicit learning is abolished (see below).

Registration of implicit memory during anesthesia

There is considerable conflict about the possibility of registering new implicit memory of intraoperative events. Ghoneim and Block[35] listed 14 papers showing implicit memory during anesthesia, whereas Merikle and Rondi[36] concluded that 'there is not a single consistent finding indicating that inadequately anesthetized patients do in fact remember events during anesthesia'. More recently, Merikle and Daneman[37] carried out a meta-analysis on 44 studies of memory for unconsciously perceived events by anesthetized patients. They showed that positive suggestions had no effect on postoperative recovery, but specific information can be registered as implicit memories so long as postoperative testing was not delayed longer than 36 hours. However, they suggested that unconsciously perceived information may have a longer lasting impact if the material is personally relevant and meaningful, i.e. the *salience of the stimulus* is important.

Memory and the salience of the stimulus

In the study of Newton et al.,[28] a subject's memory for a list of neutral words was lost at 0.2 MAC while they were still able to respond normally to commands, yet the memory of a 'shock' word was present at this concentration.

In many studies of memory during anesthesia, a neutral auditory stimulus is presented in the face of the far more salient (and frightening) stimulus of surgery. Andrade et al.[38] have shown that memory for events during anesthesia is more likely during surgery than when anesthetics are given for laboratory studies in volunteers.

Effects of surgery and depth of anesthesia on implicit memory

Bethune et al.[39] gave a taped message to anesthetized patients during cardiac surgery and again during the postoperative recovery period. The tape was also played to a different group of patients in the postoperative period only. Only those patients who were exposed to the tape during surgery showed evidence of implicit recall, suggesting that suppression of auditory awareness is a function of both the degrees of sedation and of surgical stimulation.

Until fairly recently it was impossible to determine whether auditory stimuli were presented to the patients at equivalent depths of anesthesia. Schwender et al.[40] studied anesthetized patients undergoing cardiac surgery. They measured the middle latency part of the auditory evoked potential (MLAEP). During the operation a short version of the Robinson Crusoe story was played to the patients and postoperatively they were asked to say what they associated with the word 'Friday'. Those with light anesthesia, as demonstrated by short latency/ large amplitude waves in the MLAEP, associated 'Friday' with some aspects of the Robinson Crusoe

story, whereas those with deep anesthesia and long latency/small amplitude MLAEP did not. This association with the Robinson Crusoe story was regarded as evidence of implicit memory.

This important experiment shows that the latencies of the MLAEP are related to the stepwise depression of consciousness, cognition and memory seen with surgery and general anesthesia. A very short latency, large amplitude Nb wave in the AEP is associated with wakefulness and conscious awareness with explicit recall. As the latency increases and amplitude decreases, there is loss of explicit memory of contemporary events, followed by loss of consciousness and eventually loss of implicit memory as the MLAEP wave disappears.

Fear conditioning may underlie learning during surgery. Fear conditioning is a form of Pavlovian conditioning that involves the amygdala and hippocampus. During fear conditioning, a neutral conditional stimulus (e.g. an audible tone) is followed by a painful electric shock (the unconditioned stimulus). The latter by itself routinely causes the behavioral correlates of fear.

After even one pairing of the auditory and the painful stimuli a robust memory is formed of the relationship between the two. The lateral amygdala is the critical structure in which the auditory and painful stimuli converge.[41] Fear conditioning can occur in animals during either ketamine or halothane anesthesia.[42] Thus, the psychological stress of surgery may be difficult to suppress completely by anesthetics and fear conditioning to this stress may still occur. The arousal effects from eliciting a conditional response to perioperative stimuli may well facilitate the registration of other subconscious memories.

Thus:

- A gradual increase in depth of anesthetic sedation is associated with a progressive impairment of working memory.
- Sedated patients respond to commands in a normal fashion and appear to have normal consciousness.
- At this stage of sedation, working memory may be so impaired that a word presented 2 seconds before a previous presentation is not recognized.
- In volunteers not scheduled for surgery this degree of sedation also abolished implicit learning of contemporary events.

- However, implicit learning does occur during surgery provided that light anesthesia/sedation is employed, as demonstrated by the auditory evoked potential.
- It seems that surgery itself may also be a factor and this may be via fear conditioning.[42]

On-line monitoring of the depth of anesthesia

While memory is the most sensitive measure of depth of anesthetic sedation, a suitable monitoring device must satisfy other criteria:

- Show graded changes with increasing dose of anesthetic.
- Changes must be independent of neuromuscular block.
- Changes must be independent of anesthetic agent.
- Show appropriate response to surgical stimulation.
- Reflect level of consciousness.
- Measurable on-line.
- Ideally non-invasive, cheap.

A number of methods for assessing depth of anesthesia have been proposed (Table 3.4). These may be needed to ensure adequate anesthesia in every case and standardize research into learning under anesthesia.

Table 3.4. Methods for measuring depth of anesthesia

'Gold standard'	Isolated forearm technique
Tests of autonomic function	PRST score (clinical signs)
	Esophageal motility
	Frontalis EMG
	Respiratory sinus arrhythmia
EEG methods	
Linear	Power spectrum
	Evoked potentials
	Transient
	Long latency transient
	Steady state
Non-linear	Chaos theory
	Bispectral analysis

Non-EEG methods

The isolated forearm technique (IFT)

The IFT involves introducing the neuromuscular blocking drug into one arm vein while the contra-lateral arm is free to move because it is isolated from the drug by having its arterial blood supply occluded by a blood pressure cuff. Apparently anesthetized patients who become consciously aware during surgery are able to respond to commands with the isolated arm. Jessop and Jones[43] suggest that complex motor actions indistinguishable from conscious, voluntary movements can be observed without the need for normal conscious decision making. This is not normal conscious awareness. However, despite its difficulties, the IFT is 'arguably the nearest we have to a gold standard'.

Conscious awareness and autonomic signs

CLINICAL SIGNS, PRST

Evans and Davies[44] proposed a PRST score based on blood *p*ressure, heart *r*ate, *s*weating and *t*ears. The score is affected by other drugs, e.g. anti-cholinergics, antihypertensives and adrenergics (agonists and antagonists), as well as disease processes. Using the isolated arm method, Russell[45] showed that patients could be awake during surgery and 'light' general anesthesia yet have no abnormality of PRST. Moerman *et al.*[8] found that anesthesiologists cannot correctly identify an awake patient during an 'anesthetic' by inspecting the hand written anesthetic record for evidence of clinical signs. Domino *et al.*[46] reported that, in most cases of intraoperative awareness described in the ASA Closed Claims database, there were no concomitant autonomic signs. Nevertheless, our view is that if an 'anesthetized' patient has unexplained tachycardia and hypertension, then the dose of anesthetic must be quickly reviewed.

ESOPHAGEAL MOTILITY

Lower esophageal contractions, occurring either spontaneously or provoked by inflation of an esophageal balloon, are an unreliable measure of conscious awareness during anesthesia.[47]

FRONTALIS EMG

The frontalis muscle electromyogram (EMG) is

potentially informative due to its dual innervation, voluntary and autonomic. The mean amplitude of frontalis EMG decreases by 60% on sleeping and by 85–90% under anesthesia. It rises with surgical stimulation and falls with the administration of analgesics. As consciousness is regained, there is a rapid rise to near normal levels just prior to onset of awareness. Struys et al.[48] recently pointed out that the frontalis EMG was a useful monitor of loss and recovery of consciousness, but it did not have any predictive value. There is little doubt that general anesthetics have potent effects on muscle tone. A major drawback is the use of neuromuscular blockade. For a measure of depth of anesthesia to have any real value it must operate equally effectively in the paralyzed and non-paralyzed state.

RESPIRATORY SINUS ARRHYTHMIA (RSA)

Rhythmic variations in heart rate (HR) occur at the frequency of respiration. The degree of RSA is enhanced when vagal tone is increased, so it is reduced during anesthesia. Pomfrett[49] has found that the nucleus ambiguus is very susceptible to general anesthesia. Sleigh and Donovan[50] recently pointed out that heart rate variability (HRV) has been separated into high (>0.1 Hz) and low (0.05–0.1 Hz) frequency variation in heart rate measured from the interval between R waves in the electrocardiogram (ECG). The former is due to parasympathetic regulation and caused by respiration. They surmised that changes in HRV during anesthesia could reflect brain stem effects. Several studies have demonstrated a sharp decrease in HRV at induction of anesthesia. Most have used frequency domain techniques to quantify HRV. Pomfrett[49] used statistical clusters of phase locking between HR and breathing. However, there was much inter-patient variability limiting the reliability of the technique. Large-scale validation studies are still not available. Sleigh and Donovan[50] found that apnea and hypoventilation often interfered with measurements at induction.They concluded that HRV was less reliable than any EEG index as an indicator of consciousness at induction of anesthesia.

EEG methods

The EEG is the mainstay of contemporary methods for measuring depth of anesthesia. It is recorded using electrodes on the scalp, which detect the electrical activity of large numbers of cortical cells. Only the pyramidal cortical cells are likely to contribute significantly to the EEG recording as only these are uniformly oriented with respect to the surface having dendrites long enough to form effective dipoles. Deeper pyramidal cells are particularly important since slow wave activity persists even after superficial cortical layers have been destroyed. Cortical cells respond to rhythmic discharges from the thalamus whose discharge frequency and amplitude are in some way intrinsic, giving rise to alpha waves at about 10 Hz in the conscious, relaxed, individual. Non-specific thalamic nuclei, retrieving input from the reticular formation, have been identified as the probable 'EEG pacemaker'.

With increased arousal the alpha wave pattern is disturbed, yielding 'random' fluctuations with no particular frequency and a reduced amplitude. These waves are described as 'desynchronized'. This, seemingly paradoxical, reduction in EEG amplitude with arousal may be related to the rich interconnections of cortical cells and a component of feedback into the system.

The thalamus acts as a relay station for sensory input en route to the primary sensory areas of the cerebral cortex. It is also involved with motor and autonomic function. Combined with the brain stem and neocortex it plays a role in regulating attentional mechanisms and maintaining consciousness.

The reticular formation was originally thought to be a diffuse system regulating arousal based on experiments on deeply anesthetized animals. Stimulation of the reticular formation produced EEG changes resulting in an awake picture. However, activity of the reticular formation alone does not account for changes in level of consciousness.

The EEG undergoes a series of changes with increasing depth of anesthesia. These changes are broadly independent of the anesthetic agent and include increasing amplitude, greater relative contribution of low frequencies and burst suppression. However, there are idiosyncratic changes with different anesthetics. The EEG at recovery can be different to that prior to induction; consequently, the traces may be very difficult to interpret. It is thus necessary to perform some sort of signal processing on the recorded EEG to extract useful features, which can then be classified with respect to depth of anesthesia. A variety of methods have been investigated, the most thoroughly examined thus far are based on the EEG power spectrum including bispectral analysis and evoked potentials.

Signal processing

This subject has been extensively reviewed by Rampil,[51] although he gives no consideration to evoked potentials. He discusses artifact recognition, time domain analysis and frequency domain methods, including fast Fourier transforms and the bispectrum. One example of fast Fourier transformation is the power spectrum.

POWER SPECTRUM

The EEG power spectrum is derived by fast Fourier transforming the raw EEG. This has given rise to several possible indices, including the median frequency and 90 and 95% spectral edge (Figure 3.3).

Schwilden[52] concluded that the median frequency was the most useful feature derived from the power spectrum for assessment of depth of anesthesia. He showed a correlation between median frequency, signs of awareness and anesthetic concentrations in the blood and brain by means of pharmacokinetics. The median frequency corresponding to 95% suppression of response to stimulation is stimulus specific, e.g. verbal (6.8 Hz) and venipuncture (3.0 Hz).

Recent papers have not endorsed the use of power spectrum methods in measuring depth of anesthesia. Struys et al.[48] studied a number of indexes using propofol anesthesia and found very limited usefulness of spectral edge frequency (SEF), median frequency and the power in the delta band. Sleigh and Donovan[50] showed that SEF overlapped at different stages of induction. Their results were similar to those of Gajraj et al.[53] who showed that a SEF of 16 Hz was 100% specific but only 9% sensitive for unconsciousness.

The difficulties encountered with power spectrum derivatives in relation to depth of anesthesia may be attributable to the assumptions made regarding EEG properties for the purpose of such analysis, namely: stationarity and linearity. The first assumes that the statistical properties of the signal are constant over time. This is overcome by splitting the signal into discrete epochs so that the statistical properties are approximately constant over these periods. However, there is no apparent justification for assuming linearity in physiological systems where there are large elements of feedback and they are thus likely to exhibit non-linear behavior.

Bispectral analysis

Bispectral analysis is a method of signal processing which accommodates quadratic (second order) interactions between wave components making up the EEG trace by quantifying phase coupling. This

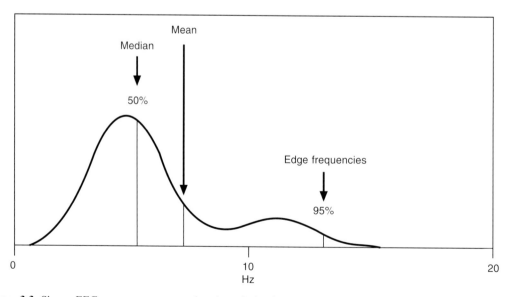

Figure 3.3. Shows EEG power spectrum and various derivatives.

bispectrum (third order) was initially used to study phenomena such as ocean waves, atmospheric pressures and seismic activity. One of the earliest to study the bispectrum in the EEG was Barnett *et al.* in 1971.[54] Significant bicoherence in the awake EEG was shown and 50% of the power spectrum at 20 Hz (beta rhythm) was harmonically coupled to that at 10 Hz (alpha rhythm). During sleep, no clear bicoherence pattern was seen. The bispectrum peaks were low and diffuse indicating that the interactions were between broad, weakly coupled regions. The changes in the power spectrum with anesthesia are well established, but how is coupling affected? Sigl *et al.*[55] have devised a bispectral index (BIS), 'using a set of features that included EEG bispectrum, real triple products and bi-coherence, as well as time domain features such as the level of burst suppression' to predict response to surgical stimulation. This index runs at 92–97 in the awake, alert state, and falls with anesthesia.

In an editorial in *Anesthesiology*, Todd[56] pointed out that, hitherto the commercial version of the EEG bispectrum, the Aspect instrument, was a black box that gave a signal, the bispectral index or BIS, that ranged from 0 to 100 with neither units nor any obvious physiological meaning. He asked the questions, 'Where does the number come from?' and 'What is the box doing?' In an accompanying article Rampil[51] described in detail how the signal was derived.

In brief outline, the BIS version 3 is derived empirically from a database of 1500 anesthetics.

1 ECG artifact is first removed and missing data interpolated.
2 Eyeblink artifacts are then removed.
3 Noisy signals are rejected.
4 Burst suppression ratio and 'QUAZI' suppression index were removed.
5 FFT is then applied to a data sample.
6 The bispectrum is calculated.

Frequency domain variables such as the 'beta ratio' and 'synch fast slow' are then derived. The *beta ratio* parameter is the log of (power 30–47 Hz band) over (power 11–20 Hz band). The *synch fast slow* parameter is the contribution from the bispectral analysis and is the log of the sum of all bispectral peaks in 0.5–47 Hz range over the sum of all bispectral peaks in the 40–47 Hz range.

With increasing depth of anesthesia, different parameter values are applied to the processed BIS signal. Thus the beta ratio (power) is weighted most heavily when EEG shows light anesthesia. The synch fast slow (bispectral component) predominates the BIS signal during the excitement phase and surgical levels of anesthesia. Burst suppression ratio (BSR) and QUAZI (not defined) were used to detect deep anesthesia.

RELATIONSHIP BETWEEN BIS SCORE AND MENTAL PERFORMANCE

Much of the early work on BIS was concerned with relating the BIS score to predicting movement in response to a painful stimulus in an anesthetized patient. This was because of the preoccupation, particularly in North America, with MAC. As we pointed out in the beginning of this chapter, this is the anesthetic concentration needed to prevent movement and is almost double the concentration to produce unconsciousness. However, we are concerned in our clinical practice more with the cognitive effects of general anesthetics rather than with effects mediated at spinal level.

More recently there has been a change of emphasis to compare BIS with cognitive effects, although many of the studies are not very satisfactory because of the poor choice of psychological test. Thus Leslie *et al.*[57] examined the effect of propofol on the performance of a Trivial Pursuit task (e.g. How tall was the world's tallest hairdo!). The study was carried out in volunteers who, for no obvious reason, had been given an epidural local anesthetic! Targets of 1 and 2 µg/ml blood propofol level were used and these achieved concentrations ranging from 0 to 8 µg/ml. They found that the BIS was 91 ± 1 when learning had been reduced by 50%, i.e. when 50% of the answers to the trivial questions were wrong. However, this BIS value is within the normal range.[50]

Kearse *et al.*[58] used the Modified Observer's Assessment of Alertness/Sedation Scale to look at the response to verbal commands during propofol infusion. This score is insensitive to the effects of anesthetics on memory and depends upon the subject's response to their name being spoken with or without shouting or shaking and to instructions to move a limb. A logistic regression showed that a 50% probability of response was achieved with a BIS value of 65. There was no response at a BIS value of 45. When 30% N_2O was added the BIS value rose to 75 for 50% probability of response and 65 for no response. They claimed that their study did not support our view[31,32] that anesthetic sedation caused a gradual loss of cognitive function. However, a change of score from 5 to 4 (in their five point sedation scale) encompassed almost the entire experimental range of our WLR studies.[31,32] We found a progressive loss of working memory from the normal to the point where a word presented 2 sec before testing could not be recognized. These changes, as were those described by Newton et al.,[29] were reflected by changes in the auditory evoked potential.

Glass et al.[59] showed that the BIS50 and 90 values (when 50% and 90% of patients were unconscious) were 67 and 50 respectively. They used either propofol, isoflurane, midazolam or alfentanil. No subject lost consciousness with alfentanil, although a BIS value as low as 46 was seen! The BIS50 value for loss of consciousness with propofol was 65 and the BIS95 was 51. For midazolam and isoflurane it was 70 and 51. Glass et al.[59] also tested their subjects for memory of events during the study period. BIS values less than 64 were associated with a low probability of recall.

For loss of consciousness with midazolam alone, Liu et al.[60] suggested a BIS50 value of 79. For loss of consciousness with propofol alone, Iselin-Chaves et al.[61] found a BIS50 value of 60 and for a combination of propofol with 100 μg/ml of alfentanil they suggested a BIS50 value of 70. In all of these studies the BIS value for loss of recall was greater than the BIS50 for unconsciousness. This is consistent with the results of evoked potential studies.[29,31,32]

A fascinating recent study by Lubke et al.[17] examined the effect of the hypnotic state, as reflected by BIS, on explicit and implicit memory of words presented during isoflurane/fentanyl anesthesia following trauma. There were three conclusions:

1 There was no reliable evidence of explicit memory.
2 There was evidence of implicit memory at BIS values between 60 and 40.
3 The occurrence of implicit memory was related to hypnotic depth.

EFFECTS OF OPIOIDS AND NITROUS OXIDE ON BIS

Opioids attenuate the rise in BIS in response to a painful stimulus.[61] However, opioids on their own have little or no effect on the BIS. This mimics the lack of effect of opioids on the AEP and will be discussed below.

Nitrous oxide is exceptional for its effects on the EEG. Barr et al.[62] showed that 70% N_2O caused loss of consciousness in 10 volunteers but no change whatsoever in BIS. Thus N_2O exemplifies a mechanism of loss of consciousness to which BIS is not sensitive. Barr et al.[62] also noted that when N_2O was added to a midazolam/fentanyl anesthetic for cardiac surgery there was no effect on BIS either with or without surgical stimulation. However, in contrast to this observation, when N_2O is added to propofol it increases the BIS value at which a subject does not respond to a verbal command.[58]

Compared with the lack of effect on BIS of N_2O on its own, the effects of N_2O on the auditory evoked potential (AEP) are significantly less than equivalent concentrations of isoflurane.[63] In this regard it is particularly interesting that N_2O has a considerably greater effect on the somatosensory than the auditory evoked response.[64]

The mechanism of action of N_2O is not fully understood. Part of its action is mediated via a release of endogenous neuromediators such as endorphin and norepinephrine.[65]

EFFECT OF SLEEP AND COMA ON BIS

One of the earliest studies of bicoherence was on the effect of normal sleep.[54] Sleigh et al.[66] recently described changes in BIS in five subjects, first awake then during normal sleep, which was staged using EEG criteria.

- Awake. BIS values 92 ± 3 (SD).
- Light sleep (stages 1 and 2) with high frequency/low amplitude EEG signals, sleep spindles or K complexes. BIS values 75–90 (mean 81 ± 9).
- Slow wave sleep (stages 3 and 4) with high amplitude/low frequency waves (delta and theta bands). BIS values 20–70 (mean 59 ± 10).
- Rapid eye movement (REM) sleep. BIS values 75–92 (mean 83 ± 6).

We[67] also studied patients during normal sleep (n = 6), anesthesia (n = 6) and unsedated patients recovering from head injury (n = 5). In sleeping subjects mean BIS (s.d) was 42 ± 10, anesthetized patients 38 ± 6 and head injury 28 ± 5. All the sleeping subjects awoke immediately (BIS 92.8 ± 1.4) when their name was spoken (Figure 3.4). This was independent of the sleeping BIS value. The anesthetized patients recovered to baseline (93.6 ± 1.5). All the post-head-injured patients responded to verbal command with BIS increasing to 46 ± 5.7. We conclude that the BIS value can only be interpreted with adequate knowledge of the clinical context.

Transient auditory evoked potentials

The limited success of EEG analysis and the dependence of EEG changes on anesthetic agent led us, in 1981, to develop auditory evoked potentials to measure depth of anesthesia.[68] Evoked potentials arise in the EEG following the delivery of a stimulus. They are small in magnitude relative to the background EEG and are therefore extracted by signal averaging. The three main types of evoked potential are visual, somatosensory, and auditory, depending on the stimulus modality. The auditory evoked potential (AEP) consists of a series of waves, the shape, latency and amplitude of which depend on stimulus parameters, electrode position, the differential effects of drugs on the neuraxis and the background EEG.

Thornton and Sharpe[69] (and Chapter 6) have reviewed the changes in the AEP under anesthesia. In outline the middle latency (early cortical) AEP or MLAEP, shows dose-related changes with general anesthetics. These changes are agent independent, namely increased latency and reduced amplitude of the MLAEP waves, Pa and Nb with increasing dose (Figure 3.5). The intravenous agents propofol, althesin, thiopentone and etomidate and the inhalation agents enflurane, halothane, isoflurane, sevoflurane and desflurane all depress the early cortical auditory evoked potentials of Pa and Nb. This depressant effect was partially reversed by the noxious stimulation of tracheal intubation and surgical incision in that more inhalation agent is required to return the AEP to pre-stimulus levels. The arousal effect of stimulation can be attenuated by opioids. Thus the AEP reflects the balance between the hypnotic effect of anesthetics and the arousal effect of noxious stimulation.

Some 'anesthetic' drugs have surprising results. Opioids, benzodiazepines and nitrous oxide have little or no effect on the MLAEP. Increasing doses of the alpha adrenergic agonist anesthetic, dexmedetomidine, produce an increase in MLAEP. Even more surprisingly, the stepwise increase of isoflurane to subjects previously given dexmedetomidine showed the normal effect of isoflurane, i.e. Pa amplitude decreased – there being no difference between the effects of zero and high dose dexmedetomidine.[70]

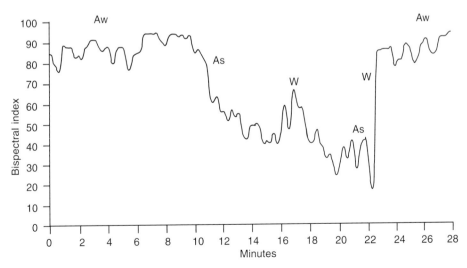

Figure 3.4. Shows the bispectral index (BIS) in an awake subject (Aw) who then falls asleep (As), partially wakens (W) when his pager is activated briefly, falls asleep again (As) and finally wakens (W) when the pager is activated near his ear.

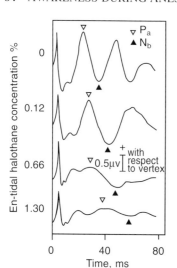 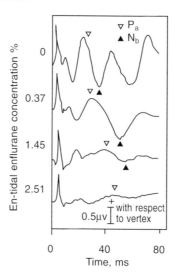 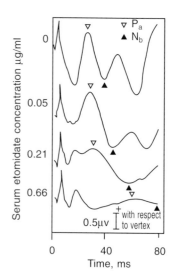

Figure 3.5. Shows the similarity of changes in auditory evoked potential pattern with graded concentrations of different anesthetics.

THE AEP AND COGNITIVE FUNCTION

Short Nb latencies with sub-MAC levels of anesthetic agent were associated with response to commands but impaired subsequent recall from word-lists but not of 'shock' words.[29] In anesthetized, paralyzed patients, response to commands with the isolated forearm technique was also associated with short Nb latency but without explicit recall postoperatively.[71] The measure is further substantiated by Schwender et al.[40] who showed that implicit memory of intraoperative events is preserved when Pa and Nb latencies are close to awake values but not with increased latencies. It seems that the Nb latencies in the AEP can be related to the four previously mentioned stages of general anesthesia[33] (see above).

THE AEP AS A GUIDE TO CONSCIOUSNESS

Davies et al.,[72] from the Glasgow group, reported the changes in latencies of AEP waves Na, Pa, Nb in 11 subjects during repeated transitions from consciousness to unconsciousness achieved with propofol (Table 3.5).

These results are consistent with the study of Tooley et al.[73] There was an almost linear relationship between plasma propofol and Na latency, the Nb latency showing a non-linearity at high doses. An Na latency greater than 24 ms gave a 95% probability of no response to eyelid stimulation and an Nb latency greater than 60 ms did likewise.

DOES THE 'AEP INDEX' INCLUDE MUSCLE ARTEFACT?

Later the Glasgow group[74] described an 'AEP index' derived from the raw AEP signal, which reflected the morphology of the signal. It was not stated what segment of the signal was analyzed (e.g. from 15 to 70 ms). They claimed that the 'AEP index' was the most sensitive processed EEG method for detecting transitions to consciousness. What is surprising in their data is the non-linearity in the relationship between 'AEP index' and calculated propofol concentration. Thus, in contrast to the linear relationship in their data between 'AEP index' and

Table 3.5. Latency of MLAEP; transitions from unconsciousness (Uncon) to consciousness (Con)

	Baseline	Uncon 1	Con 1	Uncon 2	Con 2	Uncon 3	Con 3
Na (ms)	20.0	22.5	21.3	23.2	21.7	23.1	21.3
Pa (ms)	31.7	39.3	33.5	39.2	39.2	39.7	33.3
Nb (ms)	42.8	57.8	44.6	58.9	58.9	59.1	46.3

(After Davies et al. Ref 72)

calculated propofol concentration when their subjects were unconscious, the 'AEP index' showed a very large increase when the calculated plasma propofol value was less than 2 μg ml⁻¹. This was also in sharp contrast with the linear relationship found between AEP amplitude and latency at low anesthetic dose in Tooley et al.'s study.[73] It seems possible that this effect is due to post-auricular muscle artifact in non-paralyzed patients when they are waking up. To reduce this problem Thornton[75] and Tooley et al.[73] not only use a by-eye analysis of the data to reject signals with artifact, but also a vertex-mastoid electrode placement in contrast with frontal-mastoid placements described by Kenney's Group.[74] Working with Thornton we found considerable post-auricular muscle artifact contamination with the latter placement when recording the AEP (unpublished observations). This is considerably reduced by the vertex-mastoid placement. Tooley et al.[73] also use a vertex electrode placement, but they also comment on the problem of muscle artifact. Because of this they had to discard the AEP (awake) data from 19 out of 35 subjects.

The Glasgow group[74] use filtering to remove artifacts. The post-auricular muscle artifact can have a large amplitude (>10 μV) so a low cut-off filter would be needed to reduce it substantially. Such a filter is also likely to alter the subsequent MLAEP, particularly during light anesthesia. Tooley et al.[73] said of their data 'many of the incidents in the EEG have frequency contents so close to the important frequencies in the AER that it is not feasible to remove them by filtering.' This raises the possibility that the waking 'AEP index' contains an appreciable element of muscle artifact that is either rejected by Tooley et al.[73] or Thornton's,[75] by-eye analysis and minimized by their electrode placement. This would explain the apparent sensitivity of the 'AEP index' to transitions to consciousness in non-paralyzed patients and it would be expected that this would not be the case in patients with neuromuscular blockade.

Somatosensory evoked potentials

The dose-related effects of anesthetics on the auditory evoked potential (AEP) contrast in an interesting way with the effects of these agents on the somatosensory evoked potential (SEP). Langeron et al.[76] showed that in the SEP the amplitude of the P40/N50 complex was decreased by nitrous oxide but this complex was not effected by propofol or midazolam. The effect of nitrous oxide on the somatosensory evoked potential is opposite to its effect on the auditory evoked potential. Propofol, remifentanil and dexmedetomidine produced a dose-related depression of SEP waves P15–N2O, P20 and P25 respectively.[77] McPherson et al.[78] showed a 50% reduction of SEP waves P15–N₂O with nitrous oxide which was greater than equivalent concentrations of isoflurane. It is suggested that the different effects of anesthetics on the somatosensory compared to the auditory evoked potentials reflect the *hypnotic* component of anesthetic action on AEP and an *analgesic* effect on the shorter latencies of the SEP.

Steady state (40 Hz) AEPs

The transient AEP is produced by stimulation at low frequencies (6–10 Hz), so that the response of one pulse has decayed before the arrival of the next. When stimuli are presented at higher frequencies (up to 60 Hz) the sequential responses superimpose. At a particular frequency, typically 40 Hz in the awake individual, a large amplitude stable response appears,[79] termed the steady state response (SSR). Galambos, (personal communication to J.G. Jones) suggested that the 40 Hz SSR might be due to phase locking of the Pa and Pb waves of the transient AEP. With increasing anesthetic dose the latencies of Pa and Pb increase and the frequency for phase locking should decrease.

A recent monograph[80] has extensively reviewed the subject of stimulus-induced 40 Hz oscillations (gamma oscillations) in the EEG. In their review Whittington et al.[81] showed that the inhalational anesthetics halothane, enflurane, isoflurane and the intravenous anesthetics thiopentone and propofol all disrupt gamma oscillations by increasing the duration of GABA_A receptor mediated synaptic events. With clinically relevant concentrations of these anesthetic agents the oscillation frequency can fall from 40–50 Hz to as low as 15 Hz. It was postulated by Whittington et al.[81] that, because the function of the gamma oscillation may time, precisely, a given neurone's response to afferent input, this decrease in frequency alone may constitute a mechanism by which these agents produce anesthesia.

Lisman[82] in an intriguing article entitled ' What

makes the brain's tickers tock' has also described how the 40 Hz oscillations underlie working memory by binding together the elementary features of an object. Gamma oscillations themselves are not evidence of binding. This binding, or synchronization, of gamma oscillations can only be demonstrated by measuring phase synchrony between electrode pairs. These ideas are extended by Singer[83] who goes on to summarize two very important studies on phase synchronization of gamma oscillations in man. Rodriguez et al.[84] were the first group to show that gamma phase synchrony (and de-synchrony) is directly involved in human cognitive integration and not just local visual feature binding. Miltner et al.[85] showed an increase in gamma coherence in a narrow band around 40 Hz that associated the visual cortex with the cortical area representing the hand. This followed a conditioned association between a visual and a tactile stimulus. This coherence was lost when the learned association was lost.

THE COHERENT FREQUENCY AND COGNITIVE FUNCTION

Although we have not measured phase synchrony in our experiments in man,[31,32] we propose a parallelism between the reduction in frequency of the SSR produced by a gradually increasing dose of anesthetic and the progressive loss, first of explicit memory then of consciousness itself.

Our experiments are briefly described. We measured the auditory SSR using varying stimulating frequencies from 5 to 60 Hz with sedative doses of either isoflurane or propofol.[31,32] We found the maximum power in the processed EEG to be near 40 Hz in our non-sedated, awake subjects. With increasing sedation in non-stimulated patients the maximum power fell by less than 50% at the point that consciousness was lost.

In order to describe the frequency at which maximum power was achieved we derived the coherence index (CI) which was the power in the first harmonic (Pf_1) divided by the power in subsequent harmonics (Pf_{1-n}). CI has a range of values from 0 to 1. The coherence frequency (CI max) is the stimulating frequency at which a polynomial fitted through the CI values reaches a maximum (Figure 3.6).

Using this system we showed a shift in CI max from an awake value of near 40 Hz to progressively lower values with either isoflurane or propofol sedation.[31,32] As described in the beginning of this chapter we used, at the same time, the Within List Recognition test to measure the effect of sedation on working memory. Just at the point where subjects failed to recognize words that they had heard a few seconds before, the CI max had fallen to 27 Hz (Figure 3.7). Further increase in anesthetic dose caused a further fall in CI and loss of consciousness. With cessation of isoflurane or propofol administration there was a recovery of cognitive function and an increase in CI max. The coherent frequency of the AER correlates strongly with psychological performance at sedative doses of propofol and isoflurane.

In the case of propofol the relationship between CI max and Within-list Recognition (WLR) score is similar across subjects despite large individual variations in the dose of propofol needed to bring about the required changes in psychological performance.

Recently, Dutton et al.,[86] in an excellent paper, showed that a 40 Hz index, which was a combination of AEP amplitude and latency variables, predicted wakeful responses such as hand squeezing rather

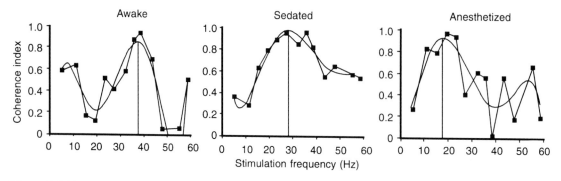

Figure 3.6. The Coherent Index is fitted by a polynomial to show the maximum coherent index (CI max) in a patient being anesthetized for surgery. Awake (48 Hz), sedated (34 Hz) and anesthetized during surgery (18 Hz).

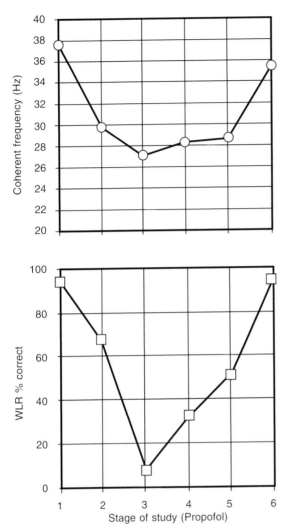

Figure 3.7. Comparison of CI max with Within-list Recognition test in a group of 10 volunteers[32] before, during and after propofol sedation. Stages of study are those described in Figure 3.2. (See text.)

than eye opening, in volunteers during induction of either propofol or desflurane anesthesia. They commented that sometimes subjects appeared wakeful but did not respond to a command. From this type of work it is becoming clear that measurements of depth of anesthesia are far superior to pharmacokinetic measures as a guide to cognitive function during anesthesia.

Use of various methods for measuring depth of anesthesia

What can the various methods for measuring depth

of anesthesia tell us? There is now a very large body of experimental data with the BIS and a smaller, but well-conducted, series of studies with auditory evoked potentials. BIS and AEP have been compared by Gajraj *et al.*[53] during repeated transitions from consciousness to unconsciousness using propofol. They compared AEP, BIS, spectral edge frequency and median frequency. Of the four measurements only the AEP index demonstrated a significant ($P < 0.05$) difference between all mean values 1 min before recovery of consciousness and all mean values 1 min after recovery of consciousness. Some BIS values during unconsciousness were higher than the mean value during consciousness and some conscious values were also lower than the mean value during unconsciousness. In contrast, all mean and awake values of AEP index 1 min after return of consciousness were significantly higher than all mean unconscious values 1 min before. As discussed above, it is possible that the greater discrimination of the AEP index than BIS, in determining the transition between consciousness and unconsciousness, may be due to the inclusion of post-auricular muscle artefact in the waking non-paralyzed patients. Studies are needed of the AEP index in paralyzed patients using the isolated forearm technique to measure responses. However, because of the poor signal to noise ratio in the AEP, it is preferable not to derive an index without having the raw signal available in each case, so that signals with excessive artefact can be identified.

It is believed by some that as anesthetic concentration is increased the BIS has a greater range of response than the AEP. In the case of the *transient* AEP the response tends to flatten only at about 1 MAC. The steady state AEP presented as the *coherent frequency* falls to a median value of 13 Hz at 1 MAC during surgery. We have argued, at the beginning of this chapter, that the ideal cognitive state during general anesthesia is achieved somewhere between 0.5–1 MAC equivalent dose of either inhalation or intravenous anesthetics. This is well within the sensitive range of transient or steady state AEP measurements. The BIS, while appearing to produce a continuously changing signal is, as described earlier, made up of several distinct segments, which are weighted computationally with increasing depth of anesthesia. This index may equally well reflect the cognitive stages of deepening anesthesia but, in the case of both AEP and BIS, there should normally be little interest in clinical anesthesia greater than 1 MAC. Such a depth may be better reflected by EEG burst suppression.

Both the BIS and AEP are insensitive to the effects of nitrous oxide and opioids but both are sensitive to the effects of sleep. It appears that both the AEP and BIS reflect cortical activity, but it is of interest that the BIS is unaffected in a subject rendered unconscious by 70% N_2O. We are now at a stage where comparisons of methods are needed but there is a need to standardize the EEG methods[87] as well as the clinical end points. Now that we have abandoned movement as an end point we can concentrate on the more relevant cognitive effects of changing depth of anesthesia.

Conclusions

- It is rare for patients to wake up during a general anesthetic and have explicit memories of intraoperative events. From 1996 to 1999 in one large region in the UK only 1 in 80,000 patients complained to the legal department.
- The incidence of patients having a vague memory of an intraoperative event is about 1 or 2 per 1000. Patients remember this only when prompted and it does not appear to present a problem for them.
- The use of monitoring devices to detect conscious awareness during anesthesia cannot be justified on the grounds of rarity of the disorder and cost (£10 per patient for disposable BIS electrodes alone). About 80,000 patients would need to be monitored to pick up one case.
- This casts doubt on the need to develop devices to monitor awareness routinely during general anesthesia.
- However, Song et al.[88] have shown that patients with high BIS values (> 75) at the end of surgery using propofol or desflurane anesthesia more rapidly achieve discharge criteria from a Post-Anesthesia Care Unit than those with lower BIS values.
- EEG measures of depth of anesthesia provide very useful tools to examine the effects of anesthetics on cognitive processes.
- The most promising measures to date relate to the bispectral analysis, the auditory evoked potential particularly the Pa/Nb amplitudes and latencies such as mid-latency waves and the coherent (gamma) frequency. These have been correlated with learning under anesthesia, and the gamma (40 Hz) frequency is implicated in attentional mechanisms.

- Deriving the auditory evoked potential is technically more demanding than bispectral (BIS) index.
- Comparisons are needed of the different methods with careful standardization of the EEG methods as well as the cognitive end points.

References

1. Jones J.G. Perception and memory during general anesthesia. *Br J Anaesth* 1994; **73**:31–37.
2. Andrade J, Jones J.G. Is amnesia for intraoperative events good enough? Editorial. *Br J Anaesth* 1998; **80**:575–576.
3. Antognini JF, Schwartz K. Exaggerated anesthetic requirements in the preferentially anaesthetized brain. *Anesthesiology* 1993; **79**:1244–1249.
4. Rampil IJ. Anesthetic potency is not altered after hypothermic spinal cord transection in rats. *Anesthesiology* 1994; **80**:606–610.
5. Evans JM. Patients' experiences of awareness during general anesthesia. In Rosen M, Lunn JN (eds). *Consciousness, Awareness and Pain in General Anesthesia*, Boston: Butterworths, 1987; 184–192.
6. Anonymous. On being aware. *Br J Anaesth* 1979; **51**:711–712.
7. Schwender D, Kunze-Kronawitter H, Dietrich P, Klasing S, Forst H, Madler C. Conscious awareness during general anesthesia: Patients perceptions, emotions, cognition and reactions. *Br J Anaesth* 1998; **80**:133–139.
8. Moerman N, Bonke B, Oosting J. Awareness and recall during general anesthesia: Facts and feelings. *Anesthesiology* 1990; **79**:454–464.
9. Russell IF. Comparison of wakefulness with two anesthetic regimens; total i.v. vs balanced anesthesia. *Br J Anaesth* 1986; **58**: 965–968.
10. Schultetus RR, Hill CR, Dharamraj CM, Banner TE, Berman LS. Wakefullness during cesarean section after anesthetic induction with ketamine, thiopental or ketamine thiopental combined. *Anesthesia and Analgesia* 1985; **64**:723–728.
11. Blacher RS. On awaking paralyzed during surgery. *JAMA* 1975; **234**:67–69.
12. Lyons G, Macdonald R. Awareness during caesarean section. *Anesthesia* 1991; **46**:62–64.
13. Pederson T, Johansen SH. Serious morbidity attributable to anesthesia. *Anesthesia* 1989; **44**: 504–508.
14. Hargrove RL. Awareness under anesthesia. *J Med Defence Union* 1987; **3**:9–11.
15. Liu WHD, Thorp AS, Graham SG, Aitkenhead AR.

Incidence of awareness with recall during general anesthesia. *Anesthesia* 1991; **46**:435–437.

16. Baddely A. Working memory. *Science* 1992; **255**:556–559.

17. Lubke GH, Kerssens C, Phaf H, Sebel PS. Dependence of explicit and implicit memory on hypnotic state in trauma patients. *Anesthesiology* 1999; **90**:670–680.

18. Andrade J. Investigations of hypesthesia: Using anesthetics to explore relationships between consciousness, learning, and memory. *Consciousness Cogn* 1996; **5**:562–580.

19. Schacter DL. The cognitive neuroscience of memory: Perspectives from neuro-imaging research. *Phil. Trans. R. Soc. Lond.B* 1997; **352**:1689–1695.

20. Schacter DL. Memory and awareness. *Science* 1998; **280**:59–60.

21. Elliot R, Dolan RJ. Neural response during preference and memory judgements for subliminally presented stimuli: A functional neuroimaging study. *J Neurosci* 1998; **18**:4697–4704.

22. Morris JS, Ohman A, Dolman R. Conscious and unconscious emotional learning in the human amygdala. *Nature* 1998; **393**:467–470.

23. Berns GS, Cohen JD, Mintun MA. Brain regions responsive to novelty in the absence of awareness. *Science* 1997; **276**:1272–1275.

24. Dehaene S, Naccache L, Le Clec'h G, *et al.* Imaging unconscious semantic priming. *Nature* 1998; **395**:597–600.

25. Whalen PJ, Rauch SL, Etcoff NL, McInerey SC, Lee MB, Jenike MA. Masked presentations of emotional facial expressions modulate amygdala activity without explicit knowledge. *J Neurosci* 1998; **18**:411–418.

26. Saharie A, Weiskranz L, Barbur JL, Simmons A, Williams SC, Brammer MJ. Pattern of neuronal activity associated with conscious and unconscious processing of visual signals. *Proc Natl Acad Sci. USA* 1997; **94**:9406–9411.

27. Artusio JF. Ether analgesia during major surgery. *JAMA* 1955; **157**:33–36.

28. Newton DEF, Thornton L, Koniezcko K, *et al.* Levels of consciousness in volunteers breathing sub MAC concentrations of isoflurane. *Br J Anaesth* 1990; **65**:609–615.

29. Newton DEF, Thornton C, Koniezcko KM, *et al.* Auditory evoked response: a study in volunteers at sub-MAC concentrations of isoflurane. *Br J Anaesth* 1992; **69**:122–129.

30. Block RI, Ghoneim MM, Sum Ping ST, Ali MA. Human learning during general anesthesia and surgery. *Br J Anaesth* 1991; **66**:170–178.

31. Munglani R, Andrade J, Sapsford DJ, Baddeley A, Jones JG. A measure of consciousness and memory during isoflurane administration: the coherent frequency. *Br J Anaesth* 1993; **71**:663–641.

32. Andrade J, Sapsford DJ, Jeevaratnam D, Pickworth AJ, Jones JG. The coherent frequency in the electroencephalogram as an objective measure of cognitive function during propofol sedation. *Anesth Analg* 1996; **83**:1279–1284.

33. Jones JG, Koniezcko K. Hearing and memory in anaesthetised patients. *Br Med J* 1986; **292**: 1291–1293.

34. Thornton C, Koniezcko K, Jones JG, Jordan C, Dore CJ, Heneghan C. Effect of surgical stimulation on the auditory evoked potential. *Br J Anaesth.* 1992; **76**:892–898.

35. Ghoneim MM, Block RI. Learning and consciousness during general anesthesia. *Anesthesiology* 1992; **76**:279–305.

36. Merikle PM, Rondi G. Memory for events during anesthesia has not been demonstrated; a psychologist's viewpoint. In Sebel PS, Bonke B, Winograd E (eds). *Memory and Awareness in Anesthesia.* Englewood Cliffs: Prentice-Hall, 1993; 476–497.

37. Merikle PM, Daneman M. Memory for unconsciously perceived events; evidence from anaesthetised patients. *Consciousness Cogn* 1996; **5**:525–541.

38. Andrade J, Stapleton CL, Harper C, Englert L, Edwards ND. The contribution of surgery to learning and memory in anaesthesia. In Memory and Awareness in Anaesthesia IV. *Proceedings of the Fourth International Symposium on Memory and Awareness in Anaesthesia.* Eds Jordan C, Vaughan DJA, Newton DEF. Imperial College Press, London. 2000; 141–163.

39. Bethune DW, Ghosh S, Gray B, *et al.* Learning during general anesthesia: implicit recall after methohexitone or propofol infusion. *Br J Anaesth.* 1992; **69**:197–199.

40. Schwender D, Kaiser NW, Klasing S, Peter K, Poppel E. Mid-latency auditory evoked potentials and explicit and implicit memory in patients undergoing cardiac surgery. *Anaesthesiology* 1994; **80**:663–641.

41. Malenka RC, Nicholl RA. Never fear LTP is here. *Nature* 1997; **390**:552–553.

42. Jones JG. Awareness during anesthesia – What are we monitoring? In Memory and Awareness in Anaesthesia IV. Eds Jordan C, Voughn OJA, Newton DEF. London: Imperial College Press, 2000; 3–40.

43. Jessop J, Jones JG. Conscious awareness during general anesthesia – What are we attempting to monitor? Editorial. *Br J Anaesth* 1991; **66**:635–636.

44. Evans JM, Davies WL. Monitoring anesthesia. *Clin Anaesthes* 1984; **2**:242–263.

45. Russell IF. Conscious awareness during general anesthesia: relevance of autonomic signs and isolated arm movements as guides to depth of anesthesia. In Jones JG (ed.) *Clinical Anaesthesiology,* London: Baillière Tindall. **3**:511–532.

46. Domino KB, Posner KL, Caplan RA, Cheney FW. Awareness during anesthesia. *Anesthesiology* 1999; **90**:1053–1061.

47. Raftery S, Enever G, Prys-Roberts C. Oesophageal contractility during total intravenous anesthesia with and without glycopyrronium. *Br J Anaesth* 1991; **66**:566–571.

48. Struys M, Versichelen L, Mortier E, *et al.* Comparison of spontaneous frontal EMG, EEG power spectrum and bispectral index to monitor propofol drug effect and emergence. *Acta Anaesth Scand* 1998; **42**:629–636.

49. Pomfrett CJD. Heart rate variability, BIS and depth of anesthesia. *Br J Anaesth* 1999; **82**:659–662.

50. Sleigh JW, Donovan J. Comparison of bispectral index, 95% spectral edge frequency and approximate entropy of the EEG, with changes in heart rate variability during induction of general anesthesia. *Br J Anaesth* 1999; **82**:666–671.

51. Rampil IJ. A primer for EEG signal processing in anesthesia. *Anesthesiology* 1998; **89**:980–1002.

52. Schwilden H. Use of median EEG frequency and pharmacokinetics in determining the depth of anesthesia, In Jones JG (ed.) *Clinical Anaesthesiology*. Baillière Tindall, London 1989; **3**:603–622.

53. Gajraj RJ, Doi M, Mantzaridis H, Kenney GNC. Analysis of the EEG bispectrum, auditory evoked potentials and the EEG power spectrum during repeated transitions from consciousness to unconsciousness. *Br J Anaesth* 1998; **80**:46–52.

54. Barnett TP, Johnson LC, Naitoh P, Hicks N, Nute C. Bispectrum analysis of EEG signals during waking and sleeping. *Science* 1971; **172**:401–402.

55. Sigl JC, Chamoun NG. An introduction to bispectral analysis for the electroencephalogram. *J Clin Monitr* 1994; **10**:392–404.

56. Todd MM. EEGs, EEG processing, and the bispectral index. *Anesthesiology* 1998; **89**:815–817.

57. Leslie K, Sessler DI, Smith Larson NW, Ozaki M, Blanchard D, Crankshaw DP. Prediction of movement during Propofol/nitrous oxide anesthesia. *Anesthesiology* 1996; **84**:52–63.

58. Kearse LA, Rosow C, Zaslavsky A, Connors P, Dershwitz M, Denman W. Bispectral analysis of the EEG predicts conscious processing of information during propofol sedation and hypnosis. *Anesthesiology* 1998; **88**:25–34.

59. Glass PS, Bloom M, Kearse L, Rosow C, Sebel P, Manberg P. Bispectral analysis measures sedation and memory effects of propofol, midazolam, isoflurane and alfentanil in healthy volunteers. *Anesthesiology* 1997; **86**:836–847.

60. Liu JL, Singh H, White PF. EEG bispectral analysis predicts the depth of midazolam-induced sedation. *Anesthesiology* 1996; **84**:64–69.

61. Iselin-Chaves IA, Flaishon R, Sebel S, *et al.* The effect of the interaction of propofol and alfentanil on recall, loss of consciousness and the bispectral index. *Anesthesiology* 1998; **87**:941–948.

62. Barr G, Jackobsson JG, Owall A, Anderson RE. Nitrous oxide does not alter bispectral index: study with nitrous oxide as sole agent and as an adjunct to iv anesthesia. *Br J Anaesth* 1999; **82**:827–830.

63. Newton D, Thornton C, Creagh-Barry P, Dore CJ. Early cortical evoked response in anaesthesia: comparison of the effects of nitrous oxide and isoflurane. *Br J Anaesth* 1989; **62**:61–65.

64. Thornton C, Creagh-Barry P, Jordan C, *et al.* Somatosensory and auditory evoked responses recorded simultaneously: different effects of nitrous oxide and isoflurane. *Br J Anaesth* 1992; **68**: 508–514.

65. Fang F, Guo T-Z, Davies F, Maze M. Opiate receptors in the periaqueductal gray mediate analgesic effect of nitrous oxide in rats. *Eur J Pharmacol* 1997; **336**:137–141.

66. Sleigh JW, Andrzejowski J, Steyn-Ross A, Steyn-Ross M. The bispectral index: A measure of depth of sleep? *Anesth Analg* 1999; **88**:654–658.

67. Driver IK, Watson BJ, Menon DK, Aggarwal SK, Jones JG. Bispectral index is a state-specific measure of cortical arousal. *Br J Anaesth* 1996; **77**: 694P–695P.

68. Thornton C, Catley DM, Jordan C, Royston D, Lehane JR, Jones JG. Enflurane increases the latency of early components of the auditory evoked response in man. *Br J Anaesth* 1981; **53**:1102–1103.

69. Thornton C, Sharpe RM. Evoked responses in anesthesia. *Br J Anaesth* 1998; **81**:771–781.

70. Thornton C, Lucas MA, Newton DEF, Dore CJ, Jones RM. Effects of dexmedetomidine on isoflurane requirements in healthy volunteers. 2: Auditory and somatosensory evoked responses. *Br J Anaesth* 1999; **83**:381–386.

71. Thornton C, Barrowcliffe M, Koniezcko KM, Ventham P, Dore C, Newton DEF. The auditory evoked response as an indicator of awareness. *Br J Anaesth* 1989; **63**:113–115.

72. Davies FW, Mantzaridis H, Kenny GN, Fisher AC. Middle latency auditory evoked potentials during repeated transitions from consciousness to unconsciousness. *Br J Anaesth* 1996; **51**:107–113.

73. Tooley MA, Greenslade GL, Prys-Roberts C. Concentration-related effects of propofol on the auditory evoked response. *Br J Anaesth* 1996; **77**:720–726.

74. Mantzaridis H, Kenney GNC. Auditory evoked potential index: a quantitative measure of changes in auditory evoked potentials during general anesthesia. *Anesthesia* 1997; **52**:1030–1036.

75. Thornton C. Assessment of graded changes in the central nervous system during general anesthesia and surgery in man using the auditory evoked

response. *Ph.D Thesis*. University of London. England 1990.

76. Langeron O, Vivien B, Paqueron X, *et al.* Effects of propofol, propofol-nitrous oxide and midazolam on cortical somatosensory evoked potentials during sufentanil anesthesia for major spinal surgery. *Br J Anaesth* 1999; **82**:340–345.

77. Crabb I, Thornton C, Koniezcko KM, *et al.* Remifentanil reduces auditory and somatosensory evoked responses during isoflurane anesthesia in a dose dependent manner. *Br J Anaesth* 1996; **76**:795–801.

78. McPherson RW, Mahla M, Johnson R, Traystman J. Effect of enflurane, isoflurane, and nitrous oxide on somatosensory evoked potentials during fentanyl anesthesia. *Anesthesiology* 1985; **62**:626–633.

79. Plourde G. Auditory evoked potentials and 40 Hz oscillations. *Anesthesiology* 1999; **91**:1187–1189.

80. Litscher G. *Monitoring of stimulus-induced 40 Hz brain oscillations*. Berlin, Pabst Science Publications, 1998, 1–246.

81. Whittington MA, Traub RD, Jeffreys JGR. Experimental gamma (40Hz) oscillations: mechanisms of generation, function and effects of general anesthetics. In Litscher G. (ed.) *Monitoring of stimulus-induced 40 Hz brain oscillations*. Berlin: Pabst Science Publications, 1998; 108–143.

82. Lisman J. What makes the brain's tickers tock. *Nature* 1998; **394**:132–133.

83. Singer W. Striving for coherence. *Nature* 1999; **397**:391–393.

84. Rodriguez E, George N, Lachaux J-P, Martinerie J, Renault B, Varela FJ. Perception's shadow: long distance synchronization of human brain activity. *Nature* 1999; **397**:430–433.

85. Miltner WHR, Braun C, Arnold M, Witte H, Taub E. *Nature* 1999; **397**:434–436.

86. Dutton RC, Smith WD, Rampil IJ, Chortkoff BS, Eger EI. Forty-hertz midlatency auditory evoked potential activity predicts wakeful response during desflurane and propofol anesthesia in volunteers. *Anesthesiology* 1999; **91**:1209–1220.

87. Smith WD, Dutton RL, Smith T. Measuring the performance of anesthetic depth indicators. *Anesthesiology* 1996; **84**:38–51.

88. Song D, van Vlymen J, White PF. Is the bispectral index useful in predicting fast-track eligibility after ambulatory anesthesia with propofol and desflurane. *Anesth Analg* 1998; **87**:1245–1248.

Chapter 4

Learning during sedation, anesthesia and surgery

Jackie Andrade

Contents

Introduction: is there evidence for learning during anesthesia but not sedation?

The majority of studies of learning during anesthesia have assessed learning of stimuli presented during surgery. In a typical study, words are played to patients during surgery and, on recovery from the anesthetic, patients attempt a test of implicit memory. Implicit memory is revealed as a change in behavior due to previous experience, without conscious or explicit recollection or recognition of that experience. For example, implicit memory for the word JAVELIN will increase the tendency to respond with JAVELIN rather than, say, JAM, when asked to think of a word beginning JA –. These studies have given mixed results for a variety of possible reasons, including lack of monitoring of depth of anesthesia, lack of standardization of the memory

test and anesthetic procedures, and lack of control of type of surgery.[1-3] However, approximately half these studies appeared to demonstrate learning during surgery, revealed as above-chance performance on tests of implicit memory despite lack of recollection of surgery itself. Following a meta-analysis of this literature, Merikle and Daneman[4] concluded that there is evidence for learning during anesthesia, providing memory is tested reasonably soon after recovery, preferably within 12 h (see also Chapter 2).

This conclusion contrasts with the findings from volunteer studies of learning during sedation with general anesthetic agents. These studies tend to show learning during sedation only when very small doses of anesthetic are administered. For example, learning persists during infusion of 1.27 $mg.kg^{-1}h^{-1}$ of propofol,[5] inhalation of 30% nitrous oxide,[6] and inhalation of approximately 0.3 MAC isoflurane.[7,8] However, it ceases at doses of isoflurane that are just sufficient to prevent volunteers responding to commands to squeeze the experimenter's hand.[7–10] How can these two sets of data be reconciled? A possible explanation is that learning occurs only during very light anesthesia. The volunteer studies just mentioned[9, 10] show that learning ceases when voluntary response to command ceases, suggesting that awareness is necessary for learning. Extrapolating to the studies of learning during clinical anesthesia, perhaps patients learn only when they are inadequately anesthetized. Certainly there is evidence that depth of anesthesia influences learning. In one of the earliest studies to combine monitoring of depth of anesthesia with assessment of learning, Schwender *et al.*[11] demonstrated learning during surgery only in patients whose EEG responses to auditory stimulation were similar to their responses when awake before anesthesia and surgery, suggesting that they were inadequately anesthetized. Recently, Lubke and her colleagues observed a linear increase in learning with decreasing depth of anesthesia.[12] They investigated learning in trauma patients, a group selected because they were likely to experience greater fluctuations in depth of anesthesia than in other types of surgery. This patient population provided an ethical means of testing learning at widely varying depths of anesthesia. In a neat experimental design, Lubke *et al.* presented each stimulus word repeatedly while measuring depth of anesthesia (as bispectral index). They tested memory by asking patients, on recovery, to complete word stems with the first appropriate word that came to mind. Depth of anesthesia correlated significantly with learning, thus the tendency to use previously presented words to complete stems increased as the bispectral index at which those words were presented increased (see also Chapter 5).

However, a conflict remains because the volunteer studies suggest that awareness is necessary for learning, whereas the patient studies show learning during light but apparently adequate anesthesia. For example, Lubke *et al.*[12] found learning with bispectral index between 40 and 60, which they took to be clinically adequate anesthesia. Moreover, although the correlation between bispectral index and memory was significant, it was relatively weak ($r = 0.35$), suggesting that depth of anesthesia explained only a minor portion (12%) of the variance in memory scores. If surgical stimulation affects

learning directly, as well as indirectly by altering depth of anesthesia, then it is conceivable that differences in levels of surgical stimulation may explain additional variance in memory scores in Lubke's patients. As the presence or absence of surgery is an important difference between patient and volunteer studies, it is also conceivable that surgery may contribute to the apparently greater probability of patients learning during clinical anesthesia than volunteers learning during equally deep experimental anesthesia. Our research lends tentative support to this hypothesis, although we did not directly test the effect of surgery on learning. Rather, we set out to discover how learning varied with varying depth of anesthesia. Because we wanted to ensure that some learning would occur, we began by testing healthy volunteers receiving small doses of anesthetic.

Experiment one: learning during propofol sedation in healthy volunteers[13]

Twelve volunteers were played three lists of fictitious names (e.g. Georgina Smith); one list while awake, the second while lightly sedated with propofol, and the third when deeply sedated but sufficiently conscious to raise a hand in response to command. Pilot subjects differed in their sensitivity to propofol; therefore, to achieve comparable depths of sedation across volunteers, we increased the propofol infusion rate in a stepwise fashion. At each step we checked whether a target depth of sedation had been achieved before progressing to the next step. Sedation was measured in terms of cognitive function, using a within-list recognition test[14] that required attention and short-term memory. Table 4.1 shows an example. Subjects were asked to raise their right thumb whenever a word was repeated – note that repeats occurred after varying numbers of intervening words, to avoid ceiling and floor effects during very light and very deep sedation respectively. Target performance on the within-list recognition test for the 'light sedation' condition was a score between 3 and 5 repeats identified from 7. The propofol infusion rate was increased in a stepwise fashion until subjects achieved a score within that range. Then the second list of fictitious names was played. Next, the stepwise infusion procedure was repeated until subjects correctly responded to two repeated words or fewer,

Table 4.1. Two of the word lists from the Within-List Recognition Test. The subject's task is to respond to repeated words, for example *flavor* in the example shown. The numbers show the number of words intervening between the first and second presentations of repeated words

ability		competition	
flavor		precaution	
flavor	0	friendship	
dignity		friendship	0
demonstration		humor	
member		indolence	
suggestion		fiancée	
character		subject	
suggestion	1	upheaval	
segment		bitterness	
expedition		indolence	4
quantity		wonder	
overtone		season	
expedition	2	humor	8
segment	4	question	
bayonet		mystery	
character	8	question	1
liberty		amendment	
liberty	0	precaution	16
attempt		faithfulness	
dignity	16	wisdom	
solution		wisdom	0
salvation		faithfulness	2

and the third list of names was played. This experiment was part of a study[15] that required testing of each volunteer when awake, lightly sedated, deeply sedated, lightly sedated, and awake again, in that order, therefore the order of the three conditions in the present experiment could not be counterbalanced.

On recovery from sedation, volunteers attempted two memory tests – a forced-choice recognition test sensitive to explicit (conscious) memory and a fame judgment task sensitive to implicit (unconscious) memory. Both tests comprised pairs of fictitious names. On the recognition test, volunteers picked the name they remembered hearing during the study phase of the experiment. On the fame judgment task, they selected the name they thought was famous. Filler items, of a famous name paired with a fictitious name, were included to make the task plausible. Implicit memory for fictitious names should show up as the 'false fame effect', i.e. people are more likely to attribute fame to previously

encountered fictitious names than to similar but novel names.[16–18]

Results

Figure 4.1 shows that volunteers had explicit and implicit memory for names presented before propofol infusion began (one-sample t-test: $P < 0.05$ for both tasks), but no memory for names presented during propofol sedation. During the light sedation phase, participants correctly identified a mean of 9 out of 14 repeated words on the within-list recognition test. During the deep sedation phase, they identified a mean of only one repeated word, but remained able to raise their hand in response to command.

The lack of memory for words played during light sedation was surprising given the relatively good short-term memory performance during that phase. It demonstrates that learning ceases before loss of consciousness and short-term memory function, hence one should not assume that lack of memory on recovery from anesthesia shows lack of consciousness during anesthesia.

Experiment two: learning during propofol sedation, anesthesia and intubation in patients about to undergo surgery[19]

We were puzzled by the contrast between the results of this study and the apparent demonstrations of memory during clinical anesthesia. We speculated that patients who are alert and presumably anxious before surgery might be more attentive to their environment, and consequently to the experimental stimuli, than the volunteers we tested. Experiment two therefore investigated learning during sedation and anesthesia prior to surgery. We also assessed learning during intubation, to compare learning during light anesthesia due to a small dose of anesthetic, with learning during light anesthesia due to stimulation opposing the hypnotic effect of a larger dose of anesthetic. Propofol was the sole anesthetic used, to allow comparison with experiment one. However, the memory testing procedure was altered in the hope of finding a technique that would be more sensitive to small amounts of memory. Two tasks were used. The first was the category generation task used by Bonke and his

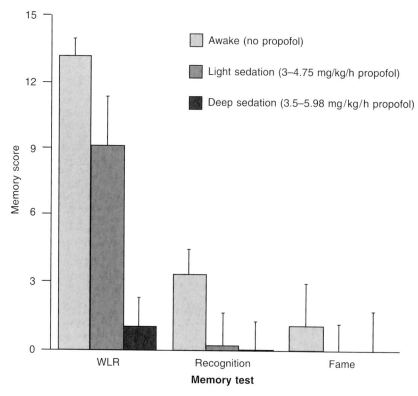

Figure 4.1. Short-term memory and learning during propofol sedation. The within-list recognition test is scored as the number of correctly identified repeats (maximum = 14), and reflects short-term memory function. The recognition test and fame judgment task respectively show explicit and implicit memory, on recovery, for fictitious names presented before and during sedation. They are scored as the number of times subjects choose a previously presented word minus the number of times they choose a distractor word, hence 0 represents chance performance (no memory). The maximum score is 10. The error bars show standard deviations.

colleagues to demonstrate learning during clinical anesthesia.[20,21] The second was a preference rating task to pick up changes in emotional responding that reflect learning.[22] The 'mere exposure effect' refers to the fact that people tend to prefer previously encountered stimuli to similar but novel stimuli. Zajonc[22,23] has argued that this emotional change persists under learning conditions that abolish the more cognitive changes that are measured by typical implicit memory tests. It may therefore provide a more sensitive test of learning during sedation.

A pilot study confirmed that people's preferences for our stimuli (auditorily presented Finnish words) increased after exposure. We asked participants in the pilot study to attend to one list of words and try to remember them. They heard a second list of words while attending to another task. This divided attention manipulation did not reduce preference for the presented words. We therefore hoped that

another manipulation of attention, i.e. propofol sedation, would also have little effect on preference, in other words that the preference rating task should be a sensitive measure of learning during sedation.

Methods

Thirty-six consenting patients took part in experiment two. Each was scheduled for laparoscopy with propofol anesthesia and took part in the experiment before surgery. None spoke or understood Finnish. Patients were randomly assigned to three groups. Each group was played a list of Finnish words 12 times before receiving propofol. Memory testing can seem rather a strange exercise for patients with no explicit recollection of experimental stimuli. The first list aimed to reduce this strangeness by ensuring that, on recovery, patients would remember some experimental stimuli. The next step varied according to the patient's group. Patients in group 1 received a sedating dose of propofol by computer-controlled infusion to a target concentration of 2 $\mu g.ml^{-1}$. The second list of Finnish words was played 12 times after 10 min of infusion. Patients were asked to listen carefully and try to remember the words. After a break of approximately 1 minute, the experimenter played the phrase 'yellow banana green pear' 30 times. Patients were then anesthetized with 5 $\mu g.ml^{-1}$ propofol, intubated (with 5 mg of vecuronium as muscle relaxant), ventilated with a 60:40 nitrous oxide:oxygen mixture, and transferred to the operating theatre. After surgery, patients were woken as normal and taken to the recovery ward.

Patients in group 2 received an anesthetic dose of propofol to a target concentration of 5 $\mu g.ml^{-1}$. After 10 minutes, they were played the second list of Finnish words 12 times. Next, they received 5 mg of vecuronium and were intubated. The 30 presentations of the 'yellow banana green pear' phrase began during intubation. The procedure for group 3 was identical except that the 'yellow banana ...' phrase was played before intubation and the Finnish words were played during intubation. Anesthesia then continued as for group 1. Bispectral index was recorded at the start and end of each set of stimuli as a measure of depth of sedation or anesthesia.

On recovery, patients were asked to name the first three examples of fruits and colors that came to mind. A control group of 12 patients, fulfilling the same criteria as the experimental sample, was asked to do likewise, but had not been played the 'yellow banana...' phrase during anesthesia. The three experimental groups then attempted the Finnish memory tests, the order of which was counter-balanced across patients. For each test, patients listened to the words they had heard before and during propofol infusion, plus distractors, presented in random order. For the implicit, preference test they rated how much they liked the sound of each word. For the explicit, recognition test they judged whether they recognized each word.

Results

Overall, the category judgment task showed no evidence of learning, patients in the control group giving 'yellow', 'green', 'banana', or 'pear' as examples of colors and fruits as often patients in the experimental groups (control mean = 1.75, experimental mean = 1.86). However, patients receiving the phrase during intubation were slightly more likely to respond with the target words than patients receiving the phrase during anesthesia (mean for intubation = 2.08, mean for anesthesia = 1.67, two-tailed t-test $P = 0.06$). The mean for the sedation group was midway between the means for intubation and anesthesia (1.83) and did not differ from either. These findings suggest that the arousing effect of intubation allowed some learning to occur, even though the bispectral index data (Table 4.2) showed no lightening of anesthetic depth during intubation. However, this suggestion is at best very tentative because responses with target words in the intubation condition were not significantly higher than in the control group.

Table 4.2 shows scores on the recognition and preference tests. Both tests revealed memory for the Finnish words presented before propofol infusion, i.e. patients rated their recognition of the presented words higher than for the distractors ($P < 0.001$) and rated their liking of the presented words higher than their liking of the distractors ($P < .05$). There was no evidence of memory for the words presented during propofol infusion.

To conclude, even relatively light sedation prevented patients learning the category examples, stimuli that had been used to demonstrate learning during surgery with general anesthesia. Propofol sedation also prevented an increase in preference for presented Finnish words, a change that should have been relatively resistant to reduced awareness. Overall, we obtained no evidence for learning during propofol infusion, an outcome that replicates that of experiment one but contrasts with that of many studies of learning during general anesthesia.[4] There was a slight hint that patients may have learned category examples presented during intubation, but not sufficient evidence to conclude that such brief stimulation enables learning. Our next experiment tested learning during propofol sedation and anesthesia with prolonged stimulation, i.e. surgery.

Experiment three: learning during surgery with propofol sedation or anesthesia[24]

This experiment tested learning during propofol sedation or anesthesia. Previous studies of learning

Table 4.2. Memory for words presented to patients when awake and during sedation, anesthesia or intubation. Bispectral index gives a measure of depth of sedation during word presentation. The recognition score is the difference between ratings of recognition for the presented and distractor words, and reflects explicit memory. The preference score is the difference in preference ratings between presented and distractor words, and reflects implicit memory. Only the scores for words presented before propofol infusion significantly exceeded zero (chance)

Group	Words played...	Recognition score	Preference score	Bispectral index during word presentation
All	before propofol	9.41	1.63	91.21
1	during sedation	−0.08	−0.13	81.75
2	during anesthesia	1.52	−1.08	51.17
3	during intubation	1.36	−0.50	55.83

during surgery with sedation have given mixed results.[25,26] When there was implicit memory of intraoperative stimuli, there was also some explicit memory.[25] We therefore used a technique called the Process Dissociation Procedure to obtain separate estimates of implicit and explicit memory. This technique is currently popular in the psychological literature as a means of separating conscious and unconscious influences on a single memory task[27,28] (although it is not without criticism).[29] It was used by Lubke *et al.*[12] in their study of learning during trauma surgery. The basic technique splits the memory test into two sets of trials. On the 'inclusion' trials, subjects are asked to respond with a word they remember or, if they remember nothing appropriate, to say the first word that comes to mind. On the 'exclusion' trials, subjects try to recall a word from the study phase so they can *avoid* responding with studied words. Thus explicit and implicit memory act in concert on the inclusion trials and in opposition on the exclusion trials. This enables estimation of explicit and implicit memory by simple algebra. Thus, explicit memory = inclusion score – exclusion score, and implicit memory = exclusion score/(1 – explicit memory) – score for distractor items (see also Chapter 2 and Chapter 5).

Methods

Seventy-two consenting patients undergoing minor gynecological surgery took part. The first 24 patients received a propofol anesthetic supplemented with alfentanil. Because of a temporary change in hospital policy, the next 36 received a sedative dose of propofol with alfentanil. The remaining 12 patients received the same anesthetic as the first 24.

Each patient was played a list of English words once before receiving the drugs and a second list (played ten times) during surgery. A third list provided distractor items for the memory test and was not played to the patient. Use of lists was counterbalanced across patients. Each study list contained 24 words, each word beginning with an audibly different syllable (the 'word stem'). Two test lists each contained the stems from half the words in each study list, in random order, making 36 test items per list.

Depth of sedation or anesthesia was assessed by recording responses to the command 'squeeze my fingers with your left hand' and eyelash reflex at the start and end of the intraoperative study list. A 5 ml venous blood sample was collected at the start and end of the list for subsequent propofol assay.[30]

Patients attempted the memory test as soon as possible after recovery. One test list was attempted under inclusion instructions, i.e. patients were asked to use the word stems to help them recall a word from before or during surgery and to use that word to complete the stem or, if they could not recall a word, to complete the stem with the first suitable word that came to mind. The other test list was completed under exclusion instructions, patients using the stems to help recall a previously heard word and then using a different, unrecalled word to complete the stem. For example, if JAVELIN were a study word, one test list would contain the stem JA -. Patients would use the stem JA- to help recall JAVELIN. If they succeeded in recalling JAVELIN, they completed the stem with that word in the inclusion condition, and avoided using that word in the exclusion condition, responding with another word such as JAM instead. The order of the instruction conditions and test lists was counterbalanced.

Results

Depth of sedation/anesthesia varied considerably across the patients. Thirty-seven patients responded to the squeeze-my-hand command at the start of the word list, 24 did so at the end. Thirty-four patients had a positive eyelash reflex at the start of the list, 18 did so at the end. The mean blood propofol concentration was 2.46 µg/ml (range 0.57 to 5.80 µg/ml). The mean alfentanil dose was 0.033 mg/kg (range 0.019 to 0.057 mg/kg).

Performance on the memory test was scored as the proportion of stems completed with a word from the corresponding list (preoperative, intraoperative or distractor). These proportions were used to estimate explicit and implicit memory using the formulae given above.[27] Table 4.3 shows the explicit and implicit memory estimates for the preoperative and intraoperative word lists.

Patients had explicit (one sample, two-tailed t-test: $P < 0.001$) and implicit ($P < 0.02$) memory for the preoperative word list. They had explicit memory for the intraoperative word list ($P < 0.02$) but no implicit memory. None of the measures of depth of sedation/anesthesia correlated with memory for the intraoperative list.

To conclude, the memory test showed evidence of memory for words played during surgery, but suggested that this memory was explicit. Explicit memory in turn suggests that patients were conscious

Table 4.3. Mean estimated explicit and implicit memory for word lists played preoperatively before propofol infusion and intraoperatively, during propofol–alfentanil sedation or anesthesia (± 95% confidence intervals)

	Memory type	Score
Preoperative list	Explicit	−0.183 (0.131–0.235)
	Implicit	−0.047 (0.011–0.084)
Intraoperative list	Explicit	−0.058 (0.012–0.104)
	Implicit	−0.026 (−0.059–0.006)

when they learned the words and, by extrapolation, that learning during anesthesia occurs only when anesthesia is light enough to permit moments of awareness. However, the finding that memory was explicit is odd because memory performance did not correlate with measures of depth of sedation, yet explicit memory is generally very sensitive to changes in level of awareness and should be reduced by increasing depth of sedation. It is possible that the process dissociation procedure becomes inaccurate with low levels of memory. For example, if patients excluded words that seemed familiar because they were implicitly remembered, as well as words they explicitly recalled, then explicit memory would have been overestimated and implicit memory underestimated. The conclusion that memory was explicit should therefore be treated with caution, but the data tentatively suggest that some learning occurred during surgery.

General discussion: a possible role of surgery in learning during anesthesia?

We examined learning during anesthesia in three experiments. The anesthetic technique was controlled as far as possible, propofol being administered alone in the first two experiments and supplemented only by alfentanil in the third. This allows comparisons between experiments that are not possible between most previously reported studies of learning during anesthesia. The method of memory testing was not controlled, however, partly for operational reasons (e.g. the volunteers in experiment one were anesthesiologists who were already familiar with several implicit memory tests) and partly in response to changes in the psychological literature on memory testing. None the less, each explicit and implicit memory test was designed to be as sensitive as possible to memory for stimuli presented during propofol infusion.

We obtained no strong evidence for learning during anesthesia or even during conscious sedation. However, experiment three showed some evidence for learning during surgery, which was surprising given the strong amnesic effects of propofol observed in the first two experiments, when stimuli were presented to volunteers or preoperatively to patients. We therefore hypothesize that surgery enables learning in conditions which would otherwise prevent it. We are not suggesting that learning always occurs during surgery. Lubke's study[12] showed clearly that relatively light anesthesia is also necessary for learning. What we are suggesting is that surgery facilitates learning during light anesthesia, therefore patients may be more susceptible to forming implicit memories of intraoperative stimuli – e.g. conversations among operating theater personnel – than might be predicted from volunteer studies.

By what mechanism might surgery affect the probability of learning during sedation or anesthesia? Candidates are the catecholamines epinephrine and norepinephrine, which play important roles in normal memory function and increase in response to stress and surgery. Increased release of epinephrine or norepinephrine is thought to underlie the exceptionally good memory that people have for shocking, threatening or otherwise emotional events.[31,32] Two studies have shown that injections of epinephrine enabled fear conditioning in rats anesthetized with pentobarbital and chloral hydrate[33,34] or thiopental.[35] However, this finding was not replicated in rabbits anesthetized with isoflurane.[36] In the rat studies, it is not clear whether epinephrine facilitated learning by lightening anesthesia or despite deep anesthesia. Future tests of the catecholamine hypothesis with humans must monitor depth of anesthesia as well as epinephrine levels.

Two studies of learning during clinical anesthesia are relevant to this hypothesis, although neither measured epinephrine levels or depth of anesthesia. Bethune et al.[37] presented words and related phrases to patients (e.g. 'Tar – tar makes a mark'), either during cardiac surgery and again in the immediate postoperative period, or only during the postoperative period. Within 48 h of surgery, patients attempted a free association task in which they listened to the phrases ('Makes a mark') and responded with the first word that came to mind. Patients who had received the phrases during surgery were more likely to respond with the target words than a control group who had not been exposed to the words. Patients who only received the words during the postoperative period showed no evidence of learning. Bethune's study therefore supports our suggestion that surgery facilitates learning. It must be weighed against data from a recent study by MacRae and colleagues,[38] in which category examples (e.g. 'peach, grape, melon') were presented during different phases of the anesthetic

procedure including periods associated with arousal, e.g. immediately after the first incision. Postoperative testing using a category generation task revealed that patients learned the category examples when they were presented pre-induction, but not when they were presented during any part of the anesthetic procedure. In this study, surgical stimulation was not sufficient to enable learning during anesthesia.

To conclude, the evidence for learning during anesthesia is equivocal, with approximately the same number of studies obtaining evidence for learning as failing to do so. Recent methodological improvements, for example monitoring depth of anesthesia[12] and manipulating the time of stimulus presentation with respect to anesthesia and the surgical procedure,[38] are very welcome but have yet to clarify the picture. We offer a possible explanation, that the probability of learning during anesthesia is a function of levels of epinephrine or norepinephrine as well as of depth of anesthesia. This hypothesis helps explain the difficulty of demonstrating learning during conscious sedation in healthy volunteers, and our observation of memory for stimuli presented during surgery despite our earlier failure to observe learning during a period of preoperative sedation. Importantly, the hypothesis is testable. We hope it will stimulate research, broadening our understanding of the mechanisms of consciousness and learning by encouraging researchers to consider the hormonal changes induced by surgery, as well as the pharmacological and cognitive changes caused by the anesthetic.

References

1. Andrade J. Learning during anaesthesia: A review. *Br J Psychol* 1995; **86**:479–506.
2. Ghoneim MM, Block RI. Learning and memory during general anesthesia: An update. *Anesthesiology* 1997; **87**:387–410.
3. Bonebakker AE, Jelicic M, Passchier J, Bonke B. Memory during general anesthesia: Practical and methodological aspects. *Conscious Cogn* 1996; **5**:542–561.
4. Merikle PM, Daneman M. Memory for unconsciously perceived events: Evidence from anesthetized patients. *Conscious Cogn* 1996; **5**:525–541.
5. Polster MR, Gray PA, O'Sullivan G, McCarthy RA, Park GR. Comparison of the sedative and amnesic effects of midazolam and propofol. *Br J Anaesth* 1993; **70**:612–616.

6. Block RI, Ghoneim MM, Pathak D, Kumar V, Hinrichs JV. Effects of a subanesthetic concentration of nitrous oxide on overt and covert assessments of memory and associative processes. *Psychopharmacology* 1988; **96**:324–331.

7. Chortkoff BS, Bennett HL, Eger EI. Subanesthetic concentrations of isoflurane suppress learning as defined by the category-example task. *Anesthesiology* 1993; **79**:16–22.

8. Dwyer R, Bennett HL, Eger EI, Heilbron D. Effects of isoflurane and nitrous oxide in subanesthetic concentrations on memory and responsiveness in volunteers. *Anesthesiology* 1992; **77**:888–898.

9. Gonsowski CT, Chortkoff BS, Eger EI, Bennett HL, Weiskopf RB. Subanesthetic concentrations of desflurane and isoflurane suppress explicit and implicit learning. *Anesth Analg* 1995; **80**:568–572.

10. Chortkoff BS, Gonsowski CT, Bennett HL, *et al.* Subanesthetic concentrations of desflurane and propofol suppress recall of emotionally charged information. *Anesth Analg* 1995; **81**:728–736.

11. Schwender D, Madler C, Klasing S, Peter K, Pöppel E. Anesthetic control of 40-Hz brain activity and implicit memory. *Conscious Cogn* 1996; **3**: 129–147.

12. Lubke GH, Kerssens C, Phaf H, Sebel PS. Dependence of explicit and implicit memory on hypnotic state in trauma patients, *Anesthesiology*. 1999; **90**:670–680.

13. Andrade J. Investigations of hypesthesia: Using anesthetics to explore relationships between consciousness, learning and memory. *Conscious Cogn* 1996; **5**:562–580.

14. Shepard RN, Teghtsoonian M. Retention of information under conditions approaching a steady state. *J Exp Psychol* 1961; **62**:302–309.

15. Andrade J, Sapsford D, Jeevaratnum RD, Pickworth AJ, Jones JG. The coherent frequency in the EEG as an objective measure of cognitive function during propofol sedation. *Anesth Analg* 1996; **83**:1279–1284.

16. Jacoby LL, Woloshyn V, Kelley C. Becoming famous without being recognized: Unconscious influences of memory produced by divided attention. *J Exp Psychol (Gen)* 1989; **118**:115–125.

17. Jelicic M, de Roode A, Bovill JG, Bonke B. Unconscious learning during general anaesthesia. *Anaesthesia* 1992; **47**:835–837.

18. Squire LR, McKee R. Influence of prior events on cognitive judgements in amnesia. *J Exp Psychol (Learn Mem Cogn)* 1992; **18**:106–115.

19. Andrade J, Englert L, Harper C, Edwards ND (submitted manuscript). Comparing the effects of stimulation and propofol infusion rate on implicit and explicit memory formation.

20. Roorda-Hrdlicková V, Wolters G, Bonke B, Phaf RH. Unconscious perception during general anaesthesia, demonstrated by an implicit memory task. In Bonke B, Fitch W, Millar K (eds). *Memory and Awareness in Anaesthesia*. Lisse/Amsterdam: Swets & Zeitlinger, 1990; 150–155.

21. Jelicic M, Bonke B, Wolters G, Phaf RH. Implicit memory for words presented during general anaesthesia. *Eur J Cog Psychol* 1992; **4**:71–80.

22. Murphy ST, Zajonc RB. Affect, cognition, and awareness: Affective priming with optimal and suboptimal stimulus exposures. *J Pers Soc Psychol* 1993; **64**:723–739.

23. Zajonc RB. On the primacy of affect. *Am Psychol* 1984; **39**:117–124.

24. Stapleton CL, Andrade J. An investigation of learning during propofol sedation and anesthesia using the process dissociation procedure. *Anesthesiology* (in press).

25. Cork RC, Heaton JF, Campbell CE, Kihlstrom JF. Is there implicit memory after propofol sedation? *Br J Anaesth* 1996; **76**:492–498.

26. Gupta P, Ghabrial N, Raab R, *et al.* Implicit and explicit memory function and stress response during general and combined general/regional anesthesia. *Anesth Analg* 1996; **82**:S148.

27. Jacoby LL, Toth J.P, Yonelinas AP. Separating conscious and unconscious influences in memory: Measuring recollection. *J Exp Psychol (Gen)* 1993; **122**:139–154.

28. Schmitter-Edgecombe M. Effects of divided attention on perceptual and conceptual memory tests: An analysis using a process-dissociation approach. *Mem Cognition* 1999; **27**:512–525.

29. Curran T, Hintzman DL. Violations of the independence assumption in process dissociation. *J Exp Psychol (Learn Mem Cogn)* 1995; **21**:531–547.

30. Plummer G. Improved method for the determination of propofol in blood by high performance liquid chromatography. *J Chromatogr* 1987; **421**:171–176.

31. Cahill L, Prins B, Weber M, McGaugh JL. Beta-adrenergic activation and memory for emotional events. *Nature* 1994; **371**:702–704.

32. Roozendaal B, Carmi O, McGaugh JL. Adrenocortical suppression blocks the memory-enhancing effects of amphetamine and epinephrine. *Proc Natl Acad Sci USA* 1996; **93**:1429–1433.

33. Weinberger NM, Gold PE, Sternberg DB. Epinephrine enables Pavlovian fear conditioning under anaesthesia. *Science* 1984; **223**:605–607.

34. Gold PE, Weinberger NM, Sternberg, DB. Epinephrine-induced learning under general anesthesia: Retention performance at several training-testing intervals. *Behav Neurosci* 1985; **99**:1019–1022.

35. Dariola MK, Yadava A, Malhotra, S. Effect of epinephrine on learning under anaesthesia. *J Indian Acad Appl Psychol* 1993; **19**:47–51.

36. El-Zahaby M, Ghoneim MM, Johnson GM, Gormezano I. Effects of subanesthetic concentrations

of isoflurane and their interactions with epinephrine on acquisition and retention of the rabbit nictitating membrane response. *Anesthesiology* 1994; **81**: 229–237.

37. Bethune DW, Ghosh S, Gray B, *et al.* Learning during general anaesthesia: Implicit recall after methohexitone or propofol infusion. *Br J Anaesth* 1992; **69**:197–199.

38. MacRae WJ, Thorp JM, Millar K. Category generation testing in the search for implicit memory under general anaesthesia. *Br J Anaesth* 1998; **80**:588–593.

Chapter 5

BIS and memory during anesthesia

Chantal Kerssens and Peter S. Sebel

Contents

Memory during anesthesia

Surgical patients undergoing general anesthesia should not be aware of any events during anesthesia, nor are they supposed to have any postoperative memory for surgical events. Traditionally, memory for surgery is assessed by asking patients whether or not they can remember anything that occurred in the operating room while they were under the influence of anesthesia. Asking for such recall is a direct test of memory, in that explicit reference is made to the learning episode. Such tests are also referred to as explicit memory tests. Most patients are unable to report any memory for surgical events and this absence of recall is often taken as evidence that no memory for intraoperative events has been formed.

However, a simple recall question is not a sensitive method for probing intraoperative memory. Recent cognitive and neuropsychological research demonstrates that information stored in memory can influence later behavior without conscious recollection of the episode during which it was

acquired.[1–3] Patients with memory disorders, for instance, generally show poor recall for previously studied words (e.g. PENSION). However, when asked to complete word stems (e.g. PEN...) with the first word that comes to mind, the study of a word increases the probability of using that word for stem completion. Tasks like these are termed *indirect* (or implicit), in that, no reference to the learning episode is made. Memory is revealed in a facilitation or change in task performance attributable to the information acquired previously ('priming'). Numerous studies have observed priming effects in the absence of conscious recall in both amnesic and normal subjects.[3–5]

The notion of implicit (or unconscious) memory was readily adopted in anesthesia research and a variety of techniques have been applied to investigate memory under anesthesia.[6, 7] Typically, a patient is presented with verbal material some time during the anesthetic, usually shortly after induction or incision. Postoperatively, explicit memory is assessed directly with a recall question or recognition task. In addition, patients may be asked to perform an indirect task in which material presented during anesthesia can be used. Memory is evident when postoperative responses are influenced or dominated by the material presented during anesthesia. A number of studies have observed implicit memory effects in the absence of conscious recollection,[6,7] and recent meta-analysis demonstrated overall evidence of memory for specific information presented under anesthesia.[8]

Despite extensive memory assessment, it remains unclear to what extent inadequate anesthesia (i.e. moments of awareness) contributes to postoperative memory. It is generally agreed upon that performance on memory tasks is mediated by conscious as well as unconscious processes, meaning that indirect memory task performance does not necessarily reflect unconscious memory processes, nor do direct tests exclusively measure conscious memory processes.[9,10] Conversely, both types of tasks may be equally sensitive to intraoperative information processing and memories.[8] Because memory tasks are not 'process-pure,' awareness is hard to quantify in retrospect. One solution to this issue entails monitoring of hypnotic adequacy *during* stimulus presentation. Few studies investigating memory under anesthesia have done so, however, which may explain inconsistency in results.[11] Moreover, monitoring hypnotic state has been problematic in general,[12] but is becoming increasingly feasible and accurate with recent advances in analysis of the electroencephalogram (EEG).

BIS monitoring technology

The EEG is a complex signal representing electrical activity of the cerebral cortex. It is a largely random appearing signal with no obvious repetitive patterns or shapes correlating with particular underlying events. Therefore, the waveform itself is of little diagnostic value. The state of the brain is reflected, however, in some statistical attributes derived from the EEG, like the degree of synchrony in neuronal firing of cortical (pyramidal) cells. This statistical approach lies at the heart of EEG monitoring for anesthesia-related purposes.[13,14]

The EEG is an alternating voltage composed of many waveforms. After acquiring the raw EEG, the analogue signal may be translated into its digital counterpart for further analysis. On the one hand, voltage changes over time can be examined, which

is referred to as analysis in the time domain.[13] In contrast, frequency domain analysis examines signal activity as a function of frequency, which evolves around the study of sine waves. Sine waves are simple mathematical functions defined by three basic elements: *amplitude* (expressed in μV), which is one half the peak-to-peak voltage, *frequency* (expressed in Hz), which is the number of cycles per second, and *phase angle*, reflecting the waveform starting point relative to time 0. A typical sine wave starts at time 0 with amplitude 0 and deviation from this typical starting point can be expressed (in degrees between 0° and 360°) as the fraction of a full cycle that the sinusoid shifted in time (Figure 5.1). Any complex time-varying signal can be decomposed into its sine wave components (Figure 5.2) and converted into a representation of frequency and amplitude, known as a Fourier transform. The resultant power spectrum comprises a series of discrete values corresponding to particular frequency components and their power (V^2).

From the power spectrum, several parameters have been derived to indicate anesthetic depth. Frequency bands (delta, theta, alpha, beta) can be identified in the EEG and corresponding power values ('band power') have been related to psychophysiologic state. Also, the frequency below which 50% and 95% of the power in the EEG resides can be calculated, referred to as median frequency (MF) and spectral edge frequency (SEF), respectively. Power variables suffer several problems, however. They are sensitive to specific EEG patterns induced by different drugs[13] and may show biphasic response to certain anesthetics.[15] In addition, anesthesia-induced burst suppression (i.e. alternating periods of normal to high voltage activity changing to low voltage or isoelectricity) is problematic for spectral analysis,[16] nor can spectral analysis quantify the amount of phase coupling in the EEG.

Phase coupling is an important characteristic of nonlinear systems like the brain[14] and refers to interfrequency dependency. Frequency relationships may be examined by bispectral analysis of the EEG, which measures the correlation of phase between different frequency components and quantifies their bicoherence and joint magnitude. Hence, both phase and power information in the EEG is incorporated. Although the physiologic meaning of phase relationships remains unclear, strong phase coupling may imply that two components have a common

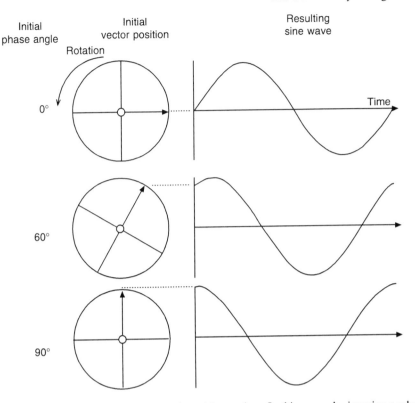

Figure 5.1. A rotating vector or spoke describes a sinusoid over time. In this example, imagine a wheel rotating counterclockwise with a light source in its rim adjacent to the marked spoke. As the wheel turns, a graph of the vertical position of the light versus time will produce the indicated sine wave. The rotational speed of the wheel determines the frequency of the resulting sine wave, and the size of the wheel determines its amplitude. The initial angle of the spoke is the phase angle of the sine wave. In this illustration, the wheel starts at three different phase angles. Note that the sine wave frequency is independent of the phase angle. (Reprinted with permission from Rampil IJ. A primer for EEG signal processing in anesthesia. *Anesthesiology* 1998; **89**: 980–1002.)

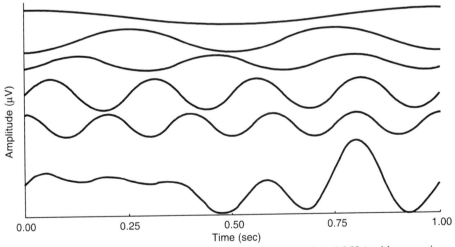

Figure 5.2. The upper five traces are five sine wave components (1, 2, 3, 4, and 5 Hz) with respective amplitudes of (1, 1.5, 1, 2, and 1.5 μV). The components have different offsets for illustrative purposes only. At the bottom is the sum of the five components. (Reprinted with permission from Kluwer Academic Publishers from Sigl JC, Chamoun NG. An introduction to bispectral analysis for the electroencephalogram. *J Clin Monit* 1994; **10**:92–404.)

generator or that the neural circuitry they drive may synthesize a new dependent component.[13] For clinical purposes, a single variable has been developed, the bispectral index (BIS), incorporating a set of EEG features, each chosen to have a specific range of anesthetic effect where they perform best.[13] Two parameters quantify the amount of burst suppression in the EEG associated with deep anesthesia. Two other features express the amount of high frequency (beta) activity, reflecting moderate or light sedation. Combining these parameters (using a nonlinear algorithm generated by an iterative process of data modeling) produces BIS, which ranges from 100 (awake) to 0 (minimal brain activity) and decreases continuously with increasing hypnosis. BIS was initially correlated with movement to surgical incision and intubation.[17–23] Although BIS predicted movement occasionally better than hemodynamic or other EEG variables, results were not uniformly positive. As movement may reflect spinal rather than cortical activity, however, relatively low correlations with cerebral parameters can be expected.[13] Therefore, BIS was recently developed in relation to cortical functions and correlated with behavioral assessments of sedation and hypnosis (for a description of studies see later).

The clinical utility of BIS monitoring is indicated by several studies where BIS was targeted to remain between 60 and 40 – referred to as adequate anesthesia. Compared to standard clinical practice monitoring hemodynamic stability, BIS guided anesthetic administration resulted in lower infusion rates of propofol[24] and lower volatile anesthetic usage in the absence of additional opioid requirement.[25] During maintenance, no significant hemodynamic responses were observed[24,26] and less intraoperative movement has been reported in BIS-guided anesthetics.[26] In addition, emergence and recovery from anesthesia may be faster.[24,25]

Auditory evoked reponses

Other monitoring techniques of central anesthetic effect have been proposed as well. Upon auditory stimulation, the EEG displays specific features representing the passage of electrical activity from the cochlea to the auditory cortex. These auditory evoked responses (AER) have been studied extensively and related to auditory information processing during general anesthesia.[27] The AER waveform has a series of peaks and troughs of different amplitudes and latencies. Midlatency auditory evoked potentials (MLAEP) arise 8 to 60 milliseconds (ms) after stimulation and appear most suitable for monitoring anesthetic depth as they show graded changes with anesthetic concentration.[28] In contrast, brain stem responses (0 to 8 ms) tend to be unaffected by anesthetics,[28,29] whereas the late cortical responses (60 to 1000 ms) are heavily attenuated.[30,31] Importantly, the AER is not affected by neuromuscular blocking drugs.[32] The MLAEP is a transient response elicited by stimulation rates near 10 clicks per second (10 Hz). When a train of stimuli is delivered at a sufficiently fast rate, however, responses to successive stimuli overlap and a steady state response occurs. This auditory steady state response (ASSR) reaches an amplitude maximum at stimulation rates near 40 Hz.[33] Furthermore, at certain stimulation frequencies, power can be observed at a particular frequency in the absence of power at other frequencies, referred to as the 'coherent frequency' (CF).[34] The next section discusses MLAEP, ASSR, and CF in relation to information processing and anesthesia.

Whereas the awake MLAEP is characterized by three periodic waveforms of high amplitude and short latency, anesthesia tends to reduce amplitudes and to lengthen the latency of specific peaks (termed Pa, Pb) and troughs (Na, Nb).[29,35] According to Davies and colleagues, Pa and Nb latency best discriminated consciousness from unconsciousness, in terms of response to command ('squeeze my hand').[36] Positive response to command has been associated with Nb latencies of 46 ms or shorter,[37,38] but sensitivity of Nb latency for detecting responsiveness appears low. When anesthesia is deepened, Nb latency increases (to 54 ms) and response to command is lost.[38] Short Nb latencies and awake MLAEP patterns have also been associated with recall.[38,39] In order to assess MLAEP characteristics for implicit memory, Schwender *et al.* played cardiac surgical patients an audiotape containing the story of Robinson Crusoe following sternotomy.[40] MLAEP was recorded shortly prior to and after audiotape presentation. In patients displaying implicit memory (free association to Friday with the Crusoe story), Na and Pa latencies resembled the awake MLAEP (20 and 36 ms, respectively). In contrast, prolonged latencies (near 55 ms and 80 ms, respectively) were observed in patients demonstrating no implicit memory effect for the Crusoe story. Villemure *et al.* observed increased Nb latencies in patients without implicit memory for words presented during abdominal hysterectomy.[41] From these studies it can be seen that it is yet difficult to separate small behavioral changes and their effects on the AER from the profound effect of anesthesia on the AER.[38] Clearly, the AER needs further refinement as a monitor of anesthesia.

Munglani *et al.* assessed responses to a series of cognitive tests in volunteers breathing increasing concentrations of isoflurane.[34,42] CF decreased as well as psychological performance and three levels were discriminated: conscious awareness with explicit memory (CF = 32.8 Hz) or without explicit memory (CF = 24.8 Hz), and no responsiveness with no implicit memory (CF = 14.8 Hz). In a different study, Andrade *et al.* found a 0.47 correlation between CF and short-term memory performance during propofol sedation.[43] Apparently, variation in immediate information processing is only partially captured by CF ($R^2 = 0.22$). With increasing concentration of isoflurane (0.26% to 0.5%), the 40-Hz ASSR amplitude tends to decrease from 0.24 µV to 0.04 µV.[44] Concordantly, responsiveness declines and a 0.95 prediction probability for loss of consciousness has been reported for the ASSR.[44,45]

The isolated forearm technique

In 1977, Tunstall first described a behavioral method for detecting consciousness, referred to as the isolated forearm technique (IFT). It comprises inflation of a pneumatic cuff around the patient's arm prior to administration of neuromuscular blocking drugs, thereby allowing the patient to communicate wakefulness by moving the arm either spontaneously or upon request.[46–48] The use of IFT has revealed that patients may respond to command in the absence of postoperative recall, demonstrating the imperfect relation between awareness and recall.

Millar and Watkinson observed response to command in 33% of patients undergoing gynecological surgery.[49] Postoperatively, patients demonstrated significant recognition of words played following first incision, in the absence of conscious recall. In contrast, King *et al.* observed patient response rates of 33% (laryngoscopy, intubation) and 97%

(incision), but no cued recall of words played during these periods.[50] In a study by Russell and Wang, no patient responded to command and no evidence of intraoperative word priming was subsequently found.[51] These studies suggest that IFT-monitoring may prevent cognitive processing and memory formation during anesthesia, but observations are limited and mixed. Also, response to command can be hard to distinguish unequivocally from spontaneous movement. The use of IFT as (on-line) monitor of anesthesia is further complicated by the fact that the technique itself relies upon the auditory channel. IFT may indicate that information is being processed, but it cannot *monitor* perception of information other than the command, like memory test material. Therefore, the technique is of limited use to memory research during anesthesia. The same applies to AER-related measures depending upon auditory clicks to be obtained.

BIS, consciousness and recall

Flaishon *et al.* examined the ability of BIS to predict return of consciousness as measured by IFT.[52] They administered 40 pre-surgical patients either a single bolus thiopental (4 mg/kg) or propofol (2 mg/kg) and assessed consciousness by asking patients to squeeze the investigator's fingers once and then twice. No response to command was observed below BIS 59. Consciousness was regained more rapidly at high BIS values than at lower values. Patients recovering in the propofol bolus group had a less than 5% chance of regaining consciousness within 50 seconds if BIS was 65. For thiopental, the probability of awareness was even smaller. Importantly, recorded times until recovery of consciousness varied widely between patients, illustrating the potential for awareness during intubation and skin incision in patients in whom drugs wear off rapidly.

To allow for more subtle assessments of sedation, other investigators observed responses to increasingly intense stimuli. Scores on an Observer Assessment of Alertness/Sedation (OAA/S) Scale typically range from 5 (alert) to 0 (deep sleep), depending upon response to one's name (score 5 to 3), to mild prodding or shaking (score 2 or 1) or to noxious stimulation (score 0). Consciousness is usually defined as OAA/S-scores of 3 and higher. Observed relations between OAA/S and BIS are displayed in Table 5.1. High correlations between OAA/S and BIS (r = 0.91) have been reported for sedation with sevoflurane, whereas SEF, MF and end tidal concentrations were found to change less consistently with level of sedation.[15] Liu and colleagues administered 4.5–20 mg midazolam in increments of 0.5–1 mg bolus to patients scheduled for elective surgery until they became unresponsive.[53] BIS showed a good relation to OAA/S scores during sedation onset (r = 0.82) and a moderately good relation to responsiveness during recovery (r = 0.60). With increasing sedation, SEF decreased (r = 0.46) as did beta power, whereas alpha power increased. During recovery, none of these variables changed significantly.[53] No consistent changes for the theta or delta power bands, or for MF were found in this study. Good correlations between BIS and OAA/S have been observed during onset and recovery of propofol sedation as well (r = 0.74 and 0.71, respectively).[54] In this study, SEF did not change significantly during sedation onset. BIS predicts consciousness versus loss of consciousness highly accurately, as expressed by prediction probabilities of 0.94–0.99, and is more accurate than other EEG parameters as well as targeted or measured concentration propofol.[15, 55–57] The accuracy is good at high BIS values, whereas patient variation in consciousness tends to increase at lower BIS levels.

With propofol, consciousness is lost in 50% of patients at BIS values near 65 and in 95% of patients at values near 50.[55,56] The addition of alfentanil may result in quicker loss of consciousness, i.e. at higher BIS values.[55] Nitrous oxide has similar effects when administered concurrently with propofol, although the agent is a weak sedative by itself.[58] Response was lost earlier in patients sedated with propofol in 30% N_2O (BIS = 70) than when sedated with propofol alone (BIS = 57).[57] BIS readings obtained by current algorithms (3.0 and higher) tend to be independent of anesthetic regimen and have been found largely insensitive to the differential effects of midazolam, propofol, isoflurane.[56] Reports that certain drug combinations alter BIS readings may reflect the use of earlier algorithms that were more sensitive to differential drug effects.

Before affecting consciousness, however, anesthetics tend to attenuate memory. Patients may respond to command in the absence of recall for information presented to them while being responsive. Apparently, information processing *per se* is not sufficient for memory to occur. Liu and colleagues assessed conscious recall for pictures shown at different levels of propofol sedation and observed 100% recall in fully alert participants, corresponding to an average BIS of 95.4.[54] Recall rapidly declined to 63% when responding was lethargic (BIS = 93.4), further to 40% when response was virtually absent (BIS = 87.3), and no recall was observed when participants were unresponsive (BIS = 80.8). Similar results were reported by Iselin-Chaves *et al.* (Table 5.2), in addition to an increased probability of recall when alfentanil had been given concordantly with propofol.[55] Because alfentanil has no known memory effects, this observation may reflect the use of behavioral indices of consciousness and not necessarily an effect of alfentanil on memory. As we have seen, consciousness may be lost quicker when alfentanil is provided. When a patient appears unresponsive, anesthetic concentration is likely decreased, resulting in an increased probability of information processing and recall.

Glass *et al.* presented volunteers with a picture or word at several drug concentrations of propofol, midazolam or isoflurane, and subsequently assessed free and cued recall.[56] The relation between BIS and recall was comparable for the different anesthetics, although the memory curve for isoflurane appeared flatter than those for propofol or midazolam, suggesting a different relation to memory function. Pooled data in this study showed a 50% probability of recall at BIS values near 86, declining to 5% at BIS values near 65. As was observed for consciousness, recall is accurately predicted at high BIS values, whereas increased interpatient variability emerges at lower values. The incidence of recall, however, is likely overestimated due to flawed memory assessment. When correct identification of presented stimuli is taken as evidence of memory, guessing and chance performance are included as well.

BIS and indirect memory assessment

An important characteristic of the aforementioned memory tasks is that participants are asked to what extent they remember or recognize material presented previously during anesthesia. In contrast, the tasks that will be discussed next can be performed without referring to the learning episode. Even if participants are instructed to remember presented

Table 5.1. BIS during sedation: overview of studies using the Observer Assessment of Alertness/Sedation (OAA/S)-scale

Study	Sedative	N	Descriptive	OAA/S						r
				5	4	3	2	1	0	
Katoh et al.[15]	sevoflurane (0.2–1.8%)	69	Median	95.8	78.3		73.1	66.1	40.1	0.911
Liu et al.[53]	midazolam (4.5–20 mg)	26	Mean (SD) *during onset*	95.4 (2.3)	90.3 (4.5)	86.6 (4.6)	75.6 (9.7)	69.2 (13.9)	—	0.815
			Mean (SD) *during recovery*	—	90.8 (6.0)	82.3 (7.3)	75.2 (10.2)	69.2 (13.9)	—	0.596
Liu et al.[54]	propofol (220–560 mg)	10	Mean (SD) *during onset*	94.5 (2.9)	93.3 (3.3)	89.0 (6.1)	80.1 (8.7)	75.6 (7.5)	—	0.744
			Mean (SD) *during recovery*	—	93.8 (0.8)	84.9 (5.9)	82.4 (10.5)	75.6 (7.5)	—	0.705
Iselin-Chaves et al.[55]	propofol (0–6 µg/ml)	40	LOC_{50} (range)				64	(61 –66)		
	+ alfentanil (50 ng/ml)		LOC_{95} (range)				49	(45 –54)		
	+ alfentanil (100 ng/ml)		LOC_{50} (range)				67	(64 –69)		
			LOC_{95} (range)				63	(57 –70)		
			LOC_{50} (range)				72	(67 –76)		
			LOC_{95} (range)				54	(45 –64)		
Kearse et al.[57]	propofol (0–4 µg/ml) + N20 (30%)	20	LOC_{50} (95%CI)				65.2	(63 –67.6)	—	
			LOC_{95} (95%CI)				53.8	(48.7–59)		
			LOC_{50} (95%CI)				75.7	(71.2–80)	—	
			LOC_{95} (95%CI)				68.3	(60.5–76)		

OAA/S-scores: 5 = patient responds readily to name spoken in normal tone, 4 = lethargic response to name spoken in normal tone, 3 = responds only after name is called loudly and/or repeatedly, 2 = responds only after mild prodding or shaking, 1 = does not respond to mild prodding or shaking/responds only after noxious stimulation, 0 = does not respond to noxious stimulation. LOC = loss of consciousness, in 50% of patients (LOC_{50}) and 95% of patients (LOC_{95}).

Table 5.2. BIS in relation to conscious recall

Study	Sedative	N	Recall					
			100%	63%	50%	40%	5%	0%
Liu et al.[54]	propofol (220–560 mg)	10	94.5 (2.9)	93.4 (3.3)		87.3 (6.1)		80.8 (8.3)
Iselin-Chaves et al.[55]	propofol (0–6 µg/ml)	40			89 (85–93)		79 (70–88)	
	+ alfentanil (100 ng/ml)				83 (77–90)		67 (51–83)	
Glass et al.[56]	propofol (0–6 µg/ml)	72			86 (83–100)		77 (72–83)	
	isoflurane (0.25–1%)				95 (81–100)		42 (13–71)	
	midazolam (0–300 ng/ml)				84 (78–89)		68 (59–78)	
	pooled				86 (83–89)		64 (57–71)	

Data are mean BIS (Sd) or (95%CI)

material, the task can be completed without conscious recollection by making use of general or implicit knowledge. In that case, participants respond with whatever comes to mind.

Most impressive is a recent study by Lubke and colleagues, investigating memory function in 96 patients with injuries varying from minor to severe trauma, thereby including a wide variety of hypnotic states.[59] After etomidate induction, patients were played 16 target words via headphones. Each word was presented consecutively for 3 min and this period was time-locked to several indicators of hypnotic state, including BIS. In that way, hypnotic state during word presentation could be related to postoperative memory performance. Mean BIS (± SD) during word presentation was 54 ± 14 (range 20–97). Postoperatively, patients performed a word stem completion task in which they were encouraged to use the word stem (e.g. fan…) as a cue to recall intraoperatively presented words (e.g. *fancy*). Otherwise, the first word coming to mind could be used for stem completion. Furthermore, they were instructed to use presented words in one part of the test (inclusion part), whereas such words should be avoided in the other (exclusion part). In the latter case, another word would have to be used for stem completion (e.g. *fantastic*). Now, a target word like *fancy* may be named by sheer chance, a probability that is reflected by the frequency with which it occurs for stem completion without prior presentation ('base rate'). Memory is evident when in the inclusion part, target words are used more often than would be expected by chance alone, i.e. when hit rates are higher than base rate. This is exactly what was found in the trauma study: patients were more prone to say *fancy* when that word had been presented to them during surgery than when it had not been presented.[59] Because both unconscious and conscious memory processes lead to responding with target words in this part of the test, however, the two sources of memory cannot be separated based on the inclusion part alone. Addition of the exclusion part indicates the extent to which subjects exert control over their responses, reflecting a more conscious level of word processing.[9,10] Whenever hit rates in the exclusion part are *lower* than base rate, the subject is capable, consciously or automatically, to avoid previously presented words.

No sign of controlled responding was observed in the trauma study, however, providing strong evidence for an unconsciously mediated memory effect. In addition, a model in which the probability of memory varied across patients provided a better data fit than a model in which the probability was equal for all patients. It seems safe to assume that depth of anesthesia was the only relevant factor varying widely in this group of patients, and consequently, that variation in memory can be best explained by individual differences in hypnotic state. This is consistent with the fact that hit rates clearly declined with deepening of hypnotic state, as reflected by categorized BIS-levels, indicating a dependency of memory function upon hypnotic state (Figure 5.3).[59] BIS proved the only significant predictor of memory, although the two correlated weakly ($R^2 = 0.12$). Hence, BIS may have limited clinical value in signaling implicit memory function.

Interestingly, trauma patients still displayed memory for words presented at BIS levels assumed to indicate adequate anesthesia (i.e. BIS between 40 and 60).[59] This contrasts with two studies where no memory effect was observed for auditory material presented at this level. Struys *et al.* played 58 female patients undergoing gynecological surgery with propofol anesthesia a 15-min audio tape.[26] It contained the story of Robinson Crusoe and was presented to 28 patients while BIS was targeted to remain between 40 and 60 (group 1), whereas classical signs of anesthetic adequacy guided anesthesia in the remaining 30 patients (group 2). Afterwards, none of the patients reported conscious recall for surgery. Average BIS readings throughout the surgical procedure did not differ for the two groups, but implicit memory for the Crusoe story was reported to occur less often in the BIS guided anesthetics ($n = 0$) than in the standard monitoring group ($n = 3$). Despite a failure to establish base rate performance (3 out of 30 people may associate Friday to Robinson Crusoe without prior presentation of the story) this study suggests abolition of information processing when BIS resides below 60. A similar observation was made by Kerssens *et al.* who presented exemplars from common word categories to 41 surgical patients (group E) while BIS remained between 40 and 60.[60] Anesthetics in the control group ($n = 41$) were monitored likewise, but here patients listened to filler sounds instead of words. BIS was targeted successfully and average BIS (± SD) values of 43.5 ± 4.6 (group E) and 46 ± 4.8 (group C) were obtained during audio presentation. Postoperatively, none of the patients

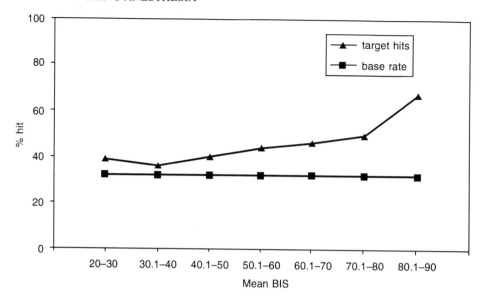

Figure 5.3. Increase of target hit rates compared with base rate performance at categorized bispectral index values. (Reprinted with permission from Lubke GH, Kerssens C, Phaf H, Sebel PS. Dependence of explicit and implicit memory on hypnotic state in trauma patients. *Anesthesiology* 1999; **90**:670–680.)

consciously recalled the surgical period, nor did groups differ in category exemplar generation. Hence, priming of category exemplars presented at adequate levels of anesthesia could not be demonstrated, whereas the same stimuli induced a clear implicit memory effect in two previous studies that did not control for hypnotic state, however.[61,62]

From these studies it cannot be concluded to what extent memory function is preserved during adequate anesthesia. As indicated above, it may be preserved in some patients but not in others, depending upon the type of patient and surgery (e.g. trauma versus elective). Vigilance and information processing are likely to be more vital to a patient who fears for his or her life than for a patient undergoing day-case surgery. Hence, the former may display signs of information processing (i.e. memory), whereas the latter may not. Circumstantial variables like psychological and physiological stress, the emotionality of the surgical setting and the relevance of information to one's survival and well-being, could make a difference when it comes to cognitive functioning during anesthesia. Clearly, additional studies are required.

In a different study, investigating memory function during a surgical procedure where anesthetic is known to be light, Lubke *et al.* presented 24 female patients undergoing cesarean section postpartum a set of words while breathing 70% N_2O in oxygen supplemented with 0.2% isoflurane and morphine.[63] The memory paradigm and stimuli were similar to the trauma study.[59] Mean BIS ($\pm$ SD) during word presentation was 76.3 ± 3. None of the patients claimed recall of intraoperative events or words, but patients were able to make correct inclusion/exclusion decisions, indicating they controlled their responses in an automatic way. This study demonstrates that information acquired during light anesthesia can be employed subsequently in the absence of conscious memory.

At light levels of anesthesia (0, 1 or 2 µg/ml propofol), Leslie *et al.* presented 14 volunteers with the answers to Trivial Pursuit type of questions.[64] After recovery from each infusion, administered on three consecutive days, questions were presented in a multiple-choice format and percentages correct were calculated after adjustment for correct guessing. All questions were answered correctly when no propofol had been given, declining to 50% correct upon infusion of 0.66 µg/ml, corresponding to a mean ($\pm$ SD) BIS value of 91 ± 1. Unfortunately, the amount of conscious recall was not reported, rendering it unclear to what extent memory performance was explicit.

Concluding remarks

From this review, it is becoming increasingly clear that multiple levels of information processing and memory function should be distinguished during anesthesia. As Lubke *et al.* suggested, the dichotomy of conscious (explicit) memory on the one hand and unconscious (implicit) memory on the other, seems too crude.[63] Anesthesia rapidly attenuates responsiveness, and a 50% deterioration in learning and conscious recall is observed at low anesthetic concentrations and BIS values near 90.[54–56,62] Response to command may be sustained during deepening of the anesthesia,[52] while memory becomes unconscious. When BIS approaches 75, intentional and controlled responding may be observed in the absence of overt memory for presented information.[63] This corresponds to the wakefulness without conscious recall reported in IFT-studies and by Munglani *et al.*[34] Further deepening of the anesthesia seems to attenuate the controlled aspect of memory, allowing only unconscious and uncontrolled memory to occur. Trauma patients demonstrated implicit memory for words presented at BIS levels below 60, without being able to exclude presented words and hence, to exert control over their responses.[59] Other studies, however, suggest absence of information processing and memory function at adequate levels of anesthesia, as reflected by BIS between 40 and 60.[26,60] It remains to be seen whether and why cognitive functioning is preserved in some patients but not in others at these levels of anesthesia.

Clearly, more research should be directed towards memory function during different levels of anesthesia. Anesthetic monitoring techniques and psychological memory assessments are becoming increasingly sophisticated and their synthesis seems a most promising tool in unraveling the relation between hypnotic adequacy, information processing and postoperative memory. In doing so, special attention should be directed towards implicit memory function, as depth of anesthesia studies have mainly focused on consciousness and recall, thereby elucidating certain aspects of memory while ignoring others. Despite growing expertise, studies are often flawed in that memory effects are not adequately distinguished from chance (base line) performance. Consequently, the incidence of memory may be overestimated. Furthermore,

presentation of auditory information should be time-locked to dynamics of the autonomic (HR, BP) and central nervous system (EEG, AER, IFT). Auditorily obtained monitors, like AER and IFT, are of limited use in this respect, as presentation of memory test material cannot coincide with assessment of hypnotic state. Also, attention may be directed towards individual differences in hypnotic state, memory function and information processing in general. So far, patients have been pooled to yield group averages, whereas their variation in the aforementioned variables could provide valuable insights into the (cognitive) dynamics of anesthesia. If we can explain why some patients seem to process information whereas others do not, and identify the variables contributing to information processing during anesthesia, our prediction of memory and awareness will become more accurate and hence, will improve patient monitoring during anesthesia.

With respect to the (CNS) monitoring techniques reviewed here, EEG bispectral analyses seem to provide for a practical and valuable on-line monitor. As it incorporates more information residing within the EEG than traditional (power) analyses, it is not surprising that BIS predicts consciousness and recall frequently better than other cortically derived measures. This seems particularly so at light levels of anesthesia, where little variation among patients and anesthetics is observed. The observation that BIS relates well to behavioral measures of sedation (i.e. responsiveness) at levels where responsiveness may be observed supports its feasibility as a measure of hypnotic state. In addition, BIS may accurately predict conscious memory during sedation as conscious memory is dependent upon attention and hence, responsiveness. When anesthesia is deepened, however, the differential anesthetic effects on memory become more apparent and responsiveness is lost. The increased variation between patients and anesthetics in consciousness and memory observed at lower BIS levels, indicates that BIS was not designed to monitor memory function during anesthesia. This notion is supported by the observation that only a low proportion of variance in (implicit) memory can be explained by BIS.[59] Memory function may be related to hypnotic state and therefore to BIS, but as anesthesia is deepened, subcortical learning and memory processes may prevail that are not well captured by parameters like BIS.

References

1. Weiskrantz L. *The unseen and the unknown, consciousness lost and found: A neuropsychological exploration.* Oxford: Oxford University Press, 1997; 7–35.
2. Schacter DL. Implicit memory: history and current status. *J Exp Psychol* (*Learn Mem Cogn*) 1987; **13**:501–518.
3. Richardson-Klavehn A, Bjork RA. Measures of memory. *Annu Rev Psychol* 1988; **39**:475–543.
4. Schacter DL, Chiu CYP, Ochsner KN. Implicit memory: a selective review. *Annu Rev Neurosci* 1993; **16**:159–182.
5. Shanks DR, St. John MF. Characteristic of dissociable human learning systems. *Behav Brain Sci* 1994; **17**:367–447.
6. Ghoneim MM, Block RI. Learning and consciousness during general anesthesia. *Anesthesiology* 1992; **76**:279–305.
7. Andrade J. Learning during anaesthesia: a review. *Br J Psychol* 1995; **86**:479–506.
8. Merikle PM, Daneman M. Memory for unconsciously perceived events: evidence from anesthetized patients. *Conscious Cogn* 1996; **5**: 525–541.
9. Jacoby LL. A process dissociation framework: separating automatic from intentional uses of memory. *J Mem Lang* 1991; **30**:513–541.
10. Jacoby LL, Toth JP, Yonelinas AP. Separating conscious and unconscious influences of memory: measuring recollection. *J Exp Psychol (Gen)* 1993; **122**:139–154.
11. Bonebakker AE, Jelicic M, Passchier J, Bonke B. Memory under general anesthesia: practical and methodological aspects. *Conscious Cogn* 1996; **5**:542–561.
12. Schneider G, Sebel PS. Monitoring depth of anaesthesia. *Eur J Anaesthesiol* 1997; **14**(Suppl. 15):1–8.
13. Rampil IJ. A primer for EEG signal processing in anesthesia. *Anesthesiology* 1998; **89**:980–1002.
14. Sigl JC, Chamoun NG. An introduction to bispectral analysis for the electroencephalogram. *J Clin Monit* 1994; **10**:392–404.
15. Katoh T, Suzuki A, Ikeda K. Electroencephalographic derivatives as a tool for predicting the depth of sedation and anesthesia induced by sevoflurane. *Anesthesiology* 1998; **88**:642–650.
16. Billard V, Gambus PL, Chamoun N, Stanski DR, Shafer SL. A comparison of spectral edge, delta power, and bispectral index as EEG measures of alfentanil, propofol, and midazolam drug effect. *Clin Pharmacol Ther* 1997; **61**:45–58.
17. Kearse LA, Manberg P, Chamoun N, deBros F, Zaslavsky A. Bispectral analysis of the electroencephalogram correlates with patient movement to skin incision during propofol/nitrous oxide anesthesia. *Anesthesiology* 1994; **81**:1365–1370.
18. Kearse LA, Manberg P, deBros F, Chamoun N, Sinai V. Bispectral analysis of the electroencephalogram during induction of anesthesia may predict hemodynamic responses to laryngoscopy and intubation. *Electroencephalogr Clin Neurophysiol* 1994; **90**:194–200.
19. Sebel PS, Bowles SM, Saini V, Chamoun N. EEG bispectrum predicts movement during thiopental/isoflurane anesthesia. *J Clin Monit* 1995; **11**: 83–91.
20. Vernon JM, Lang E, Sebel PS, Manberg P. Prediction of movement using bispectral electroencephalographic analysis during propofol/alfentanil or isoflurane/alfentanil anesthesia. *Anesth Analg* 1995; **80**:780–785.
21. Leslie K, Sessler DI, Smith WS, *et al.* Prediction of movement during propofol/nitrous oxide anesthesia: performance of concentration, electroencephalographic, pupillary, and hemodynamic responses. *Anesthesiology* 1996; **84**:52–63.
22. Sebel PS, Lang E, Rampil IJ, *et al.* A multicenter study of bispectral encephalogram analysis for monitoring anesthetic effect. *Anesth Analg* 1997; **84**:891–899.
23. Mi WD, Sakai T, Takahashi S, Matsuki A. Haemodynamic and electroencephalograph responses to intubation during induction with propofol or propofol/fentanyl. *Can J Anaesth* 1998; **45**:19–22.
24. Gan TJ, Glass PS, Windsor A, *et al.* Bispectral index monitoring allows faster emergence and improved recovery from propofol, alfentanil, and nitrous oxide anesthesia. *Anesthesiology* 1997; **87**:808–815.
25. Song D, Joshi GP, White P. Titration of volatile anesthetics using bispectral index facilitates recovery after ambulatory anesthesia. *Anesthesiology* 1997; **87**:842–848.
26. Struys M, Versichelen L, Byttebier G, Mortier E, Moerman A, Rolly G. Clinical usefulness of the bispectral index for titrating propofol target effect-site concentration. *Anaesthesia* 1998; **53**:4–12.
27. Thornton C, Sharpe RM. Evoked responses in anaesthesia. *Br J Anaesth* 1998; **81**:771–781.
28. Thornton C, Konieczko KM, Knight AB, *et al.* Effects of propofol on the auditory evoked response and oesophageal contractility. *Br J Anaesth* 1989; **63**:411–417.
29. Schwender D, Madler C, Klasing S, Peter K, Pöppel E. Anesthetic control of 40-Hz brain activity and implicit memory. *Conscious Cogn* 1994; **3**: 129–147.
30. Van Hooff JC, DeBeer NAM, Brunia CHM, *et al.* Information processing during cardiac surgery: an event related potential study. *Electroencephalogr Clin Neurophysiol* 1995; **96**:433–452.

31. Plourde G, Joffe D, Villemure C, Trahan M. The P3a wave of the auditory event related potential reveals registration of pitch change during sufentanil anesthesia for cardiac surgery. *Anesthesiology* 1993; **78**:498–509.

32. Thornton C, Jones JG. Evaluating depth of anesthesia: review of methods. In Jones JG. (ed.) *Intern. Anesth. Clinics, Depth of Anesthesia*. Boston: Little, Brown and Company, 1993; **31**:67–88.

33. Plourde G. Clinical use of the 40-Hz auditory steady state response. In Jones JG. (ed.) *Intern. Anesth. Clinics, Depth of Anesthesia*. Boston: Little, Brown and Company, 1993; **31**:107–121.

34. Munglani R, Andrade J, Sapsford DJ, Baddeley A, Jones JG. A measure of consciousness and memory during isoflurane administration: the coherent frequency. *Br J Anesth* 1993; **71**:633–641.

35. Thornton C, Creagh-Barry P, Jordan C, Newton DEF. Anaesthetic depth and auditory evoked potentials. *Acta Anaesthesiol Scand* 1993; **37**(S100):105–108.

36. Davies FW, Mantzaridis H, Kenny GNC, Fisher AC. Middle latency auditory evoked potentials during repeated transitions from consciousness to unconsciousness. *Anaesthesia* 1996; **51**:107–113.

37. Thornton C, Barrowcliffe MP, Konieczko KM, *et al.* The auditory evoked response as an indicator of awareness. *Br J Anaesth* 1989; **63**:113–115.

38. Newton DEF, Thornton C, Konieczko KM, *et al.* Auditory evoked response and awareness: a study in volunteers at sub-mac concentrations of isoflurane. *Br J Anaesth* 1992; **69**:122–129.

39. Schwender D, Klasing S, Madler C, Pöppel E, Peter K. Midlatency auditory evoked potentials and cognitive function during general anesthesia. In Jones JG. (ed.) *Intern. Anesth. Clinics, Depth of Anesthesia*. Boston: Little, Brown and Company, 1993; **31**:89–106.

40. Schwender D, Kaiser A, Klasing S, Peter K, Pöppel E. Midlatency auditory evoked potentials and explicit and implicit memory in patients undergoing cardiac surgery. *Anesthesiology* 1994; **80**:493–501.

41. Villemure C, Plourde G, Lussier I, Normandin N. Auditory processing during isoflurane anesthesia: a study with an implicit memory task and auditory evoked potentials. In Sebel PS, Bonke B, Winograd E. (eds). *Memory and Awareness in Anesthesia*. Englewood Cliffs: Prentice-Hall, 1993; 99–106.

42. Andrade J, Munglani R, Jones JG, Baddeley AD. Cognitive performance during anesthesia. *Conscious Cogn* 1994; **3**:148–165.

43. Andrade J, Sapsford DJ, Jeevaratnum D, Pickworth AJ, Jones JG. The coherent frequency in the electroencephalogram as an ojective measure of cognitive function during propofol sedation. *Anesth Analg* 1996; **83**:1279–1284.

44. Plourde G, Villemure C, Fiset P, Bonhomme V, Backman SB. Effect of isoflurane on the auditory

45. steady state response and on consciousness in human volunteers. *Anesthesiology* 1998; **89**:844–851.

45. Plourde G, Picton TW. Human auditory steady state response during general anesthesia. *Anesth Analg* 1990; **71**:460–468.

46. Tunstall ME. Detecting wakefulness during general anaesthesia for caesarean section. *Br Med J* 1977; **1**:1321.

47. Tunstall ME. The reduction of amnesic wakefulness during Caesarean section. *Anaesthesia* 1979; **34**:316–319.

48. Russell IF. Auditory perception under anaesthesia. *Anaesthesia* 1979; **34**:211.

49. Millar K, Watkinson N. Recognition of words presented during general anaesthesia. *Ergonomics* 1983; **26**:585–594.

50. King H, Ashley S, Brathwaite D, Decayette J, Wooten DJ. Adequacy of general anesthesia for cesarean section. *Anesth Analg* 1993; **77**:84–88.

51. Russell IF, Wang M. Absence of memory for intraoperative information during surgery under adequate general anaesthsia. *Br J Anaesth* 1997; **78**: 3–9.

52. Flaishon R, Windsor A, Sigl J, Sebel PS. Recovery of consciousness after thiopental or propofol: Bispectral index and the isolated forearm technique. *Anesthesiology* 1997; **86**:613–619.

53. Liu J, Singh H, White P. Electroencephalogram bispectral analysis predicts the depth of midazolam induced sedation. *Anesthesiology* 1996; **84**:64–69.

54. Liu J, Singh H, White P. Electroencephalogram bispectral index correlates with intraoperative recall and depth of sedation in propofol-induced sedation. *Anesth Analg* 1997; **84**:185–189.

55. Iselin-Chaves IA, Flaishon R, Sebel PS, *et al.* The effect of the interaction of propofol and alfentanil on recall, loss of consciousness, and the bispectral index. *Anesth Analg* 1998; **87**:949–955.

56. Glass PS, Bloom M, Kearse L, Rosow C, Sebel PS, Manberg P. Bispectral analysis measures sedation and memory effects of propofol, midazolam, isoflurane and alfentanil in healthy volunteers. *Anesthesiology* 1997; **86**:836–847.

57. Kearse LA, Rosow C, Zaslavsky A, Connors P, Dershwitz M, Denman W. Bispectral analysis of the encephalogram predicts conscious processing of information during propofol sedation and hypnosis. *Anesthesiology* 1998; **88**:25–34.

58. Rampil IJ, Kim JS, Lenhardt R, Negishi C, Sessler DI. Bispectral EEG Index during nitrous oxide administration. *Anesthesiology* 1998; **89**:671–677.

59. Lubke GH, Kerssens C, Phaf H, Sebel PS. Dependence of explicit and implicit memory on hypnotic state in trauma patients. *Anesthesiology* 1999; **90**:670–680.

60. Kerssens C, Klein J, van der Woerd A, Bonke B. Auditory information processing during adequate

propofol anesthesia monitored by EEG bispectral index. *Anesth Analg* (in press).

61. Jelicic M, Bonke B, Wolters G, Phaf RH. Implicit memory for words presented during anaesthesia. *Eur J Cogn Psychol* 1992; **4**: 71–80.

62. Roorda-Hrdlickova, Wolters G, Bonke B, Phaf RH. Unconscious perception during general anaesthesia, demonstrated by an implicit memory task. In *Memory and Awareness in Anaesthesia*. Amsterdam: Swets & Zeitlinger, 1990; 150–155.

63. Lubke GH, Kerssens C, Gershon RY, Sebel PS. Memory function in relation to hypnotic state during emergency cesarean sections. *Anesthesiology* 2000; **92**: 1029–1034.

64. Leslie K, Sessler D, Schroeder M, Walters K. Propofol blood concentration and the bispectral index predict suppression of learning during propofol/epidural anesthesia in volunteers. *Anesth Analg* 1995; **81**:1269–1274.

Chapter 6

The auditory evoked responses and memory during anesthesia

Christine Thornton and Roger M. Sharpe

Contents

Introduction

A commonly experienced scenario

How many doctors have approached a patient on the ward the day after their operation only to learn that the patient has no recollection of their conversation in the recovery room on the previous day? A similar scenario confronted us in a study[1] that we carried out on our colleagues (Figure 6.1). We gave them bolus doses of propofol until they lost response to the command 'squeeze my hand', allowed them to wake up, engaged them in conversation and gave them the name of an animal to remember. More propofol was given until they again lost response to command. At the end of the study they were then allowed to wake up.

On questioning them, following their recovery from the anesthetic, most of them could recall nothing from the middle period of wakefulness even though one or two of them had made witty statements at the time. Often they confused this middle period with the period of wakefulness before they fell asleep the first time. Similarly, the last thing patients usually remember is being put to sleep in the anesthetic room and the next thing is when they come round on the ward. In our study one subject was asked to remember the word

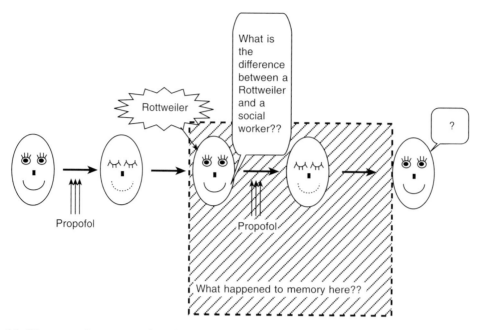

Figure 6.1. Diagrammatic representation of a subject anesthetized with propofol, then allowed to wake up. He was given the word 'rottweiler' to remember, at which point the subject spontaneously recounted a joke. The subject was then anesthetized for a second period. On awakening the subject was unable to recall the word and was unaware of telling the joke or even being awake during the study. (Reprinted with permission from Sharpe RM, Thornton C, Shannon C, Brunner MD, Newton DEF. The auditory evoked response during propofol sedation in volunteers. In Jordan C, Vaughan DJA, Newton DEF (eds). *Memory and Awareness in Anesthesia IV.* London: Imperial College Press, 2000, 75–80.)

'rottweiler'. He said 'did we know the joke – what is the difference between a rottweiler and a social worker?' On replying that we did not know it he gave us the 'punch line', which was 'it's easier to get your children back from a rottweiler than from a social worker'. He could remember nothing of the conversation when subsequently questioned and was even embarrassed when we reported it back to him, particularly in view of the fact it was being recorded for broadcast on German television.

An interesting feature of the episode described above is that during the middle period of wakefulness the subject was able to recall from long-term memory the rottweiler/social worker joke but he was not able to remember anything from this middle period when later questioned. This suggests that recall of material learned before drug administration is less sensitive to anesthetic drugs than information learned after their administration.

Scope of the review

The mechanism underlying memory formation and retrieval is the subject of ongoing research and our knowledge comes from several sources. These are: animal studies in which parts of the brain are surgically ablated;[2] clinical studies involving amnesic patients[3] (e.g. amnesia of dementia and amnesia secondary to surgery for intractable temporal lobe epilepsy); and, more recently, from functional neuroimaging techniques.[4] The amnesia produced by anesthesia provides further opportunities to extend the study of the mechanisms of memory to the 'normal' brain. Non-invasive tools, such as evoked responses, have real potential for probing brain function in relation to memory tasks.

In this chapter, following a brief introduction of memory terminology and memory testing, we will describe the auditory evoked response. We will explain its anatomical significance and relationship to cognitive processes – characteristics that have made it a tempting technique to apply to this research area. In the context of this review our interest in memory mechanisms are those involved in 'long-term memory'. This kind of memory is the basis of postoperative recall following intraoperative awareness. It is also that which is impaired when the patient cannot remember having a conversation with the doctor in the recovery room the previous day.

Short-term or working memory, on the other hand, is that which enables us to remember the first digit of a telephone number by the time we have reached the last. Impairment of short-term memory is associated with lack of concentration, confusion and, at the extreme, unresponsiveness. Intact short-term memory processes may be necessary in order for the information to be incorporated into long-term memory stores.

When reviewing the literature we have to consider whether the subject is in a state of consciousness such that the information presented will be registered in short-term memory (anesthetics are likely to inhibit registration). This is important because, if registration of the information does not take place, then retrieval is unlikely and a false conclusion concerning the point at which the memory processes are interrupted could be drawn. For example much of the work in the literature has focused on detecting intraoperative awareness during anesthesia.[5–7] Whether the patient has registered the information at the time of presentation has often not been noted and no attempt has been made to assess the depth of hypnosis. Also in order to draw conclusions on the usefulness of *evoked responses* in predicting *memory impairment* during anesthesia, these aspects (i.e. evoked responses, memory impairment and level of anesthesia) need to be included in the *same* study. Although there are a number of papers in the literature on the effect of sedatives, i.e. benzodiazepines,[8] opioids,[9] ethanol[10,11] or anesthetics, e.g. nitrous oxide,[12,13] isoflurane[14] on evoked responses, the effects of these agents on memory tasks have often been studied separately. The literature studying evoked responses together with memory is therefore sparse. Before reviewing these papers, it is worth clarifying the terminology on memory and memory testing and explaining the auditory evoked response.

Memory terminology and testing

Memory terminology

In classic models of memory, three stages are described: encoding, storage and retrieval. For the brain to develop memory of an event a sensory input is required; this may be visual, auditory or somatosensory. These inputs are then processed and laid down as memory. Retrieval of this memory may then occur implicitly (when past experiences influence current behaviour or performance, even though the original experience is not consciously recalled) or explicitly (i.e. specific and conscious memory of pictures or events). This is not to be confused with implicit and explicit *learning*. Andrade *et al.*[15] define explicit learning as learning accompanied by conscious awareness of the information that is learned, whereas implicit learning refers to learning without awareness of the information being learned. Explicit learning may lead to explicit or implicit memory, while implicit learning leads only to implicit memory. A simplified diagram of memory formation/retrieval is shown in Figure 6.2.

Memory tests

The simplest and most obvious test of long-term memory function is *spontaneous* or free *recall*, which tests *explicit memory*. The subject is simply asked to report what they remember of the test period.

Most other methods involve *priming*, where exposure to material or tasks (often repeated) changes or facilitates performance on later tests. Some examples that are commonly used in anesthetic studies are described below.

Word stem completion tests are commonly used. Subjects are given lists of words during the period of sedation. On awakening word stems are given and the subjects are then asked to complete the

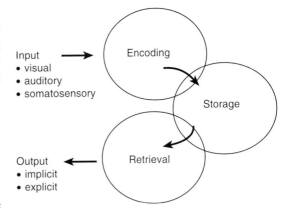

Figure 6.2. The three stages involved in memory formation and retrieval.

stem with the first word that comes to mind. A higher score of word stems completed from the list (in comparison to distracter material) suggests implicit memory.

Word association may indicate implicit memory formation during sedation. It is noted that implicit memory for previously presented names often makes a subject associate this name as being 'famous' at a later encounter. This test has been applied during anesthesia.[16] Another example of a word association test is the Robinson Crusoe/Friday test in a study by Schwender *et al.* performed in patients undergoing cardiac surgery[5] (see later). Patients were played a tape of the story during anesthesia. On recovery they were asked with what they would associate the word Friday.

Indirect methods of demonstrating cerebral processing and implicit memory formation during anesthesia include studying postoperative performance/outcomes after behavioral suggestions during anesthesia. Subjects are played commands such as 'touch your nose when you wake up' during anesthesia and observed to see whether they follow these commands postoperatively. Some studies have even demonstrated superior postoperative outcome (e.g. less analgesic use) to positive suggestions made during anesthesia.

The auditory evoked response (AER)

The AER has anatomical origins that are in proximity to those structures implicated in memory formation.

Early studies demonstrated memory processing in the hippocampus and amygdala, which are found bilaterally on the inner surface of the temporal lobes. This information came from observations in patients who developed anterograde global amnesia following damage to the hippocampus during temporal lobe surgery. It was subsequently noted that damage to the thalamus and hypothalamus resulted in organic amnesias, e.g. Korsakoff's syndrome. Neuroanatomical studies in normal subjects suggested that there were further circuits involved in memory with connections from the thalamus to the ventromedial prefrontal cortex.

Amnesic patients with damage to the medial temporal lobe are able to perform normally during implicit memory tests, suggesting that the medial temporal lobe is crucial for explicit memory but

not necessary for implicit memory formation.[3] This has been confirmed in normal subjects by functional PET neuroimaging studies that showed activation in the dorsolateral prefrontal cortex during sequence learning.[17] These observations are consistent with the view that prefrontal areas are concerned with maintenance of contextual information used 'unconsciously' during implicit memory tasks.

Recording the auditory evoked response

The principle behind AER recording is that the subjects listen to click stimuli while their EEG is recorded and an averaged response – the AER – is extracted from background 'noise' that occurs randomly with respect to the stimulus and is therefore cancelled out as the signal is averaged. We used a purpose-built system developed in our laboratory[18] to record and analyze the AER, but it is possible to buy systems 'off the shelf'.

The appearance of the AER waveform is affected by a number of factors and these have been reviewed in detail elsewhere.[19] The electrode placement and the stimulus characteristics are probably the most important to mention in the context of this review. The EEG is recorded from bipolar surface electrodes. For the middle latency responses (see later), electrodes placed at the mastoid process (over the temporal lobe) or inion bone (further back around the head but on the same level), referred to as the inactive vertex electrode, will suffice. A click or a tone pip presented at 6–9 Hz is sufficiently slow to obtain the response, which occurs between 15 and 100 ms. However, waves such as N1 and P3 (see later) are not unitary phenomena[20, 21] and the results and the cognitive processes that they reflect can vary depending on the electrode placement and the stimulus paradigm.

The AERs described above are known as 'transient' evoked responses. Derived in this way the waves are quantified by manually measuring the amplitude (peak to peak height) and latency (time from stimulus). As the rate of stimulus is increased from 6 Hz (transient response) towards 40 Hz, the peaks of the middle latency waves superimpose on one another and a much larger response is obtained. This is called the '40 Hz steady state' response[22] and its amplitude is measured manually. Because anesthesia reduces the amplitude and increases the latency of the middle latency waves the stimulus has to be slowed in order to optimize the superimposition. A series of stimulus repetition rates have to be tried and frequency analyses of these waveforms are then used to calculate the frequency (coherent frequency) that produced the maximal response.[23]

A novel approach to AER processing, namely wavelet analysis, was explored in a collaborative study that we carried out with Stockmanns *et al.*[24] This involved splitting the transient middle latency evoked response into a number of standardized waveforms or wavelets. These can be described by certain parameters, namely detail levels, approximation levels and coefficients, which are sufficient to reconstitute the waveform. Predictors of awake/asleep were extracted by feeding these parameters into a neural network and discriminant function analyses.

Anatomical significance of the auditory evoked response

The AER (Figure 6.3) is derived by averaging the response in the EEG to a click or tone stimulus.

The waves thus produced represent electrical activity from cochlea to secondary cortices and association areas. The early waves have very specific anatomical associations denoted with roman numerals I to VI.[25,26] Middle latency waves No, Po, Na, Pa, Nb have more diffuse origins but arise mainly from medial geniculate and primary cortical origins.[27] Later waves P1, N1, P2, N2 and P3, are known to be cortically generated, namely frontal cortex and association areas,[28] but their origins cannot be pinpointed to specific areas.

The AER waves are differentially sensitive to drugs, e.g. brainstem waves I–VI that occur within the first 10 ms of the stimulus being presented are only slightly affected by general anesthetics.[19] The later cortical waves P1–P3 (P3 occurs at 300 ms but is not present in the waveform in Figure 6.3) are affected by doses of sedatives and anesthetics that do not produce unconsciousness and yet produce memory impairment.[29–31] It is the proximity of the generators of these waves to anatomical locations implicated in memory processes both by animal experiments and clinical studies, which have made the midlatency waves (having a longer latency than Na) of interest to workers in the field of memory processing.

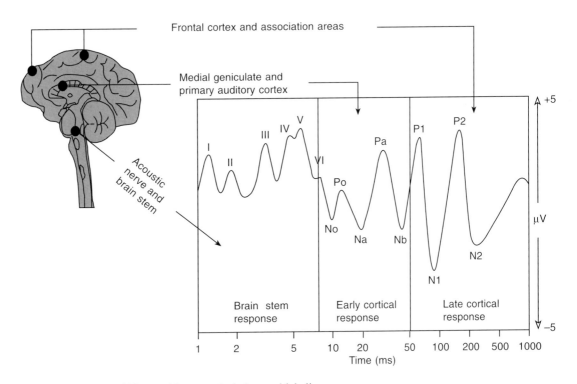

Figure 6.3. AER 1–1000 ms with anatomical sites and labeling.

Auditory evoked response and cognitive processes

Paradigms are used to extract evoked responses at the longer latencies.[32] For example, the subject is presented with a series of standard tones. Occasionally there is a deviation from this pattern because a tone of longer duration or higher pitch is presented or a tone does not occur when it is expected to occur. The AER responses to the standard and deviant stimuli are averaged separately. The difference in the waveforms in response to the standard and deviant stimuli is believed to be a measure of selective attention. This difference can be detected as early as Pa,[33] which occurs around 30 ms extending to P3, which occurs at 300 ms following the sound stimulus. The mismatch negativity is a special case of the difference that occurs at N1.

The evoked responses produced using these paradigms are proposed as measures of specific cognitive processes,[32] e.g. N1 is thought to reflect the process of excluding irrelevant information such as the standard tones and P3 to reflect matching relevant information with existing data. The ability of a patient to recall a surgeon's comment picked out from the background activity of the operating theatre could depend on the integrity of such processes.

Review of studies

Lorazepam sedation and P3

The benzodiazepine lorazepam, although not capable of producing general anesthesia alone, has strong anxiolytic and amnesic properties, which make it useful in anesthetic practice. It seems worthwhile to discuss a study by Samra et al.,[29] where the effects of lorazepam were studied, since it highlights some of the problems of interpretation in the field of investigation of memory. They tested the hypothesis that the auditory evoked response wave P3 could predict short-term or long-term memory impairment. They compared the effects of placebo (normal saline) with secobarbital (1.5 mg kg^{-1}) and lorazepam (0.05 mg kg^{-1}). Lorazepam produced good sedation, secobarbital mild sedation and placebo no sedation. Lorazepam produced incon-

sistent short-term and long-term memory loss in contrast to secobarbital and placebo where the memory loss was not significant.

In humans a proposed generator source of P3 is the hippocampus, which has been shown to be involved in memory retention. An increased P3 latency has also been suggested as a correlate of post-traumatic amnesia after closed head injury.[34] However, the amnesia in the subjects given lorazepam in the Samra study did not correspond to changes in P3. A decrease in P3 amplitude was seen in the placebo group, which was not significantly different from that seen in the lorazepam group. An increase in P3 latency was seen in both the lorazepam and the secobarbital group, which the authors attributed as effect of sedation rather than memory function. The authors concluded that the latency and amplitude of P3 could not be used as predictable indicators of auditory amnesia.

This study illustrates the value of including control groups in a study. Without a control group the reduction in P3 amplitude could have been interpreted as related to memory impairment, as would the effect of sedation on P3 latency seen in both the lorazepam and the secobarbital group.

Nitrous oxide and P3

Jessop et al.[31] carried out a study where they examined P3 with sedative and anesthetic concentrations of nitrous oxide and similarly found that P3 was not a predictor of memory impairment. P3 in response to rare tones among click stimuli was measured and reaction time (subjects were asked to press a button in response to a tone) were tested just prior to and during administration of the nitrous oxide/oxygen mixtures. There was a recovery period in between each nitrous oxide concentration during which subjects were asked about their recall of events while they were breathing the gas, e.g. hearing tones, pressing buttons. Recall of the recording period was disrupted by lesser concentrations of nitrous oxide (no subject had recall above 50%) than those concentrations that affected the ability to perform the reaction time test (no subject pressed the button above 62%). In the five subjects where P3 recordings could be made, it persisted at nitrous oxide concentrations at which subsequent recall of external events was lost.

Isoflurane and coherent frequency

Munglani *et al.*[23] examined cognitive function when volunteers breathed various doses of sub-MAC isoflurane. In the recovery period after the isoflurane was stopped, memory function was tested. Simultaneously coherent frequency of auditory evoked responses to a range of 43 frequencies at 1-Hz intervals from 47 to 5 Hz was measured.

A Within-List Recognition test was used to assess working or short-term memory while the subjects were breathing 0%, 0.2%, 0.4% and 0.8% end-tidal isoflurane. The lists were read aloud by the experimenter at a rate of one word every 2 seconds. The number of intervening words between repeated words was varied. Clearly, the smaller the number of intervening words the easier it was for the subject to register the repetitions and his task was to respond to repeated words by raising the right thumb. The experimenter recorded repetitions, which were identified correctly.

A Word Categorization test was carried out immediately after the Within-List Recognition tests while the subjects were still breathing the isoflurane. Again, lists of words were read out to the subject and his task was to raise the right thumb to those belonging to a particular category. An example of this test is if the category 'metals' was chosen, then raising the right thumb to the word 'aluminium' would be a correct response. On recovery from the anesthetic, recognition memory of words presented during anesthesia was tested. A forced choice procedure was used where pairs of words were read out, i.e. 'aluminium' and 'red', where 'aluminium' would be the correct response.

Learning under anesthesia was examined by presenting words from a different category, while the subjects were breathing 0.8% isoflurane before and following painful tetanic stimulation. On recovery the subjects were questioned as to whether they could recall the category and, having guessed or been told the correct category, they were asked to provide examples of that category. Recognition (explicit memory) for the presented words was tested using the forced choice procedure described above.

Coherent frequency reduced with increasing end-tidal isoflurane concentration. Concurrently there was a decline in the ability to perform the Within-List Recognition and Word Categorization tests. Painful tetanic stimulation applied at the 0.4% isoflurane dose reversed the effects of these declines in performance. The same pattern of decreasing performance with increasing isoflurane was seen in the results of the explicit memory tests carried out in the recovery period. For the group as a whole median coherent frequency did not show a statistically significant reversal following the application of painful tetanic stimulus (although some subjects showed reversal). So, although there was a relationship between median coherent frequency and isoflurane concentration, there is not necessarily a relationship between median coherent frequency and cognition and memory function. However, these results did at least confirm that the overall state of arousal (and cognitive processing) of a subject is determined by the balance between the depressant effects of anesthetics and the stimulation the subject receives. The implications for anesthetic practice are that a previously unresponsive patient may become responsive with surgical stimulation, which is a particularly frightening prospect in paralyzed patients.

There was no evidence of implicit memory following recovery from 0.8% end-tidal isoflurane in unstimulated or stimulated groups.

Flunitrazepam, fentanyl and isoflurane – Na and Pa latency

Schwender *et al.*[5] noted a correlation between Na and Pa latencies and implicit memory in cardiac patients given three different anesthetic regimens: flunitrazepam and fentanyl; isoflurane and fentanyl; and propofol and fentanyl. Patients were played an audiotape of the Robinson Crusoe story during their operation and postoperatively were questioned about their associations with the word Friday. The obvious association is that it is a day of the week. The patients who made the association with Robinson Crusoe or an island were assumed to have implicit recall. None of the patients experienced explicit recall. In the groups with either propofol or isoflurane, there were the least number of incidents of implicit recall. Flunitrazepam and fentanyl alone may not produce adequate anesthesia and half of the patients receiving this anesthetic regimen experienced implicit recall. Overall, the patients with implicit recall had Na and Pa latencies which were significantly shorter, i.e. 21 and 37 ms compared to those without implicit recall where the latencies were 52 and 77 ms respectively.

Isoflurane and Pa amplitude

A study by Villemure et al.[7] correlated the size of Pa amplitude with implicit memory scores. Patients had been presented lists from two categories, either birds or vegetables, while receiving 0.4% isoflurane anesthesia and fentanyl for abdominal hysterectomy. There was no evidence of explicit memory post-operatively but patients produced more target words of the category that they had been presented with compared with those who had not.

An interpretation of Villemure et al.'s results[7] and those of Schwender et al.[5] described in the previous paragraph, is that Na and Pa latencies and Pa amplitudes are predictors of implicit memory. However, it may be the case that the patients having short Na and Pa latencies were 'awake', whereas those with long latencies and reduced Pa amplitudes were adequately anesthetized. (The same comment could be made about Nb latency changes reported in our own three studies described below.) It is the belief of these reviewers (Thornton and Sharpe) that patients do not register information when they are unconscious and this is why they do not have implicit memory of it. (Learning in unconscious patients has yet to be demonstrated conclusively, although we are well aware that that does not mean it does not exist.)

Studies at Northwick Park Hospital

Using the isolated forearm technique

We recorded the AER in elective surgery in seven male patients prior to incision.[35] Following induction with propofol a tourniquet was inflated on the patient's left forearm (if right handed) to prevent blood flowing into it. The neuromuscular blocker vecuronium was given to paralyze the patients (with the exception of their 'isolated' left forearm) and their trachea intubated. Their lungs were ventilated with 70% nitrous oxide in oxygen to maintain anesthesia. The nitrous oxide concentration was then reduced to 50% and they were requested to squeeze the experimenter's fingers, which they were able to do with the isolated forearm. When the patient had woken up sufficiently and this end-point was achieved, a volatile agent was admin-istered and following a few more minutes of recording the study was finished. A specific change

in the AER occurred that distinguished response to verbal command from no response to verbal command. Namely three positive waves in a latency window of 15–100 ms were replaced by two positive waves (or less) in the same latency window. The salient feature of this change in pattern in the AER was a shift in Nb latency to above 44.5 ms. The patients had absolutely no recall of these events postoperatively.

Isoflurane and Nb latency

In another study,[6] eight volunteer anesthesiologists were given sub-MAC concentrations of isoflurane (0, 0.1, 0.2 and 0.4 MAC) and their responses to command and subsequent recall of word lists were tested. Again similar changes in Nb latency were identified as significantly associated with response to command and subsequent recall. In this study a full response to command was associated with an Nb latency of 46.1 ms increasing to 54.2 ms when there was no response to command. However, all the subjects who responded to command had subsequent recall. It was all or nothing, they had both functions or they lost both functions so we were unable to separate changes in Nb latency associated with memory impairment from those which were due to the subject losing consciousness.

Propofol sedation and Nb latency

A third study,[1] which we carried out in volunteer anesthesiologists, is that described in the first paragraph of this chapter. In this study we gave propofol boluses to produce unconsciousness, woke the volunteers up, gave them a word (an animal) to remember and made them unconscious again with propofol. We then allowed them to recover from the anesthetic and asked them whether they could remember being given a word and if so what it was. Although these subjects were clearly responsive when we gave them the information, they could remember practically nothing later. Two subjects out of 13 had slight recall of the middle awake period while the others confused the middle period with the period of wakefulness before they first lost consciousness. Nb latency plotted for the awake and anesthetized periods for all subjects is shown in Figure 6.4. An Nb latency of less than 49.5 ms was able to distinguish awake from unconscious states with a sensitivity of 95%, but the study lacked

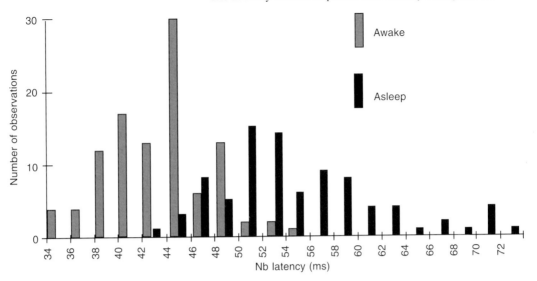

Figure 6.4. Histogram showing the number of observations at each Nb latency from subjects sedated with propofol illustrating the separation between awake and asleep data. (Reprinted with permission from Sharpe RM, Thornton C, Shannon C, Brunner MD, Newton DEF. The auditory evoked response during propofol sedation in volunteers. In Jordan C, Vaughan DJA, Newton DEF (eds). *Memory and Awareness in Anesthesia IV.* London: Imperial College Press, 2000, 75–80.)

the power to identify predictors of memory impairment.

Conclusions

Although the AER provides a wealth of information on cognitive brain function, a correlate of memory impairment remains elusive. The AER has been much investigated in the area of intraoperative awareness during anesthesia. A number of volunteer studies that model this situation have been carried out.[6,35] One factor that emerges consistently from these volunteer studies is that the ability for subsequent recall, implicit or explicit is lost before the ability to respond to command. In other words, subjects (under sedation or just awakening from anesthesia) who appear to be conscious and responding appropriately often have no memory of such interactions when they have awoken fully. Based on currently available evidence we remain convinced that memory formation does not occur in anesthetized (unconscious) patients and therefore it is unlikely that an unconscious patient will have memory for stimuli presented during unconsciousness. In this sense the AER could be used to prevent subsequent recall, because it is able to distinguish consciousness from unconsciousness. However, this

does not help in elucidating memory mechanisms where we need to distinguish between wakefulness that leads to subsequent recall, and wakefulness that does not. More efforts should be made to determine the parameters that distinguish the above situations. For instance, can the memory impairment be correlated with anesthetic blood level, duration of loss of consciousness, duration or depth of subsequent anesthesia, and significance (to the subject) of the information presented?

The studies that are helpful in the search for an AER correlate of memory impairment are few. When we reviewed those in which:

1 The AER was monitored
2 While anesthetic or associated drugs were given
3 Registration of the information at the time it was given was clearly assessed
4 Subsequent recall evaluated

there was little to suggest that the AER has value in predicting memory impairment *per se*. In Samra *et al.*'s study, changes in the latency of P3 wave with lorazepam could be explained by changes in the level of consciousness, i.e. increased sedation.[29] In Munglani *et al.*'s study there was a suggestion of a relationship between median coherent frequency and post-trial free recall of word lists, although further subjects need to be studied to ensure that this is not simply an effect of changes in the concentration of the inhalation agent.[23]

In determining the direction of future research we should try to answer a number of questions. Are we looking at the correct part of the response? For example, should we be looking at waves later than P3, i.e. readiness potentials or motor responses. This does not appear to be the answer because often when a motor response persists the patient has no recall of the experience. Should we be taking a more global view? Stimulus recognition and categorization may involve access to other modalities, e.g. visual, somatosensory and olfactory. Memory formation may depend on a number of processes being intact and, further, these may have to be fully functional for a specific time after the information is presented. It may also prove fruitful to utilize other methods of studying brain function, e.g. functional neuroimaging techniques concurrently with electrophysiological techniques in order to resolve these issues.

References

1. Sharpe RM, Thornton C, Shannon C, Brunner MD, Newton DEF. The auditory evoked response during propofol sedation in volunteers. In Jordan C, Vaughan DJA, Newton DEF (eds). *Memory and Awareness in Anesthesia IV.* London: Imperial College Press, 2000, 75–80.

2. Mishkin M, Appenzeller T. The anatomy of memory. *Sci Am* 1987; **256**:80–90.

3. Schacter D. Memory and Awareness. *Science* 1998; **280**:59–60.

4. Buckner RL, Koutstaal W. Functional neuroimaging studies of encoding, priming, and explicit memory retrieval. *Proc Nat Acad Sci USA* 1998; **95**: 891–898.

5. Schwender D, Kaiser A, Klasing S, Peter K, Poppel E. Midlatency auditory evoked potentials and explicit and implicit memory in patients undergoing cardiac surgery. *Anesthesiology* 1994; **80**:493–501.

6. Newton DEF, Thornton C, Konieczko KM, *et al.* Auditory evoked response and awareness: a study in volunteers at sub-Mac concentrations of isoflurane. *Br J Anaesth* 1992; **69**:122–129.

7. Villemure C, Plourde G, Lussier I, Normadin N. Auditory processing during isoflurane anesthesia: A study with an implicit memory task and auditory evoked potentials In Sebel PS, Bonke B, Winograd E, (eds). *Memory and Awareness in Anesthesia.*

Englewood Cliffs, New Jersey: PTR Prentice-Hall. 1993; 99–106.

8. Milligan KR, Lumsden J, Howard RC, Howe JP, Dundee JW. Use of auditory evoked responses as a measure of recovery from benzodiazepine sedation. *J R Soc Med* 1989; **82**:595–597.

9. Velasco M, Velasco R, Castaneda R, Sanchez R. Effect of fentanyl and naloxone on human somatic and auditory evoked potential components. *Neuropharmacology* 1984; **23**:359–366.

10. Teo RKC, Ferguson DA. The acute effects of ethanol on auditory event-related potentials. *Psychopharmacology* 1986; **90**:179–184.

11. Gross MM, Begleiter H, Tobin M, Kissin B. Changes in auditory evoked response induced by alcohol. *J Nerv Ment Dis* 1966; **143**:152–156.

12. Fowler B, Kelso B, Landolt J, Porlier G. The effects of nitrous oxide and P300 and reaction time. *Electroencephalogr Clin Neurophysiol* 1988; **69**:171–178.

13. Estrin WJ, Moore P, Letz R, Wasch HH. The P-300 event-related potential in experimental nitrous oxide exposure. *Clin Pharmacol Ther* 1988; **43**:86–90.

14. Plourde G, Picton TW. Long-latency auditory evoked potentials during general anesthesia: N1 and P3 components. *Anesth Analg* 1991; **72**:342–50.

15. Andrade J, Stapleton CL. Contribution of surgery to learning and memory in anesthesia. In Jordan C, Vaughan DJA, Newton DEF (eds). *Memory and Awareness in Anesthesia IV.* London: Imperial College Press, 2000, 141–163.

16. Jelicic B, De Roode A, Bovill JG, Bonke B. Unconscious learning during anesthesia. *Anaesthesia* 1992; **47**:835–837.

17. Berns GS, Cohen JD, Mintun MA. Brain regions responsive to novelty in the absence of awareness. *Science* 1997; **276**:1272–1275.

18. Jordan C, Weller C, Thornton C, Newton DEF. Monitoring evoked potentials during surgery to assess levels of anesthesia. *J Med Eng Tech* 1995; **19**:77–79.

19. Thornton C. Evoked potentials in anesthesia. *Eur J Anaesthesiol* 1991; **8**:89–107.

20. Näätänen R, Picton T. The N1 wave of the human electric and magnetic response to sound: A review and an analysis of the component structure. *Psychophysiology* 1987; **24**:375–425.

21. Johnson R Jr. On the neural generators of the P300 component of the event-related potential. *Psychophysiology* 1993; **30**:90–97.

22. Galambos R, Makeig S, Talmachoff PJ. A 40Hz auditory potential recorded from the human scalp. *Proc Nat Acad Sci USA* 1981; **78**:2643–2647.

23. Munglani R, Andrade J, Sapsford DJ, Baddeley A, Jones JG. A measure of consciousness and memory during isoflurane administration: the Coherent frequency. *Br J Anaesth* 1993; **71**:633–641.

24. Stockmanns G, Nahm W, Thornton C, Shannon C, Konecny E, Kochs E. Wavelet-analysis of middle latency auditory evoked potentials during repetitive propofol sedation. *Anesthesiology* 1997; **87**: A465 (abstr).

25. Jewett DL. Volume conducted potentials in response to auditory stimuli as detected by averaging in the cat. *Proc San Diego Biomed Symp* 1970; **28**:609–618.

26. Lev A, Sohmer H. Sources of averaged neural responses recorded in animal and human subjects during cochlear audiometry (electro-cochleogram). *Arch Klin Exp Ohren Nasen Kehlkpfheil* 1972; **201**:79–90.

27. Kaga K, Hink RF, Shinoda Y, Suzuki J. Evidence for a primary cortical origin of a middle latency auditory evoked potential in cats. *Electroencephalog Clin Neurophysiol* 1980; **50**:254–266.

28. Lovrich D, Novick B, Vaughan HG. Topographic analysis of auditory event-related potentials associated with acoustic and semantic processing. *Electroencephalog Clin Neurophys* 1988; **71**: 40–54.

29. Samra KS, Bradshaw EG, Pandit SK, Papanicolaou AC, Bartlett DM. The relation between lorazepam-induced auditory amnesia and auditory evoked potentials. *Anesth Anal* 1988; **76**:526–533.

30. Adam N, Collins GI. Alteration by enflurane of electrophysiologic correlates of search in short term memory. *Anesthesiology* 1979; **50**:93–97.

31. Jessop J, Griffiths DE, Furness P, Jones JG, Sapsford DJ, Breckon A. Changes in amplitude and latency of the P300 component of the auditory evoked potential with sedative and anaesthetic concentrations of nitrous oxide. *Br J Anaesth* 1991; **67**:524–531.

32. Picton TW, Hillyard SA. Human auditory evoked potentials II. Effects of attention. *Electroencephalog Clin Neurophysiol* 1974; **36**:191–200.

33. Woldorff M, Hansen JC, Hillyard SA. Evidence for effects of selective attention in mid-latency range of the human auditory event-related potential. Current trends in event-telated potential research. *Electroencephalog Clin Neurophysiol* 1987; **40**: 146–154.

34. Papanicolaou AC, Levin HS, Eisenberg HM, Moore BD, Goethe KE, High WM Jr. Evoked potential correlates of post-traumatic amnesia after closed head injury. *Neurosurgery* 1984; **14**: 676–678.

35. Thornton C, Barrowcliffe MP, Konieczko KM, *et al*. The auditory evoked response as an indicator of awareness. *Br J Anaesth* 1989; **63**:113–115.

Chapter 7

Memory when the state of consciousness is known: studies of anesthesia with the isolated forearm technique

Ian F. Russell

Contents

Summary

Failure to respond to command is currently the accepted indicator of the threshold between consciousness and unconsciousness. This chapter presents the results of studies into learning and memory where the conscious (responsive) state of the subject was known at the time information was presented. Data from both volunteer studies (no surgery) and investigations where responsiveness was monitored during surgery under general anesthesia by use of the isolated forearm technique are discussed. There is evidence that anesthesi-

ologists cannot assess the presence of consciousness by the use of clinical criteria alone yet, to provide reliable data, investigations of memory and recall must control for the adequacy of hypnosis. There is great variability between subjects in volunteer studies, but usually, there is inability to recall information that was presented during sedation at a time when they were still conscious. Caution is required when interpreting the results of investigations relying on brain monitoring as a guide to depth of anesthesia because, in volunteer studies, some subjects continue to respond to commands at 'EEG' values, which is accepted by some investigators as an indication of unconsciousness. The only direct method of detecting consciousness during general anesthesia in the presence of muscle relaxants is the isolated forearm technique, all other methods are indirect and require validation.

Introduction

An extensive literature has developed around the study of awareness, learning, memory and recall associated with general anesthesia. As well as the many publications there have been four international symposia on the topic.[1-4] Despite this considerable effort, the results are conflicting with evidence both for and against unconscious learning during anesthesia. In an attempt to establish some order from the chaos, Merikle and Daneman[5] performed a meta-analysis of the literature and concluded that there was 'considerable evidence that specific information is both perceived during anesthesia and remembered following surgery'. However, a fundamental assumption underlies this conclusion, namely, 'Despite the remote possibility that some patients may experience moments of awareness during anesthesia, we believe that it is reasonable to assume that patients who are undergoing general anesthesia are in fact unconscious of all external events for the entire duration of surgery.'[5] Close examination of the methodology of the studies involved in the meta-analysis[5] reveals little or no mention of how anesthesia was assessed. Herein lies the crux of the problem: the assessment of depth of anesthesia.

Despite anesthesiologists' almost universal reliance on clinical criteria (blood pressure, heart rate, sweating, tear production) to assess adequacy of anesthesia in the presence of muscle relaxants, there is no evidence to indicate that these criteria bear any predictable relationship to depth of anesthesia. Indeed, those studies that have attempted to investigate this relationship invariably conclude that clinical signs are of limited value.[6-14] Since the time when muscle relaxants were introduced into anesthetic practice to the present, it has been recognized that it is impossible to assess depth of anesthesia in their presence.[15-17] The current situation is summed up succinctly by Ghoneim and Block:[18] 'judgements of depth of anesthesia are neither quantitatively precise nor infallible' and 'there is no measurement that guarantees uncon-

sciousness in the paralysed patient'. This lack of any measurement to identify the presence of consciousness during anesthesia has considerable implications for anyone investigating memory and recall after surgery.

Detection of conscious levels during anesthesia and answers to criticisms of the IFT

In the absence of other explanations, failure to respond to command is currently the accepted indicator of the threshold between wakefulness or consciousness and unconsciousness.[19,20] To date, there is only one method that can directly detect the change from unconsciousness to consciousness during 'anesthesia' in the presence of muscle relaxants: the isolated forearm technique (IFT). The IFT (Table 7.1), first described by Tunstall,[21,22] directly assesses the patient's ability to respond to a simple command during surgery in the presence of muscle relaxants. During cesarean section Tunstall inflated a tourniquet around one of the patient's arms for some 20 minutes to prevent the muscles of that arm being paralyzed by muscle relaxants. However, since Tunstall used a succinylcholine infusion for muscle relaxation the arm became paralyzed when the tourniquet was deflated.[21,22] Russell[13,14,23-27] made some slight modifications to the basic IFT such that it could be used indefinitely for prolonged surgery in the presence of non-depolarizing relaxants (Table 7.2, Figure 7.1). Despite the many publications[13,14,21-39] which have successfully used the IFT there are ongoing criticisms of the technique.[40-50] In summary they are as follows:

Table 7.1. Description of Tunstall's original IFT[21,22]

1. Insert iv cannula in left forearm.
2. Apply BP cuff to left upper arm.
3. Apply padded tourniquet to right upper arm.
4. Induce anesthesia.
5. Inflate tourniquet.
6. Administer succinylcholine.
7. Provide maintenance anesthesia.
8. Ask patient regularly by name to 'Squeeze my fingers with your right hand'.
9. After delivery of baby deepen anesthesia and deflate tourniquet.

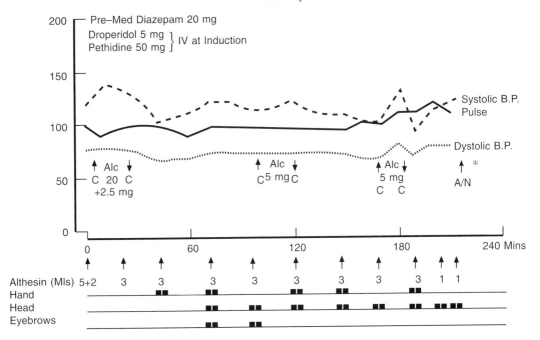

Figure 7.1. Anesthetic record illustrating prolonged use of the modified IFT during total intravenous anesthesia to enable titration of althesin requirements in a patient with grossly abnormal liver function. Ventilation of the lungs was with an air/oxygen mixture. The patient was a 56-year-old man weighing 95 kg, with alcoholic liver cirrhosis, portal hypertension, esophageal varices and diabetes mellitus.

↑ ↓
C C   inflation and deflation of the tourniquet cuff.
Alc   alcuronium (20 mg used for intubation)
A/N   atropine/neostigmine
*   awake and capable of giving date of birth
↑   althesin supplements
■   hand movements to command, spontaneous head movements, frowning
(Reprinted with permission from Russell IF. Conscious awareness during general anaesthesia: relevance of autonomic signs and isolated arm movements as guides to depth of anaesthesia. In Jones JG (ed.) *Baillière's Clinical Anaesthesiology vol 3. Depth of Anaesthesia*, London: Baillière Tindall, 1989.)

1 Response to command does not correlate with the clinical signs of light anesthesia.[40,41]
2 The IFT can only be used for 20 minutes as the arm will become paralyzed.[41,47]
3 It is difficult to distinguish purposeful arm movements from reflex movements.[42–45,47]
4 The response to command does not indicate that the patient is conscious.[44–48]
5 The IFT response does not correlate with recall.[46]
6 Patients may be awake yet not respond.[46,47]
7 The technique is complicated.[49]
8 Risk of serious side effects.[49–50]

In order to appreciate fully the utility of the IFT, it is important that the reader understands the nature

of the criticisms and below, these criticisms are answered.

Response to command does not correlate with the clinical signs of light anesthesia

This may be true, but when a patient responds to commands during surgery, then it is a clear indication that the patient is not unconscious,[19, 20] irrespective of the clinical signs. In these circumstances it is the 'normal' clinical signs that are unreliable, not the IFT. It is precisely for this reason that the IFT has been described as the 'gold standard' for assessing consciousness during 'general anesthesia' in the presence of muscle relaxants.[46]

The IFT can only be used for 20 minutes as the arm will become paralyzed

This criticism only applies to the technique as originally described by Tunstall (see Table 7.1).[21,22] It does not apply to the modified technique (Table 7.2).[13,14,23–30] If the tourniquet remains inflated for

Table 7.2. The IFT modified for prolonged surgery[13,14,23–27]

1. Insert iv cannula in left forearm.
2. Apply BP cuff to right (or left) upper arm.
3. Apply padded tourniquet to right forearm and place arm on arm board where it is visible.
4. Apply nerve stimulating electrodes to ulnar and/or median nerve at elbow.
5. Induce anesthesia, check neuromuscular integrity, intubate with succinylcholine.*
6. Provide maintenance anesthesia.
7. As effects of relaxant wear off inflate tourniquet.
8. Administer judicious dose of relaxant (e.g. atracurium 0.2 mg/kg).
9. After 20 minutes deflate tourniquet.
10. Repeat steps 7–9 as required.

Ask patient, by name, regularly throughout surgery, to 'open and close the fingers of your right hand'. In the absence of a tape recorder this can be done by the anesthesiologist at 5-minute intervals. In practice, it is much easier with a 1-minute continuous loop cassette player. The tape can be personalized for each patient before surgery.

If there appears to be a hand response then this should be verified. I reassure the patient and ask her, by name, to 'squeeze my fingers with your right hand'. If there is a squeeze to command then the patient is conscious, but for further verification the patient can be asked to 'squeeze my hand twice' or to 'squeeze my hand and keep squeezing'. At this point I continue to reassure the patient and explain how important it is for me to know if they are comfortable or in pain. Simple conditional commands are now given, e.g. 'If you are in pain squeeze my hand twice', or 'If you are comfortable squeeze my hand once'. As further verification of the pain/comfort status of the patient I will then change the conditional command, e.g. 'If you are comfortable squeeze my hand twice'.

* If succinylcholine is contraindicated then the cuff should be inflated before giving the long-acting relaxant for intubation. However, the intubating dose of non-depolarizing relaxant may weaken the arm when the cuff is deflated. (This is less of a problem today than in the past as the relatively short-acting drugs atracurium or mivacurium may be used for intubation.) Neuromuscular integrity should be checked at regular intervals to ensure that lack of response is not due to the arm being paralyzed.

much longer than 20 minutes an ischemic paralysis may ensue.[51] To prevent this, the tourniquet must be deflated after 15–20 minutes. If relaxants are used judiciously, as indicated (Table 7.2), then the arm will not become paralyzed.[13,14,23–30] When further relaxant is required the cuff is reinflated for a further 15–20 minutes. This inflation/deflation cycle can be used indefinitely (Table 7.2, Figure 7.1). However, there is one caveat: the IFT may not be reliable after tourniquet release if pancuronium is used,[52,53] because of its long duration of action and cumulative nature.

It is difficult to distinguish purposeful arm movements from reflex movements

This criticism is based on two studies where arm movements were observed but no attempt was made to distinguish between the two types of movement.[42,43] The two types of hand movement can be distinguished and categorized (Tables 7.1 and 7.3) by directly asking the patient to respond in a particular manner.

The response to command does not indicate that the patient is conscious

Several authors have suggested that a patient response to command under 'anesthesia' does not necessarily indicate the presence of consciousness.[44,46–48] Jessop and Jones[46,47] point out that subjects in reaction time experiments can respond to a simple stimulus about 200 ms after the stimulus, yet it takes 500 ms for consciousness of the stimulus to occur. In other words, they argue, the response is 'subconscious'. The neuronal pathways required for such 'subconscious' reaction times are capable of being set up and biased ('trained') in the conscious subject, but whether such 'training' can occur with the relatively infrequent commands given under anesthesia or sedation is not known. However, more importantly, even the simplest of commands is quite different in nature from a single stimulus (e.g. a tone or light flash). The latter is instantaneous and has a 'fixed' reaction, whereas a command occurs over a prolonged period of time (5–10 seconds) and the patient must concentrate and process the information during this time in order to interpret the actual command, which may not be constant.

Table 7.3. Categorization of hand responses during anesthesia when the IFT is used (after Wang)

Grade 0	No movement
Grade 1	Reflex movement not contingent on command
Grade 2*	Response to a simple command but not to a complex command or initial response to command, but the full instructions are not followed, e.g. the patient only squeezes once instead of twice
Grade 3	Response to conditional commands (capable of indicating pain or comfort)

*Grade 2 responses may consist of two subcategories: a true stable level of consciousness/responsiveness or a changing level of consciousness/responsiveness as a result of a sudden reduction in the surgical stimulus. In this latter situation, there is an initial response to a simple command during a period of intense surgical stimulation, but when this simple command is followed up with a conditional command and, at the same time the intense surgical stimulation ceases, there is no response.

Examples of commands

Simple command	'Susan, squeeze my fingers'
Complex command	'Susan, squeeze and let go my fingers three times'
Conditional command	'Susan, if you are in pain squeeze my fingers twice but if you are comfortable squeeze my fingers once'

To verify this conditional command it may be repeated with the command/responses changed, e.g. 'Susan, I need to check I have understood you properly: if you are in pain, squeeze my fingers once, but if you are comfortable, squeeze my fingers twice'.

Bonke et al.[44] draw attention to the fact that during REM sleep 'information' presented to subjects can be incorporated into the dreams or subjects may respond to commands without any conscious awareness. How this latter argument relates to anesthesia is unclear since REM sleep does not occur during anesthesia. Whatever the merits of these criticisms, they do emphasize the importance of direct communication with the patient when hand movement is seen so that either the command can be repeated with slightly altered wording or a conditional command is given. In these latter circumstances the patients cannot be described as unconscious.[19,54]

Movements and responses of the isolated arm do not correlate with recall

All anesthesiologists are aware of the fact that spontaneously breathing patients often exhibit reflex movements in response to surgery and have no recall. The 'MAC' concept of assessing potency of anesthetic agents is based on such movement (The 'MAC' is the minimum alveolar concentration of an anesthetic gas or vapor which prevents 50% of patients from moving in response to a skin incision). MAC awake (i.e. when a patient first responds to command) occurs with anesthetic concentration in the region of 0.3–0.6 MAC depending on the agent being used.[20, 55] At MAC awake patients do not have recall.[20, 55, 56] By its nature, the IFT detects the onset of consciousness (i.e. response to commands – equivalent to detecting MAC awake) and at this moment patients do not have conscious recall, thus it is not surprising that responses to the IFT do not correlate with recall. If anesthesia is permitted to become lighter then recall will begin to occur.[29,30] Although the vast majority of patients in my investigations who respond during surgery had no recall, it must be pointed out that virtually all of my patients with postoperative recall had responded to commands intraoperatively (see below). Volunteer studies provide similar results: recall is only found in patients who responded under sedation but, conversely, lack of recall does not indicate the subject was unconscious.[20,49]

Patients may be awake yet not respond

This can occur, but is unusual. In the author's experience in only one case has this been due to a technical failure of the IFT,[23] (see later for description). In earlier years the taped command did not include the patient's name and four patients (not in any of the formal investigations) who did not respond during surgery were aware of the command and were able to repeat it word for word postoperatively. When asked why they had not responded the patients gave several different reasons. Two stated they had not realized the instructions were meant for them! Another heard the tape but it kept interrupting her dream so she decided to ignore the messages and enjoy her dream. The last patient, also having a good experience, decided to play a game and do the opposite of what she was instructed: thus every time the tape asked her to open and close the fingers of her right hand she took great care to make sure she did not move her fingers at all! Over the last 3 years, since the tapes have been individualized for each patient by preceding the commands and information with the patient's preferred name these 'non-responses' have not recurred. These cases support Tunstall's assertion that, when using the IFT, wakeful women may show no spontaneous hand responses to the surgery unless they are uncomfortable (Tunstall, personal communication).

The technique is complicated

It is difficult to understand this criticism particularly as the technique has been used in children as young as 5 years old.[39] The conclusions of these latter authors should be borne in mind: The IFT 'is an easy test to apply using normal apparatus and interpretation of results is straightforward'.[39]

Risk of serious side effects

Much of the anxiety regarding potential side effects is related to the mistaken belief that the tourniquet must remain inflated for the duration of surgery. As described above this is not the case. Furthermore, tourniquets are used frequently in surgical practice and are kept inflated for much longer than the 15–20 minutes required when using the IFT. The only side effects the author has noted in 20 years of use are related to tourniquet pressure: a petechial rash over the hand and forearm if the tourniquet pressure is above venous pressure and below systolic pressure for any length of time (this seems more common in the elderly due to their increased capillary fragility); bruising/nipping of the arm under the tourniquet if padding is inadequate or creased (similar nipping/bruising may be seen under the cuff of routinely used automatic non-invasive blood pressure machines).

Obstetric anesthesia and the IFT

Since the IFT was first described in obstetric anesthesia it is pertinent to examine briefly the studies in this field. A summary of these is shown in Table 7.4. While these studies were not specifically designed to investigate memory, they demonstrate the high proportion of women who

Table 7.4. Published studies of cesarean section that used the IFT

Anesthetic	n	Responsive (n)	Recall (n)
T/N$_2$O/H[21]	12	4 (33%)	0
T/N$_2$O/H[22]	32	11 (34%)	0
T/N$_2$O/H[31]	232	95 (41%)	4
K/N$_2$O/H[32]	12	1 (8%)	0
T/N$_2$O/H[32]	13	7 (53%)	0+(1)*
K/T/N$_2$O/H[32]	11	4 (33%)	1+(1)*
T/N$_2$O/H[33]	20	14 (70%)	2
K/N$_2$O/H[33]	30	4 (13%)	0
T/N$_2$O/E[34]	50	24 (48%)	0
T/N$_2$O/I[34]	63	23 (37%)	0
K/N$_2$O/H[35]	20	3 (15%)	0
T/N$_2$O/H[36]	30	29 (97%)	0
T/N$_2$O/H[37]	25	13 (52%)	0
K/N$_2$O/H[37]	25	5 (20%)	0
Total	531	222 (42%)	9

* These two patients (marked (1)) had what were described as 'fragmentary recollections'. E, enflurane; H, halothane; I, isoflurane; K, ketamine; N$_2$O, nitrous oxide; T, thiopental. Patients in refs 21 and 22 are also included in ref 31.

were awake, yet had no explicit recall for this occurrence in the postoperative period. Out of the 531 women in these studies 222 (42%) were wakeful and responding at some stage of the operation, but only seven women had explicit recall (a further two had what were described as 'fragmentary recollections'). This wakefulness usually occurred between the intravenous induction and the establishment of adequate inhalational anesthesia. Although none of the nine women with recall had unpleasant memories, and none recalled pain, this needs to be interpreted with care. In Tunstall's[31] series he asked 26 patients who became responsive after surgery commenced if they were in pain: 17 signalled 'yes', four signalled 'no' and five stopped responding and gave no reply, while in another series,[36] 24 of the 30 women felt pain at skin incision. With this in mind, particularly as regards the very short induction to delivery interval demanded by some obstetricians, Tunstall[31] points out that an early incision in a wakeful subject is likely to be more painful than if the incision is a few minutes later after the uptake of inhalational agent.

Explicit and implicit memory after surgery while using the IFT during anesthesia

The first research project undertaken outside the obstetric suite using the IFT was a study involving total intravenous anesthesia (TIVA) with althesin.[23] Because of serious doubts regarding the assessment of unconsciousness with TIVA,[57–59] it was decided to investigate the possibility of using IFT responses as a guide to the administration of intermittent incremental doses of althesin.[23] In this study, following the induction drugs, the patients were ventilated with an air/oxygen mixture and further increments of althesin were given only after a response to command.[23]

Forty-two patients were recruited into this investigation and the general surgical procedures lasted from 35 to 225 minutes. All patients responded to commands during their surgery and received increments of althesin. There was one case of explicit recall in the series: a woman who had undergone a laparotomy described marked discomfort as her 'insides were being stretched'. She remembered being asked to move her hand/fingers but at the time was unable to do so.[23] It is not clear at what stage of the operation the awareness occurred. There was a 30-minute period during surgery when no responses occurred. From the duration of action of her previous bolus doses of althesin at least one response would have been expected during this period. This non-responsiveness coincided with a period following accidental deflation of the isolating cuff. Ulnar nerve stimulation peripheral to the tourniquet suggested there was still some neuromuscular activity, but it is possible that this did not reflect the ability of the more proximal nerves under the tourniquet to conduct stimuli. A combination of pressure ischemia from the tourniquet on the nerves of the upper arm and partial paralysis of the forearm muscles by alcuronium that leaked under the tourniquet may have prevented her from moving her fingers. During closure of the peritoneum she was noted to be moving her head vigorously without responding to the command. At this time the surgeon requested further muscle relaxation and, following inflation of the isolating cuff, increments of althesin and alcuronium were administered.

Apart from this one patient not only did this study clearly demonstrate that IFT responses could be used to determine the timing of intermittent althesin increments without the occurrence of postoperative explicit recall, but also it proved that Tunstall's original 'short-term' IFT[21,22] (see Table 7.1) could be readily modified (see Table 7.1) for use during prolonged surgical procedures (Figure 7.1).

Since the althesin study the author has used the IFT to investigate the incidence of responsiveness during surgery with a variety of anesthetic techniques involving muscle relaxants (Table 7.5). With the exception of the althesin study, the patients were all women undergoing gynecological procedures. In later studies the tape was personalized for each patient with the inclusion of her name before the command. In even later studies, where more detailed postoperative investigations of implicit memory were made, the patient was also asked by name to remember specific information.[25–27] In all these IFT studies the patients were asked the same basic questions in the immediate postoperative period and, in the case of major gynecological surgery, again on the 2nd or 3rd day (Table 7.6). In addition, in specific studies, where detailed investigation of postoperative memory was performed,[25–27] the patients were tested with direct and indirect memory tasks, e.g. to generate category exemplars, to reply with one word in a word association test, to identify a piece of music, and to identify words masked by white sound.[60]

During these studies it became obvious that clinical criteria gave no guarantee as to the conscious state of patients during surgery. Most of the studies used a PRST score[61] along with the IFT. The PRST score is based on a 0 to 2 score for the systolic blood *P*ressure, the heart *R*ate, the presence or absence of *S*weating and *T*ear formation. It is suggested that a score of <5 indicates adequate anesthesia[61] yet the majority of responses to command in the above studies occurred with PRST scores of 0 or 1 (Tables 7.7 and 7.8).

Of the 329 women in these studies (see Table 7.5), only one had any recollection of surgery: a patient (see Table 7.5, study 4[26]) awoke before surgery commenced and clearly remembers the skin incision (not painful) before she drifted off to sleep again. (Although her right arm was isolated from muscle relaxant by the tourniquet, the tape recorder was not switched on because the trial protocol specified that the tape recorder, with its commands and information should start shortly after the skin incision.) This patient's experience provides further evidence that awake patients who are not in pain may not move in response to surgery. All the other intraoperative memories that were reported in these investigations related to hearing my voice on the tape and usually occurred on prompting with questions 5–8 (see Table 7.6). Ninety-six patients

Table 7.5. Patient responses, dreams and recall in various studies conducted by the author in which the IFT was used

Anesthetic	n	Responsive n (%)	Reflex n (%)	Dreams G, B, N	Recall n
Major gynecological procedures					
Inhalational					
1. T/N$_2$O[13]	26	12 (50%)	16 (67%)	3, 1, 1	5 (+3)*
2. T/N$_2$O/F[24]	36	15 (45%)**	22 (67%)**	3, 5, 2	1
3. T/N$_2$O/F/D	30	4 (13%)	11 (37%)	0, 0, 0	0
4. T/N$_2$O/H[26]	68	0 (0%)	10 (15%)	0, 1, 2	5***
Total intravenous/air/oxygen					
5. E/F[24]	30	2 (7%)	13 (43%)	0, 2, 1	0
6. M/A[25]	32	23 (72%)	22 (69%)	1, 0, 0	3
7. P/A/Ep[27]	40	7 (18%)	2 (5%)	4, 0, 2	0
8. P/A	12	5 (42%)	7 (58)%	2, 0, 0	0
Intermediate day care gynecological laparoscopic procedures					
9. P/N$_2$O/A	30	20 (67%)	20 (67%)	3, 2, 3	4 (aware of my voice)
10. P/A	25	8 (32%)	5 (20%)	1, 0, 0	0

Studies 1–10 included muscle relaxants and the IFT

Minor and intermediate day care gynecological procedures
In the two studies below all patients breathed spontaneously and no muscle relaxants were used

11. P/N$_2$O/I[60]	54	0	0	0, 0, 0	0
12. P/N$_2$O/I	20	0	0	0, 0, 0	0

Responsive = verified responses (as described in Table 7.3). Reflex = hand/arm movements but no response to direct commands. These movements were usually non-specific hand/arm movements. Dreams G = good, B = bad, N = neutral.
* First 20 patients also included in Reference 13. One patient had succinylcholine apnea and IFT was abandoned; one patient had halothane to control blood pressure thus response percentages are based on 24 patients. On prompting, all these 8 patients remembered hearing something about moving their hand/fingers. Three of these 8 patients had no responses to command during surgery (see text for fuller description).
** Three of the 36 patients had halothane to control blood pressure thus percentage responses are based on 33 patients.
*** Four of these recalled memories were at the very beginning or end of anesthesia when the IFT was not in use: one of these women was aware of a painless skin incision before she drifted off to sleep (see above); three occurred at the end of surgery when anesthesia was discontinued. For a description of the fifth case see text. The patient with the bad dream admitted that the nightmare she experienced on this occasion, during which a voice kept repeating 'You are all alone on earth', had happened twice before: during previous surgery. At first she denied any recall but when asked the more specific questions she remembered the hand instructions.
A, alfentanil; D, droperidol; E, etomidate; Ep, epidural; F, fentanyl; H, halothane; I, isoflurane; M, midazolam; N$_2$O, nitrous oxide; P, propofol; T, thiopentone.

Table 7.6. Questions asked in the postoperative period during our IFT studies

1. What was the last thing you remember before going to sleep?
2. What was the first thing you remember on waking up?
3. Can you remember anything in between these two?
4. Do you remember what was on the tape recorder?
5. Do you remember anyone asking you to do anything?
6. Do you remember anyone asking you to do anything with your arm?
7. Do you remember anyone asking you to do anything with your hand?
8. Do you remember anyone asking you to do anything with your fingers?
9. Did you have any dreams?

More detailed investigation of memory was undertaken in some studies.

Table 7.7. PRST scores in association with various responses observed during surgery. Illustrating the unreliability of clinical monitoring in identifying responsive patients

PRST	reflex B S D	unverified B S D	verified B S D	Total
Score				
0	– 2 19	– – 4	1 6 22	54
1 – 2	– 2 16	2 1 1	– 5 11	58
>2	– – 3	– – 1	3 2 4	13
	– 4 38	2 1 6	4 13 37	105

B = before surgery; S = skin incision; D = during surgery; Reflex = not associated with command; unverified = appears to be associated with taped command but no response to direct command; verified = response to additional command to verify an unverified response. (Reprinted with permission from Russell IF. Midazolam-Alfentanil: An anaesthetic? An investigation using the isolated forearm technique. *Br J Anaesth* 1993; **70**:42–46.)

Table 7.8. PRST scores of 0 and >0 and whether or not a response occurred for each 2-minute period during surgery

Illustrating the unreliability of clinical monitoring in identifying responsive patients

	PRST = 0	PRST > 0
No response	511	286
Reflex response	22	20
Unverified response	3	6
Verified response	29	25

Reflex = not associated with command; unverified = appears to be associated with taped command but no response to direct command; verified = response to additional command to verify an unverified response. (Reprinted with permission from Russell IF. Midazolam-Alfentanil: An anaesthetic? An investigation using the isolated forearm technique. *Br J Anaesth* 1993; **70**:42–46.)

(29%) responded during surgery and, of these, 13 provided evidence of recall. Of the 233 patients who did not respond during surgery, there were four who may have had recall. Since these four women would represent false negatives for the IFT it is important to describe these women's experiences. In one case there was a problem with the IFT cuff[26] (nitrous oxide/halothane/relaxant) and three had a nitrous oxide/oxygen curare only anesthetic.

Whether these four cases represent true recall of intraoperative events is not at all clear. If the same tests are applied on two occasions then the responses on the second occasion may merely reflect memory for the first set of tests. Since none of these women expressed any recall during their immediate postoperative period this is a possibility, but there are reports of explicit recall for intraoperative events occurring several days after surgery when initially there was no such recall.[62]

With respect to my studies (see Table 7.5), if one believes that these four patients had no recall of intraoperative events, then the IFT has 100% sensitivity (all 13 cases of recall correctly identified) and 74% specificity (233 of the 316 women with no recall correctly identified). On the other hand, if these four women were expressing memory for intraoperative events, then the IFT has 77% sensitivity (13 of the 17 cases of recall correctly identified) and 73% specificity (229 of the 312 women with no recall correctly identified).

Studies in human volunteers under the influence of anesthetic drugs

There are many volunteer studies and these have

Patient 1

This patient had a halothane/nitrous oxide anaesthetic.[26] There had been six reflex responses before the cuff burst and the arm became paralyzed some 45 minutes into a 70-minute procedure. During recovery she reported no recall of surgery and no dreams but, when prompted, she remembered being asked to do something with her fingers. Three days later she was hypnotized and regressed to the time of surgery in an attempt to elicit evidence of memory. Again no evidence of recall for the surgery was obtained but, when prompted, she thought something had been said about moving her fingers as if she were 'playing a piano': she demonstrated opening and closing her fingers. At the end of the hypnotic interview, as she 'awoke' from her trance she was noted to be opening and closing the fingers of her right hand. When asked why she was doing this she stated she was sure she had been asked to do something with her right hand and had wanted to do this under hypnosis but said she had been unable to do so as her fingers would not move. Other tests of explicit and implicit memory were negative.

Patient 2

During anesthesia with nitrous oxide and curare she made one reflex response during traction on the peritoneum. During recovery she denied any recall or dreams. Two days later, when prompted, she thought someone had asked her to 'move fingers' just once. The voice seemed to linger and sounded a long way off. She did not know when she heard this voice but there was no pain associated with it. She thought it was a wonderful anesthetic and would have it again.

Patient 3

During anesthesia with nitrous oxide and curare there were no responses of any kind. In recovery she denied any recall or dreams. Two days later, when prompted, she said she remembered 'something to do with her hand' and demonstrated opening and closing movements of her right hand. She was sure this memory was from her time in the recovery ward.

Patient 4

During anesthesia with nitrous oxide and curare this patient had three reflex movements within a 5-minute period just after skin incision. On three other occasions, she opened her eyes momentarily and on six other occasions her eyebrows could be seen moving up and down. There were no responses to the taped commands.

When questioned in the recovery ward she remembered being asked to give her date of birth, open her eyes and put out her tongue: these requests were all made around the time of awakening and extubation. She also thought she had been asked to do something with her *left* hand at this time and opened and closed the fingers of her *right* hand (the IFT used her right hand). She then described a dream related to her surgery but she had experienced this same dream before coming into hospital and was not sure if she really had dreamed it a second time.

---

been reviewed in detail by Andrade.[56] In general, it would appear that explicit memory is abolished at levels of consciousness where volunteers are still capable of responding, but when the volunteers cease to respond to commands, at concentrations below that normally used in anesthesia, they no longer have explicit or implicit memory for new information.[19,56] In many of these investigations anesthetic agents, both inhalational or intravenous, are given at a particular MAC level or are titrated to a specific end point, e.g. cessation of response to command. In a study of reaction times in response to an auditory tone Jessop et al.[49] found that, although the reaction times were slowed down by increasing nitrous oxide concentration, the subjects continued to respond correctly up to a concentration of some 40% nitrous oxide and then quite abruptly the subjects lost the ability to perform the task.

Recall for performing the task was lost at lower concentrations of nitrous oxide than the ability to perform.[49] In studies involving subanesthetic doses of isoflurane, subjects began to lose the ability to respond to commands at 0.2 MAC and by 0.4 MAC none responded.[20,63] At 0.4 MAC implicit memory tests showed no evidence of recall.[20] These authors emphasized that absence of response to command guaranteed no recall, but response to command was not indicative of being able to remember.[20] One of the problems with memory studies during anesthesia is the lack of relevance of the information to the subject. Chortkoff et al.[55] attempted to repeat the original study by Levinson[64] whereby a life threatening crisis was created. These authors,[54] using concentrations of desflurane below the usual surgical MAC level, found no evidence of explicit or implicit memory for the crisis.

Other studies have investigated the intravenous anesthetic propofol with similar results, i.e. patients can be awake and responsive to commands with no evidence of explicit or implicit recall. A characteristic of the propofol studies is the wide range of propofol doses required to reach similar states of sedation or consciousness, e.g. for a specific level of 'deep sedation' doses ranged from 2 mg/kg/h to 5.98 mg/kg/h[65] and for loss of response to verbal command doses range from 6 mg/kg/h to 12 mg/kg/h.[66] These dose ranges are well within the typical propofol infusion rates used for major surgery and corroborate my own studies of propofol using the IFT where up to 42% of patients were observed to respond to command during surgery at dose rates varying from 4 mg/kg/h up to 10 mg/kg/h. None of my patients had implicit or explicit recall.

Discussion

In the studies presented above it is clear that both volunteers and patients can respond to commands at levels of consciousness associated with no subsequent recall. Thus the simple postoperative question, 'do you remember anything between going to sleep and waking up in recovery,' will detect only a small proportion of the patients who have been awake and capable of responding during surgery, and possibly in pain. This is an important concept for the reader to understand. For example, in studies of TIVA with propofol and alfentanil, a very low incidence of awareness is reported (0.2%).[62,67] However, closer scrutiny reveals that what these authors are reporting is the number of patients with recall for intraoperative events. The technique used[62,67] is almost identical to that used in my two studies of TIVA (see Table 7.5, studies 7 and 8). In my studies the incidence of intra-operative responsiveness was 18% (with additional epidural anesthesia) and 42% (without additional epidural anesthesia), but none of my patients had explicit recall for these intraoperative events. Thus, without the IFT those authors[62,67] can only speculate on how many of their patients were actually awake but had no recall. When specific prompting questions about the taped commands were put to my patients then there was evidence of explicit memory, but even this prompted memory detected only some 15% of the patients who had been awake and responsive during surgery. This result emphasizes

that during surgery with TIVA and muscle relaxants clinical monitoring will not reliably detect intraoperative wakefulness.

As described above there are occasional instances of patients who do not respond to command and who do have recall: to date the incidence of these cases approximates 1:100, but none have occurred since the taped message was personalized for each patient. In the series of studies in women undergoing gynecological surgery (see Table 7.5), except for the four patients whose recall is debatable and which is described individually above, all evidence for recall comes from patients who had been responsive during anesthesia or, as described above, who had been awake but for various reasons made a conscious decision not to respond. This is in agreement with volunteer studies where all recall came from subjects who had responded[19,20,49,56] (i.e. had been awake). In our four studies specifically designed to enable a detailed investigation of memory and recall after presenting information to patients who were known to be unresponsive, two studies involving muscle relaxants and the IFT[26,27] and two studies of spontaneously breathing patients (see Table 7.5, studies 11[60] and 12), there was no evidence of explicit or implicit memory. These results agree with the many volunteer studies that, as detailed above, show no evidence for recall, explicit or implicit, in volunteers who are unresponsive to commands.[19,20,56]

Surgical stimulation will antagonize the effects of anesthesia and evidence for such an effect can be seen in Table 7.5; studies 7 and 8 were identical (study 8 is still ongoing) with the exception that patients in study 7 had an epidural anesthetic. As yet, the numbers are small and just fail to achieve statistical significance, but it would appear that despite greater infusion rates for both propofol and alfentanil the incidence of consciousness during surgery is over 200% greater in the absence of the epidural anesthetic. Tunstall's data, discussed above, also indicate that surgical stimulation can rouse previously unconscious patients to a responsive state.[31] The fact that some patients may be awake and in pain during surgery, yet have no conscious recall for this is beginning to trouble some researchers[68-70] and is an area that deserves investigation. If one can convince an ethical committee in the years 2000+ that, with regard to cesarean section, it is still acceptable practice to continue using such light general anesthesia that women are effectively 'tied down' to the operating table with relaxants while being operated upon and that many of these women are awake, possibly in pain, but whose conscious state is such that they are unable to remember this in the postoperative period, it would seem there is scope for some intriguing studies: is there a difference in the recovery profile of women who are unconscious during surgery (i.e. make no responses) from women who do respond but are not in pain and from women who respond and who are in pain. In addition, since detailed investigations of implicit memory were not part of the design in any of the obstetric series (see Table 7.3) and almost half of the patients are responsive, there appears to be a significant potential for further study of implicit recall and/or positive suggestion in this group of lightly anesthetized patients, e.g. Lubke et al.[71]

Since the introduction of muscle relaxants into anesthetic practice, it has been recognized that it is impossible to assess depth of anesthesia in their presence.[6–11,15–18] and in 1978, shortly after the first publication of the use of the IFT[21] Lunn stated, 'the fact that auditory perception can occur during general anaesthesia, is not revealed by other clinical indicators of light anaesthesia, and yet cannot be recalled, should be noted'.[72] With the known unreliability of clinical monitoring in determining the presence of consciousness when muscle relaxants are part of the anesthetic technique and the substantial body of evidence that patients can be awake and responsive during surgery with no post-operative conscious recall for the event,[13,14,21–39] it is clear that the assumption made by Merikle and Daneman[5] that 'it is reasonable to assume that patients who are undergoing general anesthesia are in fact unconscious of all external events for the entire duration of surgery' may need to be modified.[73] Consequently, if researchers do not know the conscious state of their patients during surgery at the time when the information is provided they cannot draw conclusions from their results as regards conscious or unconscious processing of information during the 'anesthesia'.

A recent phenomenon is the growing number of memory studies correlating brain monitoring with depth of anesthesia. Of the brain monitors commercially available bispectral analysis (BIS) appears to have the best correlation with levels of sedation and consciousness. However, the data from studies using BIS need to be interpreted with care: group-average BIS values show good correlation with group-average conscious levels, but closer scrutiny of the data reveals a very wide range of individual values associated with consciousness. Flaishon et al.[38] used the IFT in conjunction with BIS monitoring and concluded that BIS can be used to predict the *probability* of recovery of consciousness: this is not the same as stating that a particular BIS value indicates consciousness. Their data show that individual patients may recover responsiveness anywhere over a range of BIS values between approximately 60 and 90.[38] Others have also shown a similar wide range of BIS values over which subjects may begin to respond, with the same BIS value associated with full consciousness in one subject and deep sedation or anesthesia in the next.[74–76] Because of this wide range of BIS values associated with consciousness, there is a risk that some statements could mislead the unwary. Rosow and Manberg,[77] in a review of the BIS monitor, state that 'a BIS value below 60 is associated with an extremely low probability of response to verbal command' and 'Free recall of word or picture cues is lost when BIS is higher than 60, suggesting that memory impairment occurs prior to loss of consciousness'. The implication of these two statements is that a BIS value of ≤60 can be assumed to indicate unconsciousness, and indeed such a definition of unconsciousness has been suggested to me on more than one occasion. When one examines the data on which Rosow and Manberg[77] base these statements it appears that a BIS of 60 is associated with a 30% probability that the subject is capable of responding! There is still a 5% probability that the subject is awake at a BIS of 50. Iselin-Chaves et al.[78] also provide data indicating that a BIS of 45 is associated with some 5% of subjects being capable of responding. A case has been reported of an unsedated, fully conscious volunteer with a BIS of 40.[79] Later EEG investigations of this volunteer revealed him to have a genetically determined low voltage EEG, defined by amplitudes not greater than 20 mv over all head regions.[79] This low voltage EEG phenomenon occurs in some 5–10% of the population[79] and must thus have serious implications for BIS monitoring and depth of anesthesia. In view of the above results care is required in specifying a specific BIS value at which unconsciousness can be assured and it is certainly not possible to specify a BIS of 75 and use this to define anesthesia as some have attempted.[80] Since a particular BIS value cannot reliably predict the transition from unconsciousness to consciousness for all individual subjects within a group,[81] it is inevitable that mixed results will be obtained from memory studies where anesthesia or sedation is targeted to a specific BIS value since some subjects will be awake while others will be unconscious.

Although the IFT has been known about for over 20 years, it is used infrequently because of the continued perpetuation of the misconceptions discussed above. While the IFT is not applicable in all anesthetic situations (e.g. head and neck surgery and ophthalmic surgery where head phones might interfere with the operative site or patient movement jeopardize surgery) it could still afford many patients direct protection from intraoperative awareness, thus answering many of the concerns of Bejenke[82] who believes 'there is no practical means to monitor levels of awareness'. Since electronic brain monitoring is, as yet, not capable of precisely identifying the point when consciousness is lost or regained, the IFT remains the most reliable method of detecting the onset of consciousness during surgery and should be a part of the methodology of any study of memory during anesthesia.

References

1. Bonke B, Fitch W, Miller K (eds). *Memory and Awareness in Anaesthesia*. Amsterdam: Swets and Zeitlinger, 1990.
2. Sebel PS, Bonke B, Winograd E. (eds). *Memory and Awareness in Anaesthesia*. Englewood Cliffs, New Jersey: Prentice-Hall, 1993.
3. Bonke B, Bovill JG, Moerman N. (eds). *Memory and Awareness in Anaesthesia III*. Assen: Van Gorcum, 1996.
4. Jordan C, Vaughn DJA, Newton DEF. (eds). *Memory and Awareness in Anaesthesia IV. Proceedings of the Fourth International Symposium on Memory and Awareness in Anaesthesia*. London: Imperial College Press, 2000.
5. Merikle PM, Daneman M. Memory for unconsciously perceived events: Evidence from anesthetized patients. *Conscious Cogn* 1996; **5**: 525–541.
6. Mushin WW. The signs of anaesthesia. *Anaesthesia* 1948; **3**:154–159.
7. Laycock JD. Signs and stages of anaesthesia. A restatement. *Anaesthesia* 1953; **8**:15–20.
8. Woodbridge PD. Changing concepts concerning depth of anesthesia. *Anesthesiology* 1957; **18**: 536–550.
9. Siker ES. Analgesic supplements to nitrous oxide anaesthesia. *Br Med J* 1956; **2**:1326–1331.
10. Eger EI. Monitoring the depth of anesthesia. In Saidman LJ, Smith NT (eds). *Monitoring in Anesthesia*. New York: John Wiley and Sons, 1978; 1–14.
11. Cullen DJ, Eger EI, Stevens WC, *et al*. Clinical signs of anesthesia. *Anesthesiology* 1972; **36**: 21–36.
12. Grantham CD, Hammeroff SR. Monitoring anesthetic depth. In Blitt CD (ed.) *Monitoring in Anesthesia and Critical Care Medicine.*, Edinburgh: Churchill Livingstone, 1985; 427–440.
13. Russell IF. The Isolated forearm technique. Relationship between movement and clinical indices. In Bonke B, Fitch W, Miller K (eds). *Memory and Awareness in Anaesthesia*. Amsterdam: Swets and Zeitlinger, 1990; 316–319.
14. Russell IF. Conscious awareness during general anaesthesia: relevance of autonomic signs and isolated arm movements as guides to depth of anaesthesia. In Jones JG (ed.) *Baillière's Clinical Anaesthesiology vol 3. Depth of Anaesthesia*, London: Baillière Tindall, 1989; 511–532.
15. Prescott F, Organe G, Rowbotham S. Tubocurarine chloride as an adjunct to anaesthesia. *Lancet* 1946; **1**:80–84.
16. Parkhouse J. Awareness during surgery. *Postgrad Med Bul* 1960; **36**:674–677.
17. Robson JG. Measurement of depth of anaesthesia. *Br J Anaesth* 1969; **41**:785–788.
18. Ghoneim MM, Block RI. Learning and consciousness during general anesthesia. *Anesthesiology* 1992; **76**:279–305.
19. Ghoneim MM, Block RI, Dhanaraj VJ. Interaction of a subanaesthetic concentration of isolfurane with midazolam: effects on responsiveness, learning and memory. *Br J Anaesth* 1998; **80**:581–587.
20. Newton DEF, Thornton C, Konieckzko KM, *et al*. Levels of consciousness in volunteers breathing sub-MAC concentrations of isoflurane. *Br J Anaesth* 1990; **65**:609–615.
21. Tunstall ME. Detecting wakefulness during general anaesthesia for caesarean section. *Br Med J* 1977; **1**:1321.
22. Tunstall ME. The reduction of amnesic wakefulness during caesarean section. *Anaesthesia* 1979; **34**: 316–319.
23. Russell IF. Auditory perception under anaesthesia. *Anaesthesia* 1979; **34**:211.
24. Russell IF. A comparison of wakefulness with two anaesthetic regimens. Total IV v balanced anaesthesia. *Br J Anaesth* 1986; **58**:965–968.
25. Russell IF. Midazolam-Alfentanil: An anaesthetic?

An investigation using the isolated forearm technique. *Br J Anaesth* 1993; **70**:42–46.

26. Russell IF, Wang M. Absence of memory for intraoperative information during adequate general anaesthesia. *Br J Anaesth* 1997; **78**:3–9.

27. Russell IF, Wang M. A randomised, double-blind investigation of post-operative memory for information presented intraoperatively during total intravenous anaesthesia. In Jordan C, Vaughn DJA, Newton DEF (eds) *Memory and Awareness in Anaesthesia IV. Proceedings of the 4th International Symposium on Memory and Awareness in Anaesthesia*. London: Imperial College Press, 2000; 280–286.

28. Wilson ME. Isolated forearm technique for detection of wakefulness during general anaesthesia. *Br J Anaesth* 1981; **53**:1234.

29. Dutton RC, Smith WD, Smith NT. Wakeful response to command indicates memory potential during emergence from general anesthesia. *J Clin Monit* 1995; **11**:35–40.

30. Dutton RC, Smith WD, Smith NT. Brief wakeful response to command indicates wakefulness with suppression of memory formation during surgical anesthesia. *J Clin Monit* 1995;**11**:41–46.

31. Tunstall ME. Wakefulness and awareness during anaesthesia for Caesarean section. *Scot Soc Anaes Newsletter* 1981; **22**:15–16.

32. Schultetus RR, Hill CR, Dharamraj CM. Wakefulness during cesarean section after anesthetic induction with ketamine, thiopental, or ketamine and thiopental combined. *Anesth Analg* 1986; **65**:723–728.

33. Baraka A, Louis F, Noueihid R, Diab M, Dabbous A, Sibai A. Awareness following different techniques of general anaesthesia for caesarean section. *Br J Anaesth* 1989; **62**:645–648.

34. Tunstall ME, Sheikh A. Comparison of 1.5% enflurane with 1.25% isoflurane in oxygen for caesarean section: avoidance of awareness without nitrous oxide. *Br J Anaesth* 1989; **62**:138–143.

35. Baraka A, Louis F, Dalleh R. Maternal awareness and neonatal outcome after ketamine induction of anaesthesia for caesarean section. *Can J Anaesth* 1990; **37**:641–644.

36. King H, Ashley S, Brathwaite D, Decayette J, Wooten DJ. Adequacy of general anesthesia for cesarean section. *Anesth Analg* 1993;**77**:84–88.

37. Gaitini L, Vaida S, Collins G, Somri M, Sabo E. Awareness detection during general anaesthesia using EEG spectrum analysis. *Can J Anaesth* 1995; **42**:377–381.

38. Flaishon R, Windsor A, Sigl J, *et al*. Recovery of consciousness after thiopental or propofol. *Anesthesiology* 1997; **86**:613–619.

39. Byers GF, Muir JG. Detecting wakefulness in anaesthetised children. *Can J Anaesth* 1997; **44**: 486–488

40. Breckenridge JL, Aitkenhead AR. Isolated forearm technique for detection of wakefulness during general anaesthesia. *Br J Anaesth* 1981; **53**:665P.

41. Breckenridge JL, Aitkenhead AR. Awareness during anaesthesia: a review. *Ann Roy Coll Surg Engl* 1983; **65**:93–96.

42. Millar K, Watkinson N. Recognition of words presented during general anaesthesia. *Ergonomics* 1983; **26**:585–594.

43. Bogod DG, Orton JK, Yau HM, Oh TE. Detecting awareness during general anaesthetic caesarean section. An evaluation of two methods. *Anaesthesia* 1990; **45**:279–284.

44. Bonke B, Jelicic M, Bonebakker AE, De Roode A, Bovill JG. (correspondence) Information processing under anaesthesia. *Anaesthesia* 1993; **48**:1122.

45. Bonebakker AE, Jelicic M, Passchier J, Bonke B. Memory during general anesthesia: Practical and methodological aspects. *Conscious Cogn* 1996; **5**:542–561.

46. Jessop J, Jones JG. (Editorial) Conscious awareness during general anaesthesia. What are we attempting to monitor? *Br J Anaesth* 1991; **66**:635–637.

47. Jessop J, Jones JG. Evaluation of the anaesthetic actions of general anaesthetics in the human brain. *Gen Pharmacol* 1992; **23**:927–935.

48. Hooper MB. Absence of memory for intraoperative information. *Br J Anaesth* 1997; **79**:143.

49. Jessop J, Griffiths DE, Furness P, Jones JG, Sapsford DJ, Breckon DA. Changes in the amplitude and latency of the P300 component of the auditory evoked potential with sedative and anaesthetic concentrations of nitrous oxide. *Br J Anaesth* 1991; **67**:524–531.

50. Jones JG. (Editorial) Memory of intraoperative events. *Br Med J* 1994; **309**:967–968.

51. Barlow ED, Pochin EE. Slow recovery from ischaemia in human nerves. *Clin Sci* 1948; **6**: 303–317.

52. Clapham MC. The isolated forearm technique using pancuronium. *Anaesthesia* 1981; **36**:642–643.

53. Russell IF. The isolated forearm technique using pancuronium. *Anaesthesia* 1981; **36**:643.

54. Wang M, Russell IF. Absence of memory for intraoperative information. *Br J Anaesth* 1997; **79**:143.

55. Chortkoff BS, Gonsowski CT, Bennett HL, *et al*. Subanesthetic concentrations of desflurane and propofol suppress emotionally charged information. *Anesth Analg* 1995; **81**:728–736.

56. Andrade J. Investigations of hypesthesia: using anesthetics to explore relationships between consciousness, learning, and memory. *J Consc Cogn* 1996; **5**:562–580.

57. Wright PJ. Attitudes to intravenous infusion anaesthesia. *Anaesthesia* 1982; **37**:1209–1213.

58. Mallon JS. Total Intravenous anaesthesia. *Can J Anaesth* 1990; **37**:279–280.

59. Dundee JW, McMurray TJ. Clinical signs of total intravenous anaesthesia: discussion paper. *J Roy Soc Med* 1984; **77**:669–672.

60. Charlton PFC. Implicit and explicit memory for general anaesthesia, MSc Thesis. Hull: University of Hull, 1991.

61. Evans JM, Fraser A, Wise CC, Davies WL. Computer controlled anaesthesia. In Prakesh O (ed). *Computing in Anaesthesia and Intensive Care*. Boston: Martinus Nijhoff, 1983; 279–291.

62. Nordström G, Engström AM, Persson S, Sandin R. Incidence of awareness in total iv anaesthesia based on propofol, alfentanil and neuromuscular blockade. *Acta Anaesthesiol Scand* 1997; **41**:978–984.

63. Newton DEF, Thornton C, Konieczko KM, *et al.* Auditory evoked response and awareness: a study in volunteers at sub-MAC concentrations of isoflurane. *Br J Anaesth* 1992; **69**:122–129.

64. Levinson B. States of awareness during general anaesthesia. *Br J Anaesth* 1965; **37**:544–546.

65. Andrade J, Jeevaratnam D, Sapsford D. Explicit and implicit memory for names presented during propofol sedation. In Bonke B, Bovill JG, Moerman N. (eds). *Memory and Awareness in Anaesthesia III.*, Assen: van Gorcum, 1996; 10–16.

66. Alkire MT, Haier RJ, Fallon JG, Barker SJ, Shah NK. In Bonke B, Bovill JG, Moerman N. (eds). *Memory and Awareness in Anaesthesia III.*, Assen: van Gorcum, 1996; 17–25.

67. Sandin R, Nordström O. Awareness during total iv anaesthesia. *Br J Anaesth* 1993; **71**:782–787.

68. Wang M. The psychological consequences of awareness. In Jordan C, Vaughn DJA, Newton DEF (eds). *Memory and Awareness in Anaesthesia IV. Proceedings of the 4th International Symposium on Memory and Awareness in Anaesthesia.* London: Imperial College Press, 2000; 315–324.

69. Mehlman MJ, Kanoti GA, Orlowski JP. Informed consent to amnestics, or: What sound does a tree make when it falls on your head? *J Clin Ethics* 1994; **5**:105–108.

70. Tinnin L. Conscious forgetting and subconscious remembering of pain. *J Clin Ethics* 1994; **5**: 151–152.

71. Lubke GH, Kerssens C, Gershon RY, Sebel PS. Bispectral index in relation to memeory function during emergency caesarean section. In Jordan C, Vaughn DJA, Newton DEF (eds). *Memory and Awareness in Anaesthesia IV. Proceedings of the 4th International Symposium on Memory and*

Awareness in Anaesthesia. London: Imperial College Press, 2000; 355–356.

72. Lunn JN. (Editorial) Auditory perception during anaesthesia. *Anaesthesia* 1978; **33**:131–132.

73. Andrade J. Learning during anaesthesia: A review. *Br J Psychol* 1995; **86**: 479–506.

74. Liu J, Singh H, White PF. Electroencephalographic bispectral index correlates with intraoperative recall and depth of propofol-induced sedation. *Anesth Analg* 1997; **84**:185–189.

75. Sleigh JW, Donovan J. Comparison of bispectral index, 95% spectral edge frequency and approximate entropy of the EEG, with changes in heart rate variability during induction of general anaesthesia. *Br J Anaesth* 1999; **82**:666–671.

76. Gajraj RJ, Doi M, Mantzaridis H, Kenny GNC. Comparison of bispectral EEG analysis and auditory evoked potentials for monitoring depth of anaesthesia during propofol anaesthesia. *Br J Anaesth* 1999; **82**:672–678.

77. Rosow C, Manberg PJ. Bispectral index monitoring. *Anesthesiol Clin N Am: Ann Anes Pharmacol* 1998; **2**:89–107.

78. Iselin-Chaves IA, Flaishon R, Sebel P S, *et al.* The effect of interaction of propofol and alfentanil on recall, loss of consciousness, and the bispectral index. *Anesth Analg* 1998; **87**:949–955.

79. Schnider TW, Luginbühl M, Petersen-Felix S, Mathis J. Unreasonably low bispectral index values in a volunteer with genetically determined low-voltage electroencephalographic signal. *Anesthesiology* 1998; **89**:1607–1608.

80. Vakkuri A, Yli-Hankala A, Linfgre L. BIS-monitored depth of anaesthesia in laparoscopic tubal ligation. In Jordan C, Vaughn DJA, Newton DEF (eds). *Memory and Awareness in Anaesthesia IV. Proceedings of the 4th International Symposium on Memory and Awareness in Anaesthesia.* London: Imperial College Press, 2000; 304–311.

81. Gajraj RJ, Doi M, Mantzaridis H, Kenny GNC. Analysis of the EEG bispectrum, auditory evoked potentials and the EEG power spectrum during repeated transitions from consciousness to unconsciousness. *Br J Anaesth* 1998; **80**:46–52.

82. Bejenke CJ. Can patients be protected from detrimental consequences of intraoperative awareness in the absence of effective technology. In Bonke B, Bovill JG, Moerman N. (eds). *Memory and Awareness in Anaesthesia III.*, Assen: van Gorcum, 1996; 125–133.

Chapter 8

The psychological consequences of explicit and implicit memories of events during surgery

Michael Wang

Contents

Introduction

Although studies conducted in the UK suggest progressive improvement in the incidence of awareness with explicit recall,[1,2] it seems unlikely that the frequency of such occurrences will ever become insignificant. At the present time estimates range between one in five hundred and one in ten thousand.[3] However, even the more conservative of these figures implies that several cases per day must occur in the UK alone. Clearly, there is great variation in the degree of trauma associated with such experiences. For example, awareness of brief episodes of intraoperative conversation between surgical staff that carries little or no meaning for the patient, who may be comfortable, free of pain and not distressed by paralysis, is unlikely to result in psychological sequelae. On the other hand, a patient enduring major surgery with full pain

perception for an hour or more is quite a different matter. It is unclear at present what proportion of awareness cases is characterized by intraoperative distress and, in turn, what proportion of such cases develops significant postoperative psychological disturbance as a consequence. It might also be possible for individuals (with some conscious intra-operative memory) to be unaware of intraoperative *distress* yet, because of subsequent *postoperative* emotional processing of the meaning and implication of the event for the patient, psychological disturbance ensues nevertheless.

The above considerations do not address an even greater potential source of psychological sequelae: that of implicit emotional learning in which there is no explicit recall of intraoperative events but, nevertheless, the anesthetic has been sufficiently light to allow some degree of emotional or other cognitive processing to take place, giving rise to

145

specific, postoperative psychological sequelae. Such sequelae may be more subtle, more difficult to demonstrate empirically and yet more psychologically insidious. I will refer to the possibility of such effects as the 'implicit emotional learning hypothesis', and much of the later part of this chapter will be devoted to this.

Psychological sequelae following awareness with explicit recall

Some 2 years ago I was referred a patient for psychological treatment immediately following an episode of anesthetic awareness. She had endured an abdominal hysterectomy in the absence of maintenance anesthetic due to anesthesiologist error: the ventilator was entraining room air instead of nitrous oxide/oxygen and enflurane. From her account it is apparent that she had been conscious with full recall for between 30 and 40 minutes of the operative procedure. It is difficult to imagine a more horrific circumstance than that of full consciousness with pain and paralysis. There was no indication of her predicament from so-called clinical signs. The intraoperative hemodynamic record was carefully examined: it was stable and unremarkable.

Although intensive cognitive-behavioral psychotherapy beginning within 48 hours of the episode may have limited the severity of the post-traumatic reaction, nevertheless, the patient suffered two to three flashback experiences per week, panic attacks and agoraphobia, sleep disturbance, night terrors and marital tension for the following $2\frac{1}{2}$ months. This was followed by a 3-month period of clinical depression. Only by 6 months were her difficulties beginning to show signs of resolving. Even at 1 year she was left with residual difficulties, including phobic avoidance of hospitals and occasional sleep disturbance.

In addition to prolonged periods of anxiety and depression, episodes of awareness with pain, distress and full recall commonly give rise to *post-traumatic stress disorder* (PTSD). The most important features fall into three distinct categories: symptoms of elevated autonomic arousal and generalized anxiety; intrusive and distressing thoughts and images recalling the trauma; and behavioral avoidance of physical cues and settings that prompt memory of the trauma.

Thus, during the months and years after their ordeal, awareness patients experience sporadic and distressing panic attacks, nightmares and daytime flashbacks in which they relive aspects of the awareness episode. Often they avoid hospitals and doctors in general, and in particular, those involved in their traumatic surgical experience. Lying in bed in the supine position cues recall of the episode and often they will have panic attacks during the night along with insomnia. Given that normal REM dream sleep is associated with a naturally occurring voluntary muscle paralysis, it is not surprising that dream content often relates to the experience of awareness and, in particular, unexpected paralysis. As discussed later, nightmares often involve ideas of being buried alive in which it is impossible to move and there is an ominous darkness. There is a devastating loss of trust in the medical profession and a sense that nothing can be taken for granted any more. The patient's conceptual world has literally been turned upside down and many of their previous assumptions about safety, competence, and trustworthiness of professions and public institutions in general are undermined.

Apart from the numerous individual case reports of traumatic psychological reactions following anesthetic awareness, there have been a small number of systematic follow-up investigations of groups of such cases.[4,5] A range of psychological problems is reported, including phobic disorder, panic disorder, clinical depression, nightmares and night terrors. Moerman and Bonke[4] followed up three patients who had experienced awareness with full recall. These patients described nightmares, night terrors, general sleep disturbance and anxiety over 3–8 months after their surgery. MacLeod and Maycock[5] provided detailed case reports of three patients. All three referred to the distressing experience of paralysis and, although in two cases pain was a significant aspect of the intraoperative experience, in the third case there was no pain whatsoever. All three developed distressing post-traumatic effects including nightmares, night terrors, insomnia, anxiety, depression, hyperarousal and impaired concentration for between 6 months and 2 years following their operations. The content of the nightmares is revealing and provides an intriguing glimpse into post-traumatic cognitive processing. This includes viewing the operation from above or from one side of the operating room, being buried alive, being dead, and being unable to breathe. Invariably the person wakes in panic and may shout out or scream.

Eight studies have been published in which larger cohorts of awareness patients have been recruited through newspaper advertisements or notification and referral from colleagues within the same hospital.[6–13] These patients' experiences have then been investigated retrospectively in a systematic fashion, commonly using structured interview techniques. Again, nightmares, sleep disturbance and other PTSD symptoms predominate. It is possible to link intraoperative perceptions and characteristics with particular postoperative sequelae in these studies. For example, Moerman *et al.*[9] provide patients' accounts of both their intraoperative experience and subsequent traumatic effects in 26 cases, and 70% describe significant post-traumatic effects. Although no formal statistical analysis of these data was undertaken, the vast majority of the intraoperative reports make reference to the experience of paralysis and the sense of power-lessness. Cundy and Dasey[11] suggest that their data support the contention that the experience of pain is the most important factor in predicting the subsequent development of PTSD. However, this is open to interpretation; their data also support a strong association between awareness of complete paralysis and subsequent PTSD. There are significant methodological difficulties with this type of study. First, recruitment via newspaper advertisement is likely to produce a biased sample of those who are only moderately disturbed by their experience, and who may be reasonably articulate and assertive. Very distressed individuals may not respond to such notices. *Ad hoc* referral by anesthesiologist colleagues may not take account of those so traumatized by their experience that they do not wish to have any further contact with treating clinicians or the hospital in which the awareness occurred. Such cases are lost at follow-up, and the anesthesiologist may be blissfully unaware that there has been a problem. Second, there is an absence of control groups. Non-wakeful patients may, for example, also experience sleep disturbance and other psychological problems. Without appropriate control comparisons, we cannot evaluate the extent to which such problems are a direct result of the awareness episode. It is therefore not surprising that there is great variation in these studies: the prevalence among those with awareness reporting psychological difficulties ranges from 20 to 80%.

Variation in response to a traumatic awareness episode is illustrated in the following anecdote. Some years ago the author was informed that two patients on the same surgical list had been fully conscious with pain and paralysis as a result of a ventilator failure. The author visited the ward some 36 hours following the surgery. The first patient, a woman, had undergone a banded gastroplexy and had felt the insertion of every single stomach staple. Despite a lengthy debriefing session, subsequently she experienced post-traumatic anxiety and depression and entered into litigation against the hospital. The second patient was a young male who had received surgery for an inguinal hernia. Despite the author's early attendance on the ward, the patient had discharged himself against medical advice, and subsequent attempts by both ward staff and the author to contact this patient failed. Although it is possible that the patient may have experienced post-traumatic disorder, he was completely lost to follow up, made no formal complaint and, unlike the first patient, certainly did not enter into litigation. This anecdote also illustrates a significant gender difference prevalent in the UK and the USA[14] in which male awareness patients much less commonly complain or take action against hospital authorities as a result of their experience. It may be that this is considered unmanly and that male patients feel they should expect to experience pain, trauma and discomfort and must 'put up with it' without complaint.

Paralysis and catastrophic misinterpretation in the genesis of PTSD

Although up to half of awareness patients also recall pain, it is not necessarily this in itself that leads to postoperative traumatic psychological disturbance. Post-traumatic stress seldom follows vaginal childbirth, for example. Despite recurrent media reports of anesthetic awareness, it remains the case that the majority of patients undergoing major surgery have no idea that a muscle relaxant will be used, or that if they are unfortunate enough to become wakeful, they will be unable to move. The realization of consciousness of which operating room staff are evidently oblivious, along with increasingly frenetic yet futile attempts to signal with various body parts, leads rapidly to the conclusion that something has gone seriously wrong.

The patient may believe that the surgeon has accidentally severed the spinal cord, or that some unusual drug reaction has occurred, rendering her totally paralyzed, not just during the surgery, *but for the rest of her life.*

It is often this kind of belief that elicits shock and traumatization. The following case example illustrates such effects. Mr A had an extensive history of sleep paralysis, the relatively common condition in which naturally occurring REM-sleep motor inhibition persists momentarily into wakefulness. Having never previously required surgery, he was scheduled for coronary artery by-pass grafting (CABG). He was concerned that his sleep paralysis might be adversely affected by anesthetic drugs, and was careful to discuss this with his anesthesiologist. The anesthesiologist consulted various texts and a psychiatric colleague, and concluded that the sleep anomaly was of no consequence. Following the operation, Mr A returned to consciousness in the recovery room only to find he could not move. Believing this to be a bout of sleep paralysis, he tried his usual strategies that would normally bring him out of this. His arm fell, hanging from the bed, but he remained paralyzed. At that moment he became severely traumatized, erroneously believing that an interaction between the anesthetic and his existing condition had resulted in permanent, irreversible paralysis. He was unaware of the use of muscle relaxants during anesthesia, or that temporary residual paralysis following CABG is not uncommon. He suffered serious and disabling PTSD and continues to have psychological difficulties. Such examples suggest that anesthesiologists need to give careful consideration as to whether such erroneous cognitive reactions could be mitigated perioperatively by the routine provision of information about the use of muscle relaxants and their effects.

Postoperative management of awareness

In the UK, improved education and, in particular, the explicit guidance of medical indemnity organizations, has resulted in generally a much more sympathetic response from medical staff[15] when, in the past, invariably it was one of denial. This is exemplified by a 66-year-old woman who wrote to us recently (1998) after a television interview that she had seen, in which the author and Dr Ian Russell

were discussing awareness. In summary, this woman had a cesarean section in 1962. On leaving the operating room she told the senior midwife that she had been awake and felt everything during the surgery. The midwife's response was 'Do not dare to ever mention such a thing to anyone again. If you do you will terrify other patients'. When we first met her she was still terrified and required considerable reassurance that she had permission to talk about her experience and that she would not 'get into trouble'. This patient had received no help for 36 years and had major psychiatric problems including chronic depression, attempted suicide and long-term PTSD symptoms. Although she had received some psychiatric treatment for her depression and suicide attempt in the 1960s, she had not told the psychiatrist about her experience. She is now receiving treatment from us, although after 36 years the chances of a successful outcome are unknown. A potential problem for the future is that she is likely to need major gynecological surgery and not surprisingly is frightened of the anesthetic.

It is not difficult to understand the devastating effects of denial on the part of hospital staff. The patient is left questioning her own sanity given the intensity and distress of her experience set alongside the dismissive reactions of expert staff she has, hitherto, trusted absolutely. Although no empirical studies have examined these effects systematically, the author has encountered tragic examples in which marital breakdown has occurred because the spouse has been unable to believe the patient's account in view of the hospital's reaction.

The nature and incidence of post-traumatic stress disorder has been widely recognized in recent years. It is now commonplace for psychological intervention in the immediate post-trauma period to be a mandatory requirement. This usually takes the form of 'psychological debriefing' in which the events, perceptions, thoughts, and emotions of the trauma are re-experienced under the guidance of the therapist.[16] The rationale here is that such intense exposure to traumatic memory aids emotional processing and ultimately, psychological assimilation and resolution. However, recent studies suggest that the routine use of psychological debriefing does not always improve psychological outcome and, in some cases, may worsen it.[17] These findings are controversial. Nevertheless, the empirical evidence in favour of psychological debriefing following trauma is at best equivocal. However, from a medicolegal point of view, case law seems to suggest that psychological consultation in the immediate aftermath of awareness with recall is essential.

Whatever the case, health authorities are more aware of the need to provide access to psychological or psychiatric expertise and treatment in the immediate postoperative period, if only to cite as mitigation in litigation suits. Clinically, there is a need to assess the premorbid personality and previous psychiatric history of the patient alongside the events surrounding the episode of awareness and its *meaning* for the patient, and it is arguable that the mental health professional is best placed to fulfil this role. However, we should not underestimate the crucial role of the anesthesiologist in the immediate aftermath of an episode of awareness. The following is some simple guidance, based on the outcome literature and clinical experience,[14] where the treating anesthesiologist's words and actions can potently determine psychological outcome.

It is important to obtain a detailed account from the patient. *Listen carefully, show concern and a desire to be clear about what the patient has experienced.* It is extremely important to acknowledge the possibility that, for a variety of reasons, the anesthetic may not have been adequate, allowing the patient to become conscious. The effects of muscle relaxants (if relevant) should be mentioned and how these may make it possible for awareness to occur because of the need to reduce potentially toxic levels of anesthetic and because of the unreliability of clinical signs. The anesthesiologist should make it clear that he or she believes the patient's account of events. The psychological condition of the patient may be made worse if hospital staff and relatives suggest that the experience was imagined. In many cases psychological sequelae are obviated if the patient's awareness memory is validated by staff. It is permissible and certainly desirable to express regret that this has occurred: this does *not* constitute an admission of liability. If no cause has been found then avoid speculation, but reassure the patient that a full investigation will take place. An accurate account of the cause of the awareness should be given to the patient as early as possible. Most lawsuits are driven by the patient's desire to find out what happened or to elicit an apology.

It is very unusual for claims of awareness to be entirely fabricated. In some cases the patient has experienced an unpleasant dream not involving specific surgical events. Such a dream could have occurred at any point in the perioperative period. Sometimes other actual events during the immediate postoperative or preoperative period are recalled and incorrectly attributed as intraoperative. It is important to confirm these events with other operating room or recovery room staff. In such cases the confusion should be addressed gently, with care and understanding of the patient's genuine experience.

All patients who believe they have been aware, however fleetingly, must be followed up, preferably by the anesthesiologist concerned, within the first 2 weeks of the operation. If it is apparent that the patient is experiencing psychological problems such as anxiety, depression, nightmares or flashbacks, he or she should be referred to a clinical psychologist or psychiatrist with expertise in the treatment of post-traumatic stress disorders, and ideally with previous experience of cases of unplanned intraoperative awareness.

Psychological sequelae without explicit recall of intraoperative events

Mrs B, a housewife aged 51, was referred to the author for treatment of dental phobia. She described episodes of anticipatory panic and, in particular, while in the dental surgeon's operating chair. These panic attacks were unusual, in that they were characterized by images and sensations as if she were 'in a coffin', buried alive and unable to move. Further investigation revealed that these difficulties had begun some 10 years previously, following a laminectomy. Mrs B had experienced a series of panic attacks *de novo* during the weeks following her operation in a variety of settings. The incidence of these then declined over time, until 3 years later when she required a laparoscopy and dilatation and curettage under general anesthesia. Again, there was a return of the panic attacks during the weeks after this second operation followed by a degree of resolution over a number of months. Much the same pattern occurred following a hysterectomy 2 years later. Since the laminectomy she had been troubled by sleep disturbance and, in particular, two recurrent nightmares. In one of these Mrs B dreamed that she had murdered her best friend and buried her in the garden. In the other, she found herself at the bottom of her garden and began to notice moving hands coming up from the soil as if a number of individuals had been buried alive. This theme of being buried alive clearly has echoes with the accounts of those with full explicit recall with distress, who describe nightmares, discussed previously. In this case the patient had no explicit memory of any intraoperative aspect of her laminectomy, or of any of the other operations. Subsequent examination of the anesthetic record for the laminectomy revealed that no volatile agent had been used. No *expired* gas concentration monitoring had been available. A technique involving muscle relaxant (pancuronium) and reliance on 60% nitrous oxide in oxygen and intermittent intravenous opioid for maintenance anesthesia had been employed. Studies conducted in Hull have demonstrated that about 60% of patients are sufficiently conscious to signal meaningfully using the isolated forearm technique with this type of 'anesthetic'.[18] Moreover, the patient had been markedly anxious preoperatively (noted in the anesthetic record), arguably increasing the risk of inadequate anesthesia without adjustment of anesthetic dose.

Remarkably there are more published studies reporting psychological disturbance following an operation *in the absence of explicit or conscious recall of intraoperative awareness* (like the above) than those in which there is full recollection of such an episode.[19–24] Typically the nature of the postoperative problems is suggestive of intraoperative wakening and associated trauma, such as recurrent nightmares related to paralysis, preoccupation with death, sleep anxiety and initial insomnia. Often it is someone other than the patient who connects the onset of psychological difficulties with the surgery. Despite the lack of knowledge of awareness on the part of the patient, subsequent examination of the intraoperative anesthetic record may yield evidence suggestive of lightness or inadequate anesthesia. These studies are now reviewed in detail.

In 1961, Meyer and Blacher[19] described a postoperative 'traumatic neurosis' in a series of patients who appeared to have awakened while paralyzed during heart surgery. The main features of this traumatic reaction were anxiety and irritability, repetitive nightmares, a preoccupation with death, and a reluctance to discuss the symptoms lest the patients be thought insane. These symptoms correspond closely with those associated with the contemporary psychiatric diagnosis of post-traumatic stress disorder. The significant point here is that, according to Meyer and Blacher's account, these patients were uncertain of the cause of their difficulties, and had no clear recollection of intraoperative wakefulness.

Bergstrom and Bernstein[20] investigated six patients who had received nitrous oxide/oxygen alone and a further 11 who received the same regimen preceded by a barbiturate induction. Although no patient had any immediate postoperative recollection, all six of the first group recalled terrifying intraoperative dreams one week later. These six patients (but not the 11 who had also received barbiturate) described distressing psychological sequelae for up to one year after their operations, including fears associated with the dream content that, in one case, precipitated a psychosis. It is unclear whether or not this latter patient had a previous psychiatric history.

Blacher[21] presented six case reports in which surgical patients experienced recurrent nightmares involving paralysis, and a preoccupation with death. For example, one patient had a recurrent dream of being tied down, while another dreamt of being strapped down by the Mafia who stuck wires into her chest. None of these patients had conscious recall of intraoperative wakefulness, but it was clear that their difficulties had begun immediately following surgery. These patients had been referred to Blacher, a psychiatrist, by anesthetic and surgical colleagues. In these cases, explanation of the likelihood that the patient had been wakeful during surgery, and how this related to the dream content, was often sufficient to prompt resolution of the nightmares.

Tunstall[22] reported a case in which a woman presented with *de novo* panic disorder that was associated with going to bed at night. The family physician (rather than the patient herself) noticed that the onset of this problem coincided with previous surgery. Investigation of anesthetic records indicated the possibility of intraoperative wakefulness. The patient was referred to Tunstall for assistance. Tunstall gave the patient a general anesthetic with muscle relaxant, but used the isolated forearm technique to communicate with her when deliberately lightening the anesthetic. The patient was asked to indicate whether this was the condition she found herself in during the previous operation.

Using the isolated forearm, she indicated that this indeed was the case. Tunstall then proceeded to provide verbal reassurance to the effect that this would not happen again, and that she would recover from the panic disorder, now that the cause had been ascertained. The panic disorder is reported to have remitted following this intervention.

Howard[23] describes two further case examples in which apparent intraoperative perception without explicit recall gave rise to psychological problems: in the first, a case of chronic insomnia, which persisted for 3 years, and in the second, relapse and return of an eating disorder. In both these cases, Howard obtained evidence of episodes of intra-operative wakefulness by means of regression under hypnosis. In the insomnia case, the patient under hypnosis recalled hearing someone say, 'She will sleep the sleep of death' during her operation. Subsequently the anesthesiologist concerned confirmed that he did indeed make this unfortuitous casual remark.

Tinnin[24] was referred a 61-year old patient who was refusing potentially life-saving surgery for uterine cancer. The author describes how, using hypnosis, he uncovered evidence of intraoperative wakefulness, paralysis, pain and trauma during previous orthopedic operations to repair leg-crush injuries. The patient had no conscious recollection of this experience, which appeared to have led to phobic avoidance of surgery. Further psychotherapy using the material recovered under hypnosis was sufficient to allow the patient eventually to undertake the surgery.

Clearly these reports do not constitute meth-odologically rigorous evidence of intraoperative effects; nevertheless, it is the close correspondence of the content of the emotional disturbance, whether nightmares or phobias, which is impressive, particularly given the context of apparent absence of knowledge on the part of the patient of a direct connection with intraoperative events. In an extensive review published elsewhere,[25] the author has argued that such implicit effects are the result of intraoperative episodes of wakefulness in which anesthetic and sedative drugs impair subsequent explicit (but not implicit) recall. Hence, postoperatively, certain cues are able to evoke emotional responses that correspond to distressing intraoperative states, but there is no conscious recollection of the intraoperative learning episode itself.

Implicit emotional learning

There are numerous, intriguing anecdotal reports of apparent instances in which intraoperative conversation (without explicit recall) has led to specific psychological or psychosomatic distur-bance. Cheek[26] described many such examples that he claimed were, at the time, being sys-tematically ignored by anesthesiologists. Howard's insomniac patient who had heard the words 'she will sleep the sleep of death'[23] has already been discussed. Levinson[27] describes a case of Cheek's in which, under hypnosis, a patient reported hearing a surgeon say, 'Look at the lung. Have you ever seen anything as black as that?' during surgery immediately prior to the onset of asthma. Bennett[28] reviews a number of similar cases. However, such examples remain anecdotal with attendant meth-odological limitations. In order to examine the implicit emotional learning hypothesis in a more rigorous manner, we initiated several double-blind studies within the limitations of ethical acceptability. The main purpose has been to investigate the post-operative emotional effects of uncontrolled episodes of wakefulness in the absence of explicit recall. Two such studies are summarized below.

In one study, a cohort of patients with intra-operative indications of wakefulness (in the absence of recall) was compared with patients identified as non-wakeful. Eighty consecutive hysterectomy cases were investigated. Patients with a psychiatric history and/or who were taking psychotropic medication were excluded from the study. Hemodynamic variables, inspired gas and vapor concentrations were obtained and analyzed. Each anesthesiologist completed a detailed questionnaire on their observations of the patient and whether there was any indication of lightening of the anesthetic state. Fifteen of the 80 patients also were monitored using the isolated forearm technique. Two of us (IFR and MW) rated the intraoperative data from each case independently on a 5-point scale ranging from 'no evidence at all of lightening of anaesthesia' (1) to 'episode of wakefulness highly probable' (5). Postoperatively, all patients were asked if they had any conscious recollection of intraoperative events: none did.

The patients were contacted at 1 month and 3 months after the operation and asked to complete and return a number of mental state screening questionnaires, including the General Health

Questionnaire 28 (GHQ-28), the Hospital Anxiety and Depression Scale (HADS) and a sleep questionnaire that asked about sleep disturbance and nightmares. The patients had also completed these measures following admission, the night before their operation, providing baseline data. Once follow-up data collection was completed, the cohort was divided in half on the basis of the ratings of lightness of anesthetic, with one half designated 'unlikely to have been light' and the other 'likely to have been light'. Follow-up mental state scores from each of these groups were compared using repeated measures analysis of variance.

On the majority of psychopathology indices, the group mean scores were in the predicted direction, with higher mean scores in the 'likely to have been light' group. In particular, statistically significant differences between the groups were obtained for measures of postoperative anxiety. The speculation that these findings merely reflect starting differences between the groups can be discounted on the grounds that preoperative scores did not indicate such differences. Furthermore, results from the neuroticism scale of the Eysenck Personality Inventory (again administered preoperatively), which provides an indication of existing constitutional or 'neurotic' anxiety, suggested that both groups were comparable prior to surgery. What makes these findings particularly remarkable is the fact that patients were totally unaware of their intraoperative state, i.e. as to whether they belonged to the 'light' or 'non-light' group.

This raises the intriguing possibility of implicit emotional learning, which may have important implications for the postoperative mental health of surgical patients. In effect, intermittent episodes of wakefulness (possibly with distress) without explicit recall may result in postoperative emotional disturbance, which may be all the more insidious and difficult to resolve by virtue of the absence of an accurate subjective understanding of the cause of the problem on the part of the patient. Clearly a great deal more needs to be done to confirm that this is indeed the case.

In 1990, Russell[29] reported that while conducting a trial of total intravenous anesthesia with midazolam and alfentanyl, 20 out of 30 patients indicated wakefulness and pain using the isolated forearm. None of these patients had explicit recall for these events. Recently, we followed up these patients in a double-blind manner using a structured interview that identified episodes of psychological disturbance during the postoperative period to the present, comparing patients who gave no indication of intraoperative wakefulness with those indicating pain. Some evidence of the persistence of depressed mood in the wakeful patients in comparison with the non-wakeful patients was obtained. However, there are methodological difficulties with the retrospective nature of the study and the small sample size. Nevertheless, these are likely to reduce the probability of obtaining statistically significant group differences rather than to inflate it. Furthermore, within the wakeful group there were some interesting case examples of psychological disturbance whose content was consistent with the intraoperative implicit emotional learning hypothesis. No such case examples emerged from the non-wakeful group.

Conclusion

Having reviewed the literature on the psychological consequences of explicit and implicit memories of events during surgery, it is clear that much further research is necessary before unequivocal conclusions may be drawn. Most would agree that episodes of unplanned awareness with full recall should be avoided, and the psychological disorders that occur in their wake are not surprising. However, there is considerable variability in outcome and it is unclear what factors are responsible for this. One likely candidate is that of unanticipated paralysis and associated misconceptions, and we need to consider whether patients and the public at large should be more aware of the widespread use of muscle relaxants in major surgery and their effects.

Much of the evidence for implicit emotional learning is anecdotal, although a few recent more rigorous prospective studies have been attempted. These suggest implicit emotional learning occurs when patients become wakeful (and possibly distressed) but with subsequent impaired explicit recall. This type of research is fraught with practical and ethical difficulties. However, despite these limitations, the data thus far indicate that it is unsafe to conclude that episodes of intraoperative wakefulness in the absence of explicit recall are of no consequence.

References

1. Breckenridge JL, Aitkenhead AR. Awareness during general anaesthesia: a review. *Ann R Coll Surg Eng* 1983; **65**:93–96.
2. Lui WHD, Thorp TAS, Graham SG, Aitkenhead AR. Incidence of awareness with recall during general anaesthesia. *Anaesthesia* 1991; **46**:435–437.
3. Jones JG. Perception and memory during general anaesthesia. *Br J Anaesth* 1994; **73**:31–37.
4. Moerman N, Bonke B. Psychological sequelae of 'awareness' in general anesthesia. *Ned Tidschr Geneeskd* 1990; **134**:2465–2467.
5. MacLeod A, Maycock E. Awareness during anaesthesia and post-traumatic stress disorder. *Anaesth Intensive Care* 1992; **20**:378–382.
6. Guerra F. Awareness and recall. In Hindman B (ed.) *International Anesthesiology Clinics 24: Neurological and Psychological Complications of Surgery and Anesthesia*. Boston: Little Brown, 1986; 75–99.
7. Evans J. Patients' experiences of awareness during general anaesthesia. In Rosen M, Lunn J. (eds). *Consciousness, Awareness and Pain in General Anaesthesia*. London: Butterworths, 1987; 84–192.
8. Cobcroft M, Forsdick C. Awareness under anaesthesia: the patients' point of view. *Anaesth Intensive Care* 1993; **21**:837–843.
9. Moerman N, Bonke B, Oosting J. Awareness and recall during general anesthesia: facts and feelings. *Anesthesiology* 1993; **79**:454–464.
10. Cundy G. Early intervention in the treatment of post-anesthetic stress disorders. In Sebel P, Bonke B, Winograd E (eds). *Memory and Awareness in Anaesthesia*, Englewood Cliffs: Prentice-Hall, 1993; 343–348.
11. Cundy G, Dasey N. An audit of stress disorders related to anaesthesia. In Bonke B, Bovill J, Moerman N (eds). *Memory and Awareness in Anaesthesia 3*. Assen, Netherlands: Van Gorcum, 1996;143–150.
12. Schwender D, Kunze-Kronawitter H, Dietrich P, Klasing S, Forst H, Madler C. Conscious awareness during general anaesthesia: patients' perceptions, emotions, cognition and reactions. *Br J Anaesth* 1998; **80**:133–139.
13. Ranta S, Laurila R, Saario J, Ali-Melkkila T, Hynynen M. Awareness with recall during general anesthesia: incidence and risk factors. *Anesth Analg* 1998; **86**:1084–1089.
14. Domino KB, Posner KL, Caplan RA, Cheney FW. Awareness during anesthesia: a closed claim analysis. *Anesthesiology* 1999; **90**:1053–1061.
15. Aitkenhead AR Editorial: Awareness during anaesthesia – what should the patient be told? *Anaesthesia* 1990; **45**:351–352.
16. Dyregrov A, Mitchell JT. Critical incident stress debriefing. *Tidss Norsk Psykol* 1988; **25**:217–224.
17. Bisson JI. Is post-traumatic stress disorder preventable? *J Ment Health* 1997; **6**:109–111.
18. Russell IF. Conscious awareness during general anaesthesia: relevance of autonomic signs and isolated forearm movements as guides to depth of anaesthesia. In Jones, JG (ed.) *Balliere's Clinical Anaesthesiology* 1989; **3**:511–532.
19. Meyer B, Blacher R. A traumatic neurotic reaction induced by succinylcholine chloride. *N Y J Med* 1961; **61**:1255–1261.
20. Bergstrom H, Bernstein K. Psychic reactions after analgesia with nitrous oxide for caesarean section. *Lancet* 1968; **2**:541–542.
21. Blacher R. On awakening paralysed during surgery: a syndrome of traumatic neurosis. *JAMA* 1975; **234**:67–68.
22. Tunstall M. Anaesthesia for obstetric operations. In MacGillivray I. (ed.) *Clinics in Obstetrics and Gynaecology 7, Number 3*. London: WB Saunders, 1980; 665–694.
23. Howard J. Incidents of auditory perception during anaesthesia with traumatic sequelae. *Med J Aust* 1987; **146**:44–46.
24. Tinnin L. Conscious forgetting and subconscious remembering of pain. *J Clin Ethics* 1994; **5**: 151–152.
25. Wang M. Learning, memory and awareness during anaesthesia. In Adams AP, Cashman JN (eds). *Recent Advances in Anaesthesia and Analgesia, volume 20*. Edinburgh: Churchill Livingstone, 1998; 83–106.
26. Cheek DB. Surgical memory and reaction to careless conversation. *Am J Clin Hypn* 1964; **6**:237–240.
27. Levinson B. The states of awareness in anaesthesia in 1965. In Bonke B, Fitch W, Millar K. (eds). *Memory and Awareness in Anaesthesia*. Amsterdam: Swets & Zeitlinger, 1990; 11–20.
28. Bennett HL. Influencing the brain with information during general anaesthesia: a theory of 'unconscious hearing'. In Bonke B, Fitch W, Millar K, (eds). *Memory and Awareness in Anaesthesia*. Amsterdam: Swets & Zeitlinger, 1990; 50–56.
29. Russell IF. Midazolam-alfentanil: an anesthetic? An investigation using the isolated forearm technique. *Br J Anaesth* 1993; **70**:42–46.

Chapter 9

Medicolegal consequences of awareness during anesthesia

Karen B. Domino and Alan R. Aitkenhead

Contents

Awareness under general anesthesia is a frightening experience, which may result in serious emotional injury and post-traumatic stress disorder. For most individuals, this awareness results in no litigation. However, a few patients file a medical malpractice claim as a result of their injury. This chapter will review background information on malpractice litigation in general, the medicolegal consequences of awareness in the UK and Europe, the medicolegal consequences of awareness in the USA, and future medicolegal implications of intraoperative awareness.

General principles of malpractice litigation

Relationship between malpractice claims, adverse outcomes and negligence

The medical malpractice system is an imperfect attempt to compensate financially victims of medical accidents. In order to sustain a claim successfully for medical malpractice, the plaintiff must demonstrate that a breach in the physician's duty to the patient caused the injury.[1] Care falling below an acceptable standard comprises a breach in the duty.[1]

Appropriate care is generally defined as that which meets the standard of care for a prudent anesthesiologist practising in the community at the time of the event.[2] Substandard or inappropriate care fails to meet the acceptable standard of practice, and therefore, constitutes negligence.[2] Substandard anesthetic care usually involves the poor choice/conduct of anesthesia, use of shortcuts, lack of continuous monitoring, or serious error in judgment; all errors that adversely affected the patient's outcome.

The legal system often fails to adjudicate malpractice claims according to the above principles. Medical malpractice litigation and payment correlated with severity of patient disability, not negligence, in the Harvard Medical Malpractice Study of patients hospitalized in New York State in 1984.[3,4] There was no association between the occurrence of an adverse event (whether or not associated with negligence) and payment to the plaintiff.[4] Adverse events do not necessarily imply poor-quality care, nor does the absence of adverse events indicate good-quality care.

When there is an adverse outcome, non-negligent physicians frequently pay malpractice judgments against them.[2,5,6] Cheney et al.[2] reviewed closed US malpractice claims and found that compensation was made to the plaintiff in more than 40% of claims where the anesthesia care was judged as appropriate by impartial physician reviewers. Edbril and Lagasse[6] found that none of their departmental malpractice claims were the result of human error or negligence, as judged by peer review. Instead, all malpractice litigation was associated with adverse outcomes that were judged to be secondary to limitations of therapeutic or diagnostic standards.

Only a small fraction of negligent adverse medical events result in a malpractice claim. Less than 10% of patient injuries due to medical error resulted in a malpractice claim.[3,7,8] The Harvard Medical Practice study found that almost 4% of hospitalized patients sustained an iatrogenic injury and nearly 30% of these adverse events were due to negligence.[3] While the majority (70%) resulted in disability lasting less than 6 months, 3% of the events caused permanently disabling injuries, and 14% led to death.[3] However, only eight of the 280 patients (less than 3%) who had adverse outcomes due to medical negligence actually filed malpractice claims.[9] The investigators estimated that in New York State only one out of eight adverse events

associated with negligence resulted in a medical malpractice claim.[9] Even fewer adverse outcomes, not necessarily associated with negligence, led to malpractice claims – approximately one out of 25 adverse events.

The relationship between malpractice claims and adverse outcomes, such as intraoperative awareness, is illustrated in Figure 9.1.[9] Area A represents all medical injuries among hospitalized patients, estimated at approximately 4% of all patient admissions.[3] Area B represents all errors by health care providers, the extent of which is unknown. Area C represents the subset of adverse patient outcomes due to error or negligence (about 1% of all hospital admissions).[3] The fraction of outcomes represented by medical malpractice claims is represented by Area D. A small percentage of adverse events due to error end in a malpractice claim, and many of the claims that do occur are associated with care that was judged inappropriate.[9] Area E signifies filed claims resulting in claimant compensation, estimated at about one in 25 patients who experience an injury.[9] Therefore, malpractice litigation seldom occurs with any medical complication. As a result only a small proportion of cases of intraoperative awareness would result in litigation.

Factors influencing malpractice litigation

There are multiple factors that influence whether an adverse outcome results in a malpractice claim, including physician–patient interactions, the severity of the outcome, the expected compensation for damages and sociocultural factors.[10–13] Surveys of randomly selected patients suggest that there is a large number of patients who are dissatisfied with their medical care. Twelve to 25% of adults feel that either they or a close relative have had at least one episode of harm as a result of medical treatment.[10] However, only 10% of these patients had contacted an attorney. Patients informally consult with family members, friends, lawyers, and medical professionals in order to decide whether to pursue a lawsuit.[10,11] Many factors influence the patients' decisions to contact an attorney, including poor relationships with the providers, television advertisements, recommendations from health care providers, impressions of not being kept informed or appropriately referred by providers, and financial concerns, such as unemployment, lack of health

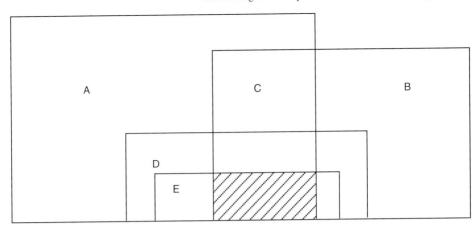

Figure 9.1. Relationship among adverse outcomes, errors during medical care and malpractice claims. A = incidence of patient injuries, B = incidence of errors during medical care, C = patient injuries due to errors during medical care, D = filed malpractice claims, E = filed claims resulting in claimant compensation. Shaded portion represents fraction of negligent adverse outcomes that receive compensation. (Reprinted with permission from Morlock LL, Lindgren OH, and Mills DH. Medical malpractice and clinical risk management. In Goldfield N. and Nash D.B. (eds). *Providing Quality Care: The Challenges to Clinicians*. 1989; Philadelphia, PA: American College of Physicians, 1989; 225–229).

insurance, outstanding medical bills, and cost of continuing medical care.[11,12]

Dissatisfaction with physician–patient communication is a key factor promoting patient calls to plaintiff attorneys[12] and filing of medical malpractice claims.[11] Over half of potential plaintiffs had a poor relationship with their physician prior to calling a plaintiff law firm.[12] The physician's failure to keep informed, to refer when needed, and to be available when needed were common concerns of the potential plaintiffs. Many families who filed a medical malpractice claim following perinatal injuries were concerned that there was a cover-up (24% of respondents), wanted more information (20%), and wanted revenge or to protect others (19%).[11] The physician was criticized for not talking openly (32%), not listening (13%), or misleading them about long-term disabilities (70%). Although the role of physician rapport has not been quantified in anesthetic malpractice claims, it is likely that excellent physician–patient communication and patient support are especially important in preventing malpractice claims for awareness and other emotional injuries. Patients experiencing awareness under anesthesia often complain of insensitivity of medical personnel to their complaints.[14] In addition, many patients do not inform their anesthesiologist about recall during general anesthesia.[15] Many awareness claims mention a lack

of interest, concern, or emotional support by the anesthesiologist.[16] The liability risk may be, therefore, decreased in awareness cases by a responsive physician.

The selection of meritorious malpractice claims is a complex process. Although plaintiff calls to attorneys are frequent, few lead to a lawsuit.[12] Huycke and Huycke found that only one out of 30 calls by disgruntled patients to plaintiff law firms resulted in the filing of a lawsuit.[12] Plaintiff attorneys screened cases for the essential components of a successful medical malpractice claim, i.e. lack of duty of the physician to provide care, negligence, causation, and damages. The most common reason for attorneys to decline a potential lawsuit was a projected insufficient compensation for damages.[12] Attorneys generally rejected claims with potentially recoverable damages of less than $50,000.[2–12] Imminent or expired statute of limitation was also an important cause for declining claims for potential plaintiffs without medical expert review.[12] Following medical expert review, a quarter of claims were declined because of the assessment of lack of negligence.[12]

The likelihood of payment and amount of payment in a claim are influenced by the appropriateness of care and the severity of patient injury. Review of closed anesthesia malpractice claims in the American Society of Anesthesiologists (ASA)

Closed Claims database (detailed description presented later in this chapter) demonstrated that the frequency of payment is linked to appropriateness of care, but not to severity of injury (Figure 9.2).[2] Payment was received in 80% of cases when the care was substandard, in contrast to 40% of the cases when the standard of care was met, regardless of the severity of injury. However, the magnitude of the payment was linked to both severity of injury and to standard of care (Figure 9.3).[2] Non-disabling physical and emotional injuries were associated with lower payments than injuries producing permanent physical disabilities or death. Substandard care, especially, increased the payment for permanent disabling injuries, with a fivefold increase in median payment (see Figure 9.3).[2] Adverse outcomes judged preventable with better monitoring[2] were far more costly than those that were not considered preventable with better monitoring.[2] Therefore, the judgment of the appropriateness of care is a key factor that influences both the prospect of successful litigation as well as the magnitude of financial compensation.

However, there are several important ambiguities and biases in the judgment of standard of care. The evaluation of appropriateness of care is a complex and subjective assessment which is based upon the expert reviewer's own unstated criteria.[17] Medical experts commonly disagree on the standard of care. Anesthesiologist reviewers agreed on the appropriateness of care in 62% of claims and disagreed in 38% of claims, or chance-corrected level of agreement in the poor-to-good range.[17] Therefore, divergent expert opinions may be easily found by seeking opinions from multiple experts.

Unfortunately, the judgment of the appropriateness of care is markedly influenced by the severity of the outcome.[18] To study this question, anesthesiologist reviewers were asked to rate the appropriateness of care in cases involving adverse outcomes. The original case involved either a temporary or permanent outcome. An alternate case was constructed that was identical to the original case, except that a plausible outcome of opposite severity was substituted. Examples of these cases included brain damage after airway obstruction, brachial plexus injury, seizures, eye injury, pneumothorax, ulnar nerve injury, and aspiration of gastric contents. Knowledge of severity of injury resulted in a significant inverse effect on judgment of appropriateness of care. The proportion of ratings for appropriate care decreased by 31% when the outcome was changed from temporary to permanent and increased by 28% when the outcome was changed from permanent to temporary.[18]

The end result is that a claim for awareness

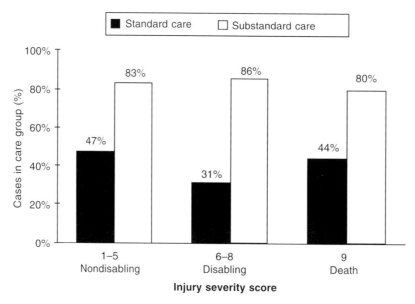

Figure 9.2. Influence of standard of care on the percentage of claims resulting in payment ($n = 4183$ claims in the ASA Closed Claims database). Payment is made in a greater proportion of claims when care is judged to be substandard, regardless of severity of injury.

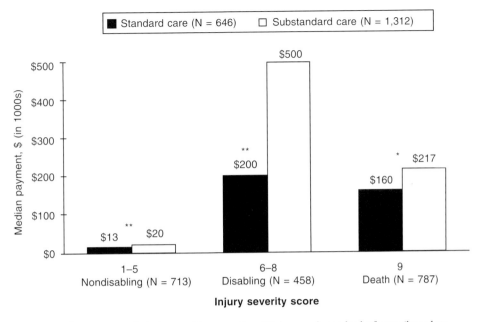

Figure 9.3. The median payment is influenced by severity of injury and standard of care (based on 1958 out of 4183 claims in the ASA Closed Claims database in which standard of care was possible to judge). Payment was greatest for permanently disabling injuries when care was judged to be substandard. $*P < 0.05$, $**P < 0.01$.

under anesthesia is more likely to be pursued by a plaintiff's attorney when the injury is more severe (e.g. post-traumatic stress disorder) and the anesthesia care was substandard. Because of the implicit bias that emotional injuries are less severe and less documentable than physical injuries, the relatively low payment for an emotional rather than physical injury may deter plaintiff's attorneys from pursuing claims for intraoperative awareness.

Sociocultural factors also influence whether an adverse outcome results in malpractice litigation. Patients with high incomes are more likely to file malpractice claims after adverse outcomes.[13] A case-control study of malpractice claims in New York State found that poor patients were five times less likely and uninsured patients were ten times less likely to file a malpractice claim when injured.[13] The elderly were also five times less likely to file a claim.[13] Gender and race were not associated with risk of malpractice claims. Payments for awareness claims also show interesting variability from one country to another, as is subsequently described in this chapter. These facts suggest that cultural factors are important in awareness claims.

In summary, awareness during anesthesia infrequently may result in medical malpractice litigation. Factors that may increase the anesthesiologist's liability include a more severe, permanent injury, substandard anesthetic care, poor physician–patient communication, and higher patient income and sociocultural factors.

Medicolegal consequences of awareness in the UK and Europe

Litigation and health care

In the UK, it has been estimated that there are between 15,000 and 40,000 outstanding claims relating to medical negligence in National Health Service hospitals alone, with an estimated liability of £1.8 billion. In addition, there may be liabilities of £1 billion for incidents that have occurred but that are not yet the subject of legal action.[19] This total liability represents 7.5% of the annual cost of the entire National Health Service in England.

Litigation is much more common in the UK and the Republic of Ireland than in any other countries in Europe. Although the number of claims per 100 000 population is lower in the UK than in the USA, the number of hospital-based claims per 100 whole-time equivalent hospital doctors is much higher in the UK than in the USA (because there are far fewer doctors per 100,000 population in the UK). In 1991, there were 10.5 new claims opened per year for every 100 hospital doctors in England, and there were 81.4 claims open (i.e. there was an 81.4% chance that there was an open claim against each hospital doctor).[20]

In contrast to the USA, civil claims in most European countries are tried by a judge, not a jury. Awards in successful claims are based on formulae which take into account pain and suffering, loss of amenity and loss of earnings; the concept of punitive damages is not recognized. However, in some European countries, including the UK, all legal costs are paid by the state for individuals with a low income, and for minors (the Legal Aid system). Although insurance can be obtained by others to cover the cost of litigation if a claim is unsuccessful, the cost is high, because the probability of success in medical negligence cases is much lower than in other civil claims. Consequently, in a number of European countries, the frequency of litigation is highest among patients with low incomes and those with very high incomes. Patients with a moderate income are disinclined to sue because of the financial risk; a successful claim in a case of awareness with mild psychological sequelae might result in an award of £15,000–£20,000 ($24,000–$32,000) plus legal costs, but an unsuccessful claim following a 5-day trial could cost the patient up to £100,000 ($160,000) because the patient would become liable for all the costs of the action.

The Legal Aid system also influences the way in which hospitals deal with claims of low financial value. Even if a claim by a legally aided patient fails in court, the hospital's own legal costs cannot be recovered from the patient or the Legal Aid Board. Consequently, in low-value cases, it is often cheaper to settle a claim before trial than to bear the costs of a trial, even when there is a very high probability of a successful defense.

Litigation and awareness

Historical context

It should not be forgotten that the principal reason for attempting to minimize the incidence of awareness should be humanitarian, not fear of litigation. Awareness during anesthesia had an incidence of 1–2% in Europe during the 1960s and 1970s (Table 9.1).[21–27] Despite this high incidence, there were only a very modest number of law suits annually in the UK and Europe. This occurred partly because the culture of medical litigation was very different to that in the present day. In addition, some patients were led to believe that awareness was an inevitable complication of anesthesia and other patients were disbelieved when they reported awareness, and became convinced that their experience must have been imaginary.

A dramatic change in the UK occurred in 1985. In that year, a patient who had experienced severe and prolonged pain during cesarean section, with serious psychological sequelae (Ackers v Wigan Health Authority, 1985),[28] sued her anesthesiologist, and was awarded damages in excess of £13,000 (approximately $21,000; current value, allowing for inflation and other changes, approximately £30,000 or $48,000). The case generated a blaze of publicity because her lawyer knew that a number of other patients treated by the same anesthesiologist were also seeking compensation. However, the trial dealt only with the magnitude of the damages, because it had already been admitted that the anesthesiologist had been negligent. The publicity

Table 9.1. Summary of incidence of awareness with recall and dreaming in studies using a structured interview 1960–2000

Authors	Date	Awareness (%)	Dreaming (%)	Sample size
Hutchinson[21]	1960	1.2	3.0	656
Harris et al.[22]	1971	1.6	26.0	120
McKenna and Wilton[23]	1973	1.5	–	200
Wilson et al.[24]	1975	0.8	7.7	490
Liu et al.[25]	1990	0.2	0.9	1000
Ranta et al.[26]	1998	0.4	13.1	2612
Sandin et al.[27]	2000	0.15	–	11 785

resulted in an enormous increase in litigation by patients who claimed that they had been aware during anesthesia. Some of the alleged experiences had occurred up to 20 years earlier, many of these claims were allowed to proceed despite the normal limitation period of 3 years. The large majority of claims were sustainable. New claims for awareness during anesthesia suddenly escalated, and have remained high. Approximately one-eighth of legal claims against anesthesiologists in the UK relate to allegations of awareness during general anesthesia (Table 9.2).[29]

In contrast, claims of compensation for awareness during general anesthesia have remained low in the rest of Europe. Ranta *et al.*[30] reviewed claims for awareness in Finland during the late 1980s to early 1990s. In Finland, compensation is paid for an injury to a patient caused by medical treatment, according to the Patient Injury Act. Out of 23,363 claims for patient injury, only 391 were for anesthesia-related injuries (1.7% of all malpractice claims). Only four claims were made for awareness under general anesthesia (1% of anesthesia claims). All of the patients sustained serious psychological sequelae. They were awarded between 4000 to 9600 Finnish Marks (about $1000–2400). The differences between the experiences in the UK suggests that claims for awareness under anesthesia are markedly influenced by cultural factors.

Incidence of awareness claims

In the UK, there is no method for collecting information about the number of claims for compensation arising from alleged awareness during anesthesia; low value claims are handled by solicitors acting for the hospital, and data are not collected centrally. Consequently, it is necessary to rely on anecdotal data from individuals with experience of handling such claims in order to identify their frequency and causes.

A cause of some alarm is that the proportion of claims against anesthesiologists that relate to awareness during anesthesia does not appear to have changed substantially in the last decade. Awareness claims have continued despite the fact that the surge of historical claims that followed the Ackers case was short-lived, and despite the fact that the deliberate use of predictably inadequate anesthetic techniques involving the use of nitrous oxide that was not supplemented by volatile or intravenous anesthetic agents had stopped in the mid-1980s. One of the authors (ARA) has reviewed 10–12 claims for awareness every year since 1988, with no obvious downward trend in the frequency. The reason for this may be that delivery systems for anesthetic gas mixtures have become more complex, with an increased potential for misuse. However, in some cases it is apparent that substandard anesthesia care occurred despite the availability and use of monitoring apparatus that can confirm that predictably adequate concentrations of inhaled anesthetics are being delivered to the patient's lungs. Some anesthesiologists fail to detect inadequate delivery resulting from leaks from the breathing system and dilution of anesthetic gases by oxygen or air used to drive mechanical ventilators, failure to deliver the anticipated concentration of volatile anesthetic agent from a vaporizer, or because of negligence to check the monitors.

Table 9.2. Pattern of injuries among claims against anesthesiologists in the UK and the Republic of Ireland

Nature of injury	Claims (% of total)
Brain/spinal cord damage	23.8
Death in postoperative period	17.0
Awareness during general anesthesia	12.2
Death during anesthesia	11.6
Pain during regional anesthesia	7.5
Peripheral nerve damage	4.1
Miscellaneous injuries	23.9

(Reprinted with permission from Aitkenhead AR. Anaesthesia. In: Jackson JP (ed.) *A Practical Guide to Medicine and the Law*. London: Springer-Verlag. 1991; 45–75.)

Common causes of awareness in litigants in the UK

Spontaneous recall of intraoperative events is, by definition, due to delivery of inadequate concentrations of anesthetic agents to the brain for the needs of the individual patient. The types of operative procedure associated with awareness, and the commonest causes, in cases reported to one of the medical defense organizations in the UK between 1982 and 1986[31] are shown in Tables 9.3 and 9.4. Seventy percent of cases of recall in these litigants were deemed to be caused by the use of an inappropriate anesthetic technique and 20% by failure to check equipment. These cases were, almost by definition, indefensible. Details of causes of awareness are discussed in the following paragraphs.

FAULTY ANESTHETIC TECHNIQUE

This is the commonest single cause of awareness with recall in the UK. A faulty technique is one that could reasonably be predicted to result in recall of intraoperative events, or in which drug doses are not adjusted when clinical signs of inadequate anesthesia become apparent. In general, the likelihood of recall is related inversely to the dose or concentration of anesthetic drug administered. However, because high concentrations of most anesthetic agents result in an increased incidence and severity of side effects, and delayed recovery, it became common in the UK in the 1960s and 1970s for anesthesiologists to use paralyzing doses of a muscle relaxant to prevent movement during surgery (in contrast to the smaller doses used in North America), and to administer nitrous oxide

Table 9.3. Types of operative procedure associated with cases of awareness with recall reported to a British medical defense organization between 1982 and 1986

Type of procedure	Percentage of cases
General surgery	31
Obstetrics	28
Gynecology	18
Orthopedic surgery	11
Miscellaneous*	12

*Miscellaneous includes dental, ear, nose, and throat, and ophthalmologic procedures (Reprinted with permission from Hargrove RL. Awareness under anaesthesia. *J Med Defense Union* 1987; (Spring):9–11.)

Table 9.4. Causes of awareness with recall reported to a British medical defense organization between 1982 and 1986

Cause	Percentage of cases
Faulty anesthetic technique	70
Failure to check equipment	20
Genuine apparatus failure	5
Spurious claims	2.5
Justified risks/unknown cause	2.5

(Reprinted with permission from Hargrove RL. Awareness under anaesthesia. *J Med Defense Union* 1987; (Spring):9–11.)

alone, or with an opioid analgesic, to maintain anesthesia.

Inhalational anesthetics: The use of unsupplemented nitrous oxide predictably results in awareness with recall in an unacceptably high proportion of patients. Utting[32] reported definite or probable recall in 2.2% of 500 patients anesthetized with unsupplemented nitrous oxide 70% in oxygen. The addition of opioids may reduce the incidence of recall slightly, but not significantly. Rosen[33] demonstrated that auditory perception occurred in some patients breathing 60–75% nitrous oxide, despite an opioid premedication. Browne and Catton[34] reported an incidence of recall of 5.3% in patients premedicated with meperidine or promethazine, and moderately hyperventilated using nitrous oxide 60% in oxygen.

The alveolar concentration of an inhalational agent is normally lower than the delivered concentration and failure to use 'overpressure' with volatile agents may result in awareness, particularly at the start of surgery. The concentration of an inhalational agent delivered to a patient may be considerably less than the concentration set on the flowmeters or vaporizer if a circle system with vaporizer outside the circle is used with low fresh gas flow rates. This discrepancy is predictable, but may not be known to the anesthesiologist if gas and vapor monitors are not employed. A number of cases of awareness have occurred because predictably inadequate anesthetic gas mixtures have been administered, usually by trainee anesthesiologists, to treat very modest decreases in arterial oxygen saturation between induction of anesthesia and the start of surgery. This is a new mechanism of awareness, attributable to the use (or abuse) of the pulse oximeter!

Intravenous anesthetics: Anesthetic drugs administered intravenously are less predictable than inhalational agents. Distribution volumes vary widely between individual patients. While distribution volume has some influence on the rate of uptake of inhalational drugs, its effect is relatively small because increased distribution is to a large extent compensated for by increased uptake from the lungs, and the total dose of anesthetic administered is increased. In contrast, the total dose of an intravenous drug is selected by the anesthesiologist, and the blood and brain concentrations are determined, at least in the short term, by redistribution to tissues that receive high blood flow. Recall may occur during tracheal intubation if a muscle relaxant has been given before clear signs of loss of consciousness have become apparent following administration of an intravenous agent for induction of anesthesia, or if inhalational anesthetics are not given between induction and tracheal intubation. This risk is highest if a non-depolarizing relaxant has been used.

There may be a higher risk of recall in the paralyzed patient if anesthesia is maintained by an infusion of an intravenous agent than if inhalational anesthetics are used. This is true particularly if the lungs are ventilated with oxygen-enriched air (total intravenous anesthesia) rather than oxygen and nitrous oxide. During inhalational anesthesia there is a reasonably predictable relationship between alveolar concentration and blood (or brain) concentration. However, blood concentration of an intravenous agent given by infusion is influenced by both the distribution volume (which varies widely among individuals) and the clearance, which may alter significantly with plasma concentration. Even when sophisticated computerized apparatus is used in an attempt to attain a 'target' concentration, based on an algorithm derived from population kinetic data, there is wide variation in the plasma concentrations achieved.[35]

One relatively frequent cause of awareness during total intravenous anesthesia is that the anesthesiologist has misinterpreted a published technique. This has resulted in a number of cases of awareness when infusion regimens for propofol, which have been demonstrated to be effective when used in conjunction with nitrous oxide and an infusion of a short-acting opioid analgesic such as alfentanil, have been used with no analgesic supplementation.

Supplements of non-anesthetic drugs: The use of opioids, butyrophenones or benzodiazepines to supplement nitrous oxide anesthesia is common. In the doses usually employed, these agents do not produce anesthesia.[36] Midazolam is often administered if the anesthesiologist suspects that anesthesia has become so inadequate that awareness is a possibility, although benzodiazepines do not appear to offer reliable retrograde amnesia.[37] There was recently an indefensible claim for awareness in the UK by a patient who received a single dose of diazepam 20 mg intravenously for an abdominal operation. No inhaled anesthetic and no analgesic drug was given. The anesthesia care in this case was clearly substandard as the only other drug that the patient received was a non-depolarizing muscle relaxant!

Cesarean section: The high incidence of recall of intraoperative events that have been reported in obstetric patients who received general anesthesia in Europe is attributable largely to a reluctance to use inhalational agents in adequate concentrations because of fears of inducing depression of the fetus and of increasing hemorrhage from the uterus. There is no evidence that these fears are justified. There is normally no good reason to discontinue administration of the volatile agent after delivery of the baby. In Europe, it was common practice until the mid-1980s to discontinue the administration of volatile agent after delivery of the baby because of fears that uterine hemorrhage might be increased. Lyons and Macdonald[38] showed that the incidence of awareness during cesarean section decreased from 1.3% to 0.4% when the anesthetic technique was changed from one in which halothane was given in 50% nitrous oxide before delivery and nitrous oxide 67% was given alone after delivery, to one in which isoflurane was used to supplement nitrous oxide throughout the operation. This change in technique occurred as a direct result of the publicity surrounding the Ackers case,[29] and is one of the very few examples of litigation resulting in improved outcome rather than simply the practice of defensive medicine.

Difficult intubation: It is often desirable to discontinue the administration of nitrous oxide and to administer oxygen alone in order to maintain adequate oxygenation if tracheal intubation is difficult. This can lead predictably to awareness with recall unless anesthesia is maintained either by administration of adequate concentrations of a volatile agent in oxygen or by giving further doses of an intravenous anesthetic agent between attempts at tracheal intubation.

Premature discontinuation of anesthesia: A desire to produce unnecessarily rapid recovery of consciousness after surgery may lead the anesthesiologist to discontinue administration of a volatile anesthetic agent or intravenous infusion of anesthetic drug several minutes before the end of the operation, or to switch off the nitrous oxide before reversal of the effects of neuromuscular blockers.

Failure to understand apparatus: Air is entrained by some mechanical ventilators if the supply of anesthetic gases from the anesthetic machine is less than the total minute volume delivered by the ventilator. Oxygen or air may dilute anesthetic gases if tubing with an inadequate volume is used to connect a ventilator to a Bain system. Failure to understand the principles of the circle system may result in delivery of inadequate concentrations of anesthetic gases. Awareness arising from any of these mechanisms cannot be defended because the anesthesiologist should have understood the dynamics of the breathing system employed.

FAILURE TO CHECK EQUIPMENT

It is universally recognized that apparatus must be checked before and during every anesthetic. Common causes of recall include failure to ensure that the anesthetic gases are delivered to a mechanical ventilator of a type that does not depend upon the supply of fresh gas for its power; loose connections in the ventilator tubing or breathing system, which result in loss of fresh gas and rebreathing or entrainment of air; failure to connect the vaporizer into the fresh gas supply at all or at least securely, or to lock the vaporizer on to a Selectatec block; failure to ensure that the vaporizer contains the anesthetic agent; and failure to notice that a nitrous oxide cylinder has become empty. The emergency oxygen flush may be switched on accidentally, diluting the concentration of anesthetic gases. An infusion of intravenous agent may become disconnected, leak into surrounding tissues, or the syringe in the infusion pump may become empty. A number of these events may occur during anesthesia, even though a pre-anesthetic check has been undertaken. There may also be misinterpretation of signs of light anesthesia if ECG monitors and automated blood pressure devices are not checked regularly. Recall may occur if an inaccurate inspired oxygen monitor or pulse oximeter causes the anesthesiologist to increase the inspired concentration of oxygen inappropriately.

A number of cases of awareness have occurred after inadvertent administration of a muscle relaxant to a conscious patient when it was intended that another drug should be given; the usual causes are failure to label the syringe, or failure to read the label.

GENUINE APPARATUS FAILURE

In some circumstances, failure of apparatus could not reasonably have been predicted by the anesthesiologist. Flexible hoses connecting the supply of anesthetic gases to the vaporizer may become perforated, resulting in a reduction in fresh gas flow rate. There may be a loss of fresh gas because of leaks in the back bar of the anesthetic machine or a damaged flowmeter. Vaporizers may very occasionally deliver grossly inaccurate concentrations of volatile agent. Infusion pumps may malfunction without sounding an alarm. Ventilators may operate incorrectly despite appropriate external connections. However, virtually all types of equipment failure should be detected before awareness occurs if monitoring of inspired and expired gases and vapors is employed, and the measurements heeded. Consequently, it is difficult to defend claims which fall into this category.

SPURIOUS CLAIMS

Very occasionally, patients complain of recall without foundation. Some patients claim recall of intraoperative events that are found on detailed questioning to be memories of the early postoperative period, or (rarely) a dream.

JUSTIFIED RISKS

In a very small number of cases, the patient is so seriously ill that there is a genuine risk to life if normally adequate doses or concentrations of anesthetic drug are administered. The commonest cause is profound hypotension caused by hypovolaemia when only surgery can effect a cure.

UNKNOWN CAUSES

Very occasionally, there may be no identifiable factor to explain a genuine case of awareness with recall. It is possible that some of these cases are attributable to the variability in response to anesthetic agents. However, in most of these cases, the standard of documentation is insufficient to exclude a predictable cause of awareness.

Is awareness always the result of negligence?

Although some anesthesiologists believe that many claims of intraoperative awareness are spurious, and are invented by aggressive litigants, it is our experience that such cases are exceptionally rare. In the UK, no case of awareness has been defended in court if both parties (the claimant and the defendant) agreed that the awareness occurred at a time when the patient should have been unconscious. Only six cases have been defended in court, and in all cases, it was the defendant's claim that the patient's memories related to events in the immediate postoperative period, usually in the operating room, and that the patient had come, quite genuinely, to believe that these memories related to the intraoperative period. Five of these six cases were defended successfully. In the sixth, there was no anesthetic record of intraoperative measurements, or of drug administration, and it was easy for the judge to find in favor of the claimant because there was no contemporaneous evidence that the anesthetic technique had been appropriate or that abnormal values of blood pressure and heart rate had not occurred (which would have been signals to increase the inspired concentrations of anesthetic drugs).

The case of Taylor v Worcester and District Health Authority[39] exemplifies some of the issues which arise in claims of awareness during anesthesia, and has become established as an important legal precedent.

Miss Taylor underwent cesarean section in 1985. Anesthesia was induced by administration of thiopental 250 mg. Succinylcholine 100 mg was administered and the trachea was intubated. Anesthesia was maintained by inhalation of nitrous oxide 50% and halothane 0.5% until delivery of the baby. On delivery of the baby, the inspired concentration of nitrous oxide was increased to 70%, the administration of halothane was discontinued because of fears about its effects on uterine contractility and the risk of postpartum hemorrhage, and the opioid analgesic papaveretum was given in a dose of 20 mg. No abnormal values of heart rate or blood pressure were recorded during the procedure. The anesthetic technique was not one that was regarded as acceptable for cesarean section at the time of the trial (1991), but it was employed in a number of hospitals at the time of the incident (1985), and was almost identical to the technique recommended for cesarean section in an obstetric anesthesia textbook published in 1987.

Miss Taylor said that, after injection of thiopental, she had gone to sleep, but that she had then awakened. She felt a sharp pain, which she described as a burning sensation. There was a feeling of something pressing down inside her. She could not open her eyes or move in any way. She felt a tugging sensation, and heard a hissing noise and people laughing. She felt terrified, and thought that she was dying.

All of these memories were consistent with intraoperative awareness. However, she had no memory of the baby crying after delivery. In addition, at the time that she was aware of the other memories, she recalled a man saying, 'We're going to leave you alone with her' and 'No. Don't leave me here'. She recalled opening her eyes, and being unable to focus. She recalled someone saying 'Wake up. Wake up'. She still felt paralyzed. A woman nearby held her hand and patted it. She remembered *saying* 'I'm paralyzed'. All of these memories, the defendant argued, were consistent with awareness during the immediate postoperative period, when she might also have experienced all of her other memories.

The judge decided that, on the balance of probabilities, Miss Taylor's memories did relate to the immediate postoperative period, when it was accepted that the recollection of memories, albeit of unpleasant sensations, was an inevitable risk. However, he did consider in detail what his response would have been if he had concluded that the memories related to the intraoperative period.

> Even if the episode of awareness was during the operation, I entirely acquit [the anesthesiologist] of negligence. She adopted a widely used technique, which she carried out in a careful and competent manner. That technique carried with it a small statistical risk of awareness during the operation, a risk which arose from respectable and responsible medical opinion that halothane affected contraction of the uterus.

This judgment conforms to the 'Bolam' principle,[40] that a doctor is not guilty of negligence simply because a complication arises, provided that the doctor's actions are supported by a respectable and responsible body of opinion. Consequently, in the UK, it is possible to defend cases of intraoperative awareness provided that a respectable and responsible body of anesthesiologists supports the anesthetic technique employed.

The fact is, of course, that there are now very few circumstances in which a technique that would be supported by respectable and responsible anesthesiologists carries a predictable incidence of intraoperative awareness, if the technique is applied correctly and monitored appropriately. It is probable that intraoperative awareness would now be regarded as acceptable only if considered to be a 'justified risk' in a patient so seriously ill that administration of predictably adequate concentrations of anesthetic drugs could reasonably be expected to result in death or permanent injury.

Medicolegal consequences of awareness in the USA

The medicolegal ramifications of intraoperative awareness in the USA in the 1970s–1990s have been recently described by ASA Closed Claims Project and are summarized below.[16]

ASA Closed Claims Project

The ASA Closed Claims Project is a structured evaluation of adverse anesthetic outcomes obtained from the closed claim files of 35 professional liability insurance companies in the USA. One company processes claims from more than 40 states. The other sources mainly are statewide organizations that include both physician-owned and private companies. These organizations insure approximately 14,500 anesthesiologists. Over three-fourths of the claims in the ASA Closed Claims database originated in the Northeast, upper Midwest, and West Coast. Relatively few claims originate in Southern States due to the lack of access to insurance company files in these states. Currently, there are a total of 4183 claims for adverse outcomes that originated between 1961 and 1996 in the closed claims database. Sixty-eight percent of the claims occurred between 1980 and 1990.

To collect data, one or more trained practicing anesthesiologists visited each insurance company office to review all files for claims against anesthesiologists. A standardized data collection instrument was completed for claims in which there was enough information to reconstruct the sequence of events and determine the nature and causation of injury. The closed claims files typically consisted of relevant hospital and medical records, narrative statements from involved health care personnel, expert and peer reviews, deposition summaries, outcome reports, and the cost of settlement of jury award. The reviewer used standardized instructions to fill out a standardized form which records information on patient characteristics (age, sex, weight, and physical status), date of procedure, surgical procedures, anesthetic agents and techniques, monitors employed, sequence and location of events, critical incidents, clinical manifestations of injury, complications and outcomes, whether a lawsuit was filed, and the amount of award. The review assessed the overall appropriateness of anesthetic care and its contribution to the injury. Reviewers also wrote a brief summary of each case that summarized the sequence of events. Each data collection focus was reviewed and approved by the three practicing anesthesiologists of the Closed Claims Study Committee in Seattle, Washington.

Each claim was assigned a severity of injury score that was designated by the on-site reviewer using the insurance industry's 10-point scale. This ordinal scale rates severity in injury from 0 (no injury) to 9 (death).[2] A value of 1 represents temporary emotional injury, 2 through 4 reflect temporary physical injuries, 5 reflects permanent, non-disabling emotional and physical injuries, and 6 through 8 reflect permanent and disabling emotional and physical injuries. For purposes of analysis, injuries were grouped into two categories: temporary/non-disabling (0 to 4) and disabling/permanent/death (5 to 9).

Awareness claims

Awareness accounted for 79 out of 4183 claims (1.9%) in the ASA Closed Claims Project database, a similar proportion in the database as burns, aspiration pneumonia, and myocardial infarction, hepatic dysfunction, and renal failure. Compared to all other claims, awareness claims more often involved females (77% of awareness claims *versus* 59% of all other claims), patients younger than 60 years of age (89% for awareness claims *versus* 79% for all other claims), and patients undergoing elective surgery (87% of awareness claims *versus*

72% for all other claims, Table 9.5). The severity of injury in claims for awareness during anesthesia was lower than the severity in the other claims, with over 90% involving temporary injury (score = 0 to 5) in contrast to 32% of anesthesia malpractice claims resulting in temporary injuries.

In the entire database, a greater proportion of claims by women for all cases involved temporary injuries than among those for males. The trend for claims by females to involve a lower severity of injury was evident whether obstetrical claims were included or excluded. Forty-eight percent of claims by females were for a temporary or non-disabling injury compared to 42% of claims by men. A smaller proportion of awareness claims originated in the 1970s and a greater proportion originated in the 1990s (Figure 9.4).

Claims for awareness were divided for subsequent analysis into two categories: *awake paralysis,* i.e. the inadvertent paralysis of an awake

Table 9.5. Demographic characteristics of patients filing claims for awareness in the USA

	Awareness claims (n = 79) (%)	All other claims (n = 4104) (%)
Gender		
Female	60 (77%)	2412 (59%)*
Male	18 (23%)	1656 (41%)*
ASA status		
1–2	32 (68%)	1789 (70%)
3–5	15 (32%)	761 (30%)
Age		
<60 years	62 (89%)	3039 (80%)*
≥60 years	8 (11%)	810 (21%)*
Emergency surgery		
Yes	7 (13%)	782 (28%)*
No	47 (87%)	2041 (72%)*
Procedure		
Inpatient	45 (82%)	1900 (78%)
Outpatient	10 (18%)	521 (22%)
Surgery		
Obstetrics- gynecology	29 (37%)	951 (23%)*
Other	50 (63%)	3153 (77%)*

* $P < 0.05$ compared to awareness claims by Chi square test. (Reprinted with permission from Domino KB, Posner KL, Caplan RA, Cheney FW. Awareness during anesthesia. A closed claims analysis. *Anesthesiology* 1999; **90**:1053–1061.)

patient, and *recall under general anesthesia,* i.e. patient recalled events while receiving general anesthesia. The claims for recall during anesthesia represent typical cases of awareness during anesthesia.

Awake paralysis claims

Most claims for awake paralysis were related to intravenous infusion errors or syringe swaps. The periods of highest risk were in the preinduction and induction periods, when a muscle relaxant was administered instead of a sedative or hypnotic agent. Follow-up care by the anesthesiologist was described as adequate in most claims. Reviewers considered most cases of awake paralysis to be examples of substandard anesthesia care, although the paralysis was promptly recognized and appropriately managed. Ninety-four percent of awake paralysis closed claims were judged to represent substandard care by the anesthesiologist, in contrast to 40% of all other closed claims. The one case for which the care by the anesthesiologist was judged to be appropriate involved mislabeling of a syringe in the pharmacy. Payments were made in a greater proportion of awake paralysis claims (78%) compared to all other claims (55%, Table 9.6). However, consistent with the judgment of substandard care, payments for awake paralysis claims were lower than all other claims, with a median payment of only $9500 (range $1000 to $75,000), reflecting the low severity of injury.

Recall under general anesthesia claims

Claims for recall during general anesthesia were a more diverse group of claims. Most of the cases of recall originated during the maintenance phase of anesthesia. The anesthesia care was judged to be substandard in 43% of the recall claims and appropriate in 33%, in the remainder of claims, the standard of care was impossible to judge (see Table 9.6). The standard of care was commonly judged to be appropriate with a planned nitrous-narcotic-relaxant technique or if the recall was associated with hypotension requiring discontinuation of anesthetic agents. Recall associated with vaporizer problems, inadequate doses of drugs, and during difficult intubation predominantly represented

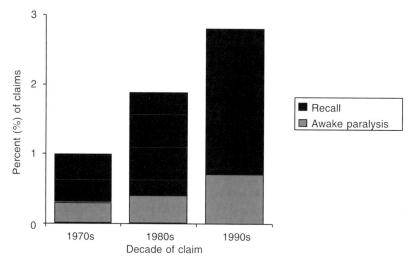

Figure 9.4. Proportion of claims as percent of total claims in each decade for recall under general anesthesia (solid bar) and awake paralysis (hatched bar). The proportion of other claims is not shown. A smaller proportion of awareness claims originated in the 1970s and a greater proportion originated in the 1990s ($P = 0.023$). (Reprinted with permission from Domino KB, Posner KL, Caplan RA, Cheney FW. Awareness During Anesthesia: a closed claims analysis. *Anesthesiology* 1999; **90**:1053–1061.)

substandard care. The judgment of appropriateness of care was similar to that for all other claims in the database but different from awake paralysis claims (see Table 9.6). Follow-up care was described as adequate in most claims. However, three claim files explicitly described a lack of concern and attention by the anesthesiologist.

A similar proportion of recall under general anesthesia claims resulted in a law suit (82%), a settlement prior to court (67%), and in payment (49%), as for all other anesthesia malpractice claims. However, the amount of payment was similar to awake paralysis claims and less than for all other claims (see Table 9.6). The median payment was $18 000 compared to a median payment of $100 000 for all other claims. The lower median payment is consistent with the lower severity of injury and is similar to compensation for awake paralysis, back pain and emotional distress. The marked variability in range of compensation (see Table 9.6) reflects

Table 9.6. Standard of care and claim payment for awake paralysis, recall under general anesthesia, and all other claims in the USA

Type of claim	Standard of care.* No. (%)		Payment		
	Standard	Substandard	Yes no. (%)	Median amount ($)	Minimum–maximum amount ($)
Awake paralysis (n = 18)	1 (6%)[†]	17 (94%)[†]	14 (78%)[†]	9500[‡]	1000–75,000
Recall under general anesthesia (n = 61)	20 (33%)	26 (43%)	30 (49%)	18 000[‡]	1700–600,000
All Other Claims (n = 4104)	1882 (46%)	1645 (40%)	2271 (55%)	100 000	15–23 200,000

* These data represent claims where standard of care could be judged. The remainder was impossible to judge.
[†] $P < 0.001$ compared to recall under general anesthesia claims. [‡] $P < 0.001$ compared to all other claims.
(Reprinted with permission from Domino KB, Posner KL, Caplan RA, Cheney FW. Awareness during anesthesia. A closed claims analysis. *Anesthesiology* 1999; **90**:1053–1061.)

differences in the geographic distribution, severity of injury, standard of care, and presence of additional injuries (e.g. aspiration pneumonia with substandard care). Higher payments have been reported for more severe injuries in which care was substandard.

Interestingly, the classic cues for light anesthesia (hypertension, tachycardia, and patient movement) were absent in most cases. One claim alleged recall despite use of an intraoperative electroencephalograph.

Logistic regression analysis demonstrated that five factors were significantly associated with claims for recall under general anesthesia compared to other general anesthesia claims: no volatile anesthetic agent, female gender, obstetric or gynecologic procedure, intraoperative narcotic, and intraoperative muscle relaxant (Table 9.7). Age, ASA status, anesthesia personnel, standard of care, and use of benzodiazepines, barbiturates, and nitrous oxide were not associated with claims for recall during general anesthesia.

After adjusting for the other factors using multiple logistic regression analysis, female gender and anesthetic techniques using intraoperative narcotic and muscle relaxants without a volatile anesthetic increased the relative frequency of claims for recall under general anesthesia by two to three times when compared to all claims under general anesthesia (Table 9.7). Obstetric or gynecologic procedures alone were not independently associated with an increased relative frequency of a claim for recall.

The association of claims for recall during general anesthesia with anesthetic techniques using opioids, muscle relaxants, and little or no volatile anesthetic is consistent with the known increased incidence of intraoperative awareness with these light anesthetic techniques.[26] However, it is unclear why female gender was associated with a three times higher rate of a recall claim than other claims. This could represent a gender-related increase in propensity for recall during general anesthesia or a greater likelihood to file a claim for recall. Although many reports of intraoperative awareness involve a preponderance of women, this is most likely secondary to light anesthetic techniques, especially for cesarean section. However, gender-related differences in the requirements for intravenous anesthetics have been reported.[41,42] Women wake up faster from propofol/alfentanil anesthesia.[41] Plasma remifentanil levels, titrated to ensure the lack of a hemodynamic response to a surgical stimulus, were almost twice as high in women than in men.[42]

Women may also file claims for emotional injury more often than men. Claims for females in the Closed Claims database involved a lower severity of injury than those for males. For instance, the frequency of claims by females for emotional injury was nearly double of that of men (13% vs. 7%, respectively). These data suggested that women may be more likely than men to file a claim for recall under general anesthesia.

Summary of section

Claims for awareness under anesthesia in the ASA Closed Claims database consisted of two varieties of claims. Awake paralysis represented error in labeling and vigilance. Alternatively, claims for

Table 9.7. Risk factors for malpractice claims for recall under general anesthesia in the USA

Factor	Univariate logistic regression		Multivariate logistic regression	
	OR	**(95% CI)**	**OR**	**(95% CI)**
No volatile anesthetic	3.33***	(1.97, 5.63)	3.20***	(1.88, 5.46)
Female gender	3.21***	(1.89, 6.05)	3.08***	(1.58, 6.06)
Obstetric/gynecologic procedure	2.66***	(1.57, 4.50)	–	
Intraoperative narcotic	2.48***	(1.42, 4.32)	2.12**	(1.20, 3.74)
Intraoperative muscle relaxant	2.47***	(1.35, 4.53)	2.28**	(1.22, 4.25)

Abbreviations: OR = odds ratio (an OR of unity [1.0] means no difference in odds for recall claims versus other claims); 95% CI = 95% confidence interval; ***$P < 0.001$, **$P < 0.01$. (Reprinted with permission from Domino KB, Posner KL, Caplan RA, Cheney FW. Awareness during anesthesia. A closed claims analysis. *Anesthesiology* 1999; **90**:1053–1061.)

recall under general anesthesia were more diverse and they were more likely in women and with nitrous-narcotic-relaxant techniques. Claims for awareness frequently resulted in compensation to the plaintiff, although the magnitude of payment was relatively low, consistent with the low severity of injury. However, there was marked variability in the range of compensation, reflecting differences in geographic distribution, severity of injury, standard of care, and presence of additional injury.

Future medicolegal implications of awareness

The pattern of litigation related to awareness during anesthesia over the last 20 years has not been the same in the USA and Europe. The incidence of litigation varies widely in different European countries. In the UK, claims related to awareness are much more frequent as a proportion of all claims against anesthesiologists than is the case in the USA. This may be a result of differences in anesthetic techniques, but may, alternatively, relate to the fact that low-value claims are much more likely to be pursued if the patient is able to obtain all legal costs from the State (as in the UK) than if the risk of litigation is assumed by the plaintiff's lawyer, whose reimbursement will be restricted if the outcome is a low settlement. In addition, the media coverage of awareness during anesthesia in the UK has probably peaked, and the number of claims relating to awareness appears to have reached a plateau.

In contrast, it is likely that malpractice claims for awareness during anesthesia will increase in quantity and payment in the USA. The ASA Closed Claims project has demonstrated an increase in proportion of awareness claims in the 1990s, compared to the 1970s (see Figure 9.4). There is a trend for most of the increase in these claims to be claims for recall under general anesthesia, rather than mistakenly paralyzing an awake patient. The trend for an increase in awareness claims may represent an increase in public knowledge about and intolerance for intraoperative awareness. Recent prominent discussion in the news media and on television is likely to increase the risk of litigation.

The proportion of claims for awareness may also be influenced by improvements in anesthetic safety and a decrease in events associated with death or serious physical injury. A decrease in the number of severe adverse outcomes from anesthesia is bound to result in a proportional increase in claims for less severe outcomes, including awareness. This may, in part, explain the continuing increase in the proportion of awareness claims in the USA, and the high proportion of awareness claims in the UK. The severity of injury in patients recorded in the ASA Closed Claims database has been decreasing since the 1970s.[43] The proportion of claims for death and brain damage has decreased from 56% of anesthesia malpractice claims in the 1970s to 31% in the 1990s.

In addition, partly in response to criticism of medical practice by the media and by politicians, patients are likely to become increasingly intolerant of any complication arising from medical treatment. This intolerance is likely to affect anesthetic practice particularly because anesthesia is not a therapeutic procedure, and because the practice of anesthesia is perceived by most patients as being easy. Consequently, while many patients expect that complications may arise from surgery, they expect anesthesia to be free of complications, and are more likely to complain or litigate if any complication attributable to anesthesia occurs.

Introduction of a potential monitor for awareness may also increase the risk of litigation and magnitude of payment. Bispectral analysis of the electro-encephalogram (BIS monitoring) predicted responsiveness to verbal commands during sedation and hypnosis with propofol or propofol plus nitrous oxide.[44] Although it has not been, nor can it be, shown to be a monitor of 'awareness', as a monitor of 'hypnosis' or 'anesthetic depth', expert reviewers may suggest that its use might have prevented awareness. In addition, if BIS monitoring becomes widespread in the community, plaintiff's attorneys may argue that lack of its use constitutes negligence, although in law, negligence could be proved only if it could be demonstrated that awareness would not have occurred if the monitor had been employed. Current knowledge indicates that this cannot be demonstrated. The use of 'depth of anesthesia' monitors is not without risk. Some anesthesiologists may try to achieve lighter levels of anesthesia, either to save on drug costs or to produce more rapid recovery, on the false assumption that the monitor can differentiate between light anesthesia and consciousness. Consequently, it is even possible that the use of these devices might increase the incidence of awareness. As with all monitoring devices, the information provided must be collated with all other available and relevant information, and interpreted appropriately.

In conclusion, the commonest cause of intra-operative awareness is error by the anesthesiologist. The frequency of litigation related to intraoperative awareness will be minimized by improved education and training of anesthesiologists in understanding the minimum requirements of anesthetic drugs, by increased vigilance in detecting differences between the doses or concentrations of drugs that it is anticipated that the patient is receiving and those which the patient is actually receiving, and by identifying patients who have suffered awareness, so that appropriate explanations can be given and psychological counseling offered. No 'awareness' monitor exists, or is likely to within the foreseeable future. The vast majority of cases of awareness can be avoided using current knowledge and technologies.

References

1. Liang BA, Cullen DJ. The legal system and patient safety: Charting a divergent course. The relationship between malpractice latigation and human errors. (Editorial) *Anesthesiology* 1999; **91**:609–611.
2. Cheney FW, Posner K, Caplan RA, Ward RJ. Standard of care and anesthesia liability. *JAMA* 1989; **261**:1599–1603.
3. Brennan TA, Leape LL, Laird NM, *et al.* Incidence of adverse events and negligence in hospitalized patients. Results of the Harvard Medical Practice Study I. *New Engl J Med* 1991; **324**:370–376.
4. Brennan TA, Sox CM, Burstin HR. Relationship between negligent adverse events and the outcomes of medical-malpractice litigation. *New Engl J Med* 1996; **335**:1963–1967.
5. Taragin MI, Willett LR, Wilczek AP, Trout R, Carson JL. The influence of standard of care and severity of injury on the resolution of medical malpractice claims. *Ann Intern Med* 1992; **117**:780–784.
6. Edbril SD, Lagasse RS. Relationship between malpractice litigation and human errors. *Anesthesiology* 1999; **91**:848–855.
7. Leape LL, Brennan TA, Laird N, *et al.* The nature of adverse events in hospitalized patients. Results of the Harvard Medical Practice Study II. *New Engl J Med* 1991; **324**:377–384.
8. Localio AR, Lawthers AG, Brennan TA, *et al.* The nature of adverse events in hospitalized patients. Results of the Harvard Medical Practice Study II. *New Engl J Med* 1991; **325**:245–251.

9. Morlock LL, Lindren OH, Mills DH. Medical malpractice and clinical risk management. In Goldfield N, Nash DB (eds). *Providing Quality Care, Second Edition: Future Challenges.* Ann Arbor, MI: Health Administration Press, 1995; 163–183.
10. Meyers AR. 'Lumping it': The hidden denominator of the medical malpractice crisis. *Am J Public Health* 1987; **77**:1544–1548.
11. Hickson GB, Clayton EW, Githens PB, Sloan FA. Factors that prompted families to file medical malpractice claims following perinatal injuries. *JAMA* 1992; **267**:1359–1363.
12. Huycke LI, Huycke MM. Characteristics of potential plaintiffs in malpractice litigation. *Ann Intern Med* 1994; **120**:792–798.
13. Burstin HR, Johnson WG, Lipsitz SR, Brennan TA. Do the poor sue more? A case-control study of malpractice claims and socioeconomic status. *JAMA* 1993; **270**:1697–1701.
14. Cobcroft MD, Forsdick C. Awareness under anaesthesia: The patients' point of view. *Anaesth Intensive Care* 1993; **21**:837–843.
15. Moerman N, Bonke B, Oosting J. Awareness and recall during general anesthesia. *Anesthesiology* 1993; **79**:454–464.
16. Domino KB, Posner KL, Caplan RA, Cheney FW. Awareness during anesthesia. A closed claims analysis. *Anesthesiology* 1999; **90**:1053–1061.
17. Posner KL, Caplan RA, Cheney FW. Variation in expert opinion in medical malpractice review. *Anesthesiology* 1996; **85**:1049–1054.
18. Caplan RA, Posner KL, Cheney FW. Effect of outcome on physician judgments of appropriateness of care. *JAMA* 1991; **265**:1957–1960.
19. *Public Accounts – Fifth Report.* London: House of Commons, 1999.
20. Dingwall R, Fenn P. Is NHS indemnity working and is there a better way? *Brit J Anaesth* 1994; **73**:69–77.
21. Hutchinson R. Awareness during surgery. *Brit J Anaesth* 1960; **33**:463–469.
22. Harris TBJ, Brice DD, Hetherington RR, Utting JE. Dreaming associated with anaesthesia: the influence of morphine premedications and two volatile adjuvants. *Brit J Anaesth* 1971; **43**:172–178.
23. McKenna J, Wilton TNP. Awareness during endotracheal intubation. *Anaesthesia* 1973; **28**: 599–602.
24. Wilson S, Vaughan R, Stephen C. Awareness, dreams and hallucinations associated with general anesthesia. *Anesth Analg* 1975; **54**:609–619.
25. Liu D, Thorp S, Graham S, Aitkenhead AR. Incidence of awareness with recall during general anaesthesia. *Anaesthesia,* 1991; **46**:435–437.
26. Ranta SOV, Laurila R, Saario J, Ali-Melkkilä T, Hynynen M. Awareness with recall during general

anesthesia: Incidence and risk factors. *Anesth Analg* 1998; **86**:1084–1089.

27. Sandin RH, Enlund G, Samuelsson P, Lennmarken C. Awareness during anesthesia: a prospective study. *Lancet* 2000; **355**:707–711.

28. Ackers v Wigan Health Authority. *Med L R* 1991; **2**:232–233.

29. Aitkenhead AR. Anaesthesia. In Jackson JP (ed.) *A Practical Guide to Medicine and the Law*. London: Springer-Verlag, 1991; 45–75.

30. Ranta S, Ranta V, Aromaa U. The claims of compensation for awareness with recall during general anesthesia in Finland. *Acta Anesthesiol Scand* 1997; **41**:356–359.

31. Hargrove RL. Awareness under anaesthesia. *J Med Defense Union* 1987; (Spring):9–11.

32. Utting JE. Awareness: clinical aspects. In Rosen M, Lunn JN (eds). *Consciousness, Awareness and Pain in General Anaesthesia*. London: Butterworths, 1987; 12–17.

33. Rosen J. Hearing tests during anaesthesia with nitrous oxide and relaxants. *Acta Anaesthesiol Scand* 1959; **3**:1–8.

34. Browne RA, Catton DV. Awareness during anaesthesia: a comparison of anaesthesia with nitrous oxide-oxygen and nitrous oxide-oxygen with Innovar. *Can Anaesth Soc J* 1973; **20**:763–768.

35. White M, Kenny GMC. Intravenous propofol anaesthesia using a computerized infusion system. *Anaesthesia* 1990; **45**:204–209.

36. Aitkenhead AR. Awareness during anaesthesia: when is an anaesthetic not an anaesthetic? *Can J Anaesth* 1996; **43**:206–211.

37. Barr AM, Moxon A, Woolam CH, Fryer ME. Effect of diazepam and lorazepam on awareness during anaesthesia for Caesarean section. *Anaesthesia* 1977; **32**:873–878.

38. Lyons G, Macdonald R. Awareness during Caesarean section. *Anaesthesia* 1991; **46**:62–64.

39. Taylor v Worcester and District Health Authority. *Med L R* 1991 **2**:215–231.

40. Bolam v Friern Hospital Management Committee. *All England Law Reports* 1957; **2**:118.

41. Gan TJ, Glass PS, Sigl J, *et al*. Women emerge from general anesthesia with propofol/alfentanil/nitrous oxide faster than men. *Anesthesiology* 1999; **90**:1283–1287.

42. Drover DR, Lemmens HJM. Population pharmacodynamics and pharmacokinetics of remifentanil as a supplement to nitrous oxide anesthesia for elective abdominal surgery. *Anesthesiology* 1998; **89**:869–877.

43. Cheney FW. The American Society of Anesthesiologists Closed Claims Project. What have we learned, how has it affected practice, and how will it affect practice in the future? *Anesthesiology* 1999; **91**:552–556.

44. Kearse LA, Rosow C, Zaslavsky A, Connors P, Dershwitz M, Denman W. Bispectral analysis of the electroencephalogram predicts conscious processing of information during propofol sedation and hypnosis. *Anesthesiology* 1998; **88**:25–34.

Index